NURSING SERIES

Psychiatric Nursing:
Current Trends in Diagnosis and Treatment

2nd Edition

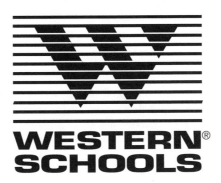

WESTERN® SCHOOLS

By
Bethany A. Murray, APRN, BC

30 contact hours will be awarded upon successful completion of this course.

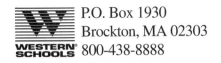
P.O. Box 1930
Brockton, MA 02303
800-438-8888

ABOUT THE AUTHOR

Bethany A. Murray, APRN, BC, is an advanced practice registered nurse with her master's degree in child and adolescent psychiatric mental health nursing. She is certified in her specialty area by the American Nurses Credentialing Center. Ms. Murray has worked in the psychiatric field since 1986. She is currently employed as the Director of Nursing and a Clinical Nurse Specialist at Centerstone in Bloomington, IN, where she sees adults and children for psychiatric medication evaluations and management. Ms. Murray is the Region One representative of the Coalition of Advanced Practice Nurses of Indiana (CAPNI), an educational and political organization that promotes advanced nursing practice at local, state, and national levels. Ms. Murray has extensive teaching experience as a part-time lecturer and adjunct faculty member of the Indiana University School of Nursing and she is a preceptor for graduate students in the clinical setting. Since 1986, Ms. Murray has been a national disaster volunteer for the American Red Cross. She was deployed in 2001 to Washington, DC, following the 9/11 terrorist attacks, and in 2005 to Baton Rouge, LA, following Hurricane Katrina, as well as to several smaller scale flood, hurricane, and tornado disasters.

> **Bethany A. Murray** has disclosed that she is on the Speaker's Bureau for Pfizer Pharmaceuticals and speaks on behalf of Lyrica.
>
> Western Schools ensures that this content is free from bias and commercial influence.

ABOUT THE CONTENT EDITOR

Lynette Jack, PhD, RN, has a BSN from the State University of New York at Buffalo and a master's degree in psychiatric and mental health nursing and a PhD in higher education from the University of Pittsburgh. Lynette has taught psychiatric nursing for more than 20 years and has been president of the International Society of Psychiatric-Mental Health Nurses (ISPN) and of the International Nurses Society on Addictions (IntNSA). She currently works as the director of RN-BSN, MSN, MSN/MBA, and DNP programs at Waynesburg University in western Pennsylvania.

> **Lynette Jack** has disclosed that she has no significant financial or other conflicts of interest pertaining to this course book.

Nurse Planners: Amy Bernard, MS, BSN, RN-BC and Anne Manton, PhD, APRN, BC, FAAN, FAEN

> Amy Bernard and Anne Manton have disclosed that they have no significant financial or other conflicts of interest pertaining to this course book.

Copy Editor: Dorothy Terry

Indexer: Sylvia Coates

Western Schools' courses are designed to provide nursing professionals with the educational information they need to enhance their career development. The information provided within these course materials is the result of research and consultation with prominent nursing and medical authorities and is, to the best of our knowledge, current and accurate. However, the courses and course materials are provided with the understanding that Western Schools is not engaged in offering legal, nursing, medical, or other professional advice.

Western Schools' courses and course materials are not meant to act as a substitute for seeking out professional advice or conducting individual research. When the information provided in the courses and course materials is applied to individual circumstances, all recommendations must be considered in light of the uniqueness pertaining to each situation.

Western Schools' course materials are intended solely for *your* use and *not* for the benefit of providing advice or recommendations to third parties. Western Schools devoids itself of any responsibility for adverse consequences resulting from the failure to seek nursing, medical, or other professional advice. Western Schools further devoids itself of any responsibility for updating or revising any programs or publications presented, published, distributed, or sponsored by Western Schools unless otherwise agreed to as part of an individual purchase contract.

Products (including brand names) mentioned or pictured in Western School's courses are not endorsed by Western Schools, the American Nurses Credentialing Center (ANCC) or any state board.

ISBN: 978-1-57801-417-0

COURSE INSTRUCTIONS
IMPORTANT: Read these instructions *BEFORE* proceeding!

COMPLETING THE FINAL EXAMINATION

Enclosed with your course book you will find a FasTrax® answer sheet. Use this answer sheet to respond to all the final exam questions that appear in this course. If the course has less than 100 questions, leave any remaining answer circles on the FasTrax answer sheet blank.

Be sure to fill in circles completely using **blue or black ink.** The FasTrax grading system will not read pencil. If you make an error, you may use correction fluid (such as Wite-Out®) to correct it.

FasTrax answer sheets are preprinted with your name and address and the course title. If you are completing more than one course, be sure to record your answers on the correct corresponding answer sheet.

A PASSING SCORE

The final exam is a multiple choice exam. You must score 70% or better in order to pass this course and receive a certificate of completion. Should you fail to achieve the required score, an additional FasTrax answer sheet will be sent to you so that you may make a second attempt to pass the course. You will be allowed three chances to pass the same course without incurring additional charges. After three failed attempts, your file will be closed.

RECORDING YOUR HOURS

Use the Study Time Log provided in this course book to monitor and record the time it takes to complete this course. Upon completion, tally your total time spent and use this information to respond to the final question of the course evaluation.

COURSE EVALUATIONS

The Course Evaluation provided in this course book is a critical component of the course and must be completed and submitted with your final exam. Responses to evaluation statements should be recorded in the right hand column of the FasTrax answer sheet, in the section marked "Evaluation." Evaluations provide Western Schools with vital feedback regarding courses. Your feedback is important to us; please take a few minutes to complete the evaluation.

To provide additional feedback regarding this course, Western Schools services, or to suggest new course topics, use the space provided on the Important Information form found on the back of the FasTrax instruction sheet included with your course. Return the completed form to Western Schools with your final exam.

SUBMITTING THE COMPLETED FINAL EXAM

For your convenience, Western Schools provides a number of exam grading options. Full instructions and complete grading details are listed on the FasTrax instruction sheet provided with this course. If you are mailing your answer sheet(s) to Western Schools, we recommend you make a copy as a back-up.

COURSE COMPLETION TIME FRAMES AND EXTENSIONS

You have two (2) years from the date of purchase to complete this course. If you are not able to complete the course within 2 years, a six (6) month extension may be purchased. If you have not completed the course within 30 months from the original enrollment date, your file will be closed and no certificate will be issued.

CHANGE OF ADDRESS?

In the event that your address changes prior to completing this course, please call our customer service department at 1-800-618-1670, so that we may update your file.

WESTERN SCHOOLS GUARANTEES YOUR SATISFACTION

If any continuing education course fails to meet your expectations, or if you are not satisfied for any reason, you may return the course materials for an exchange or a refund (less shipping and handling) within 30 days. Software, video, and audio courses must be returned unopened. Textbooks must not be written in or marked up in any other way.

Thank you for using Western Schools to fulfill your continuing education needs!

WESTERN SCHOOLS
P.O. Box 1930
Brockton, MA 02303
800-438-8888
www.westernschools.com

WESTERN SCHOOLS
STUDY TIME LOG

PSYCHIATRIC NURSING: CURRENT TRENDS IN DIAGNOSIS AND TREATMENT

INSTRUCTIONS: Use this log sheet to document the amount of time you spend completing this course. Include the time it takes you to read the instructions, take the pretest, read the course book, take the final examination, and complete the evaluation.

Date	Time Spent	
	Hours	Minutes
_____	_____	_____
_____	_____	_____
_____	_____	_____
_____	_____	_____
_____	_____	_____
_____	_____	_____
_____	_____	_____
_____	_____	_____
_____	_____	_____
_____	_____	_____
_____	_____	_____
_____	_____	_____
_____	_____	_____
_____	_____	_____
_____	_____	_____
TOTAL*	[_____]	[_____]
	Hours	Minutes

* Please use this total study time to answer the final question of the course evaluation.

WESTERN SCHOOLS
COURSE EVALUATION

PSYCHIATRIC NURSING: CURRENT TRENDS IN DIAGNOSIS AND TREATMENT

INSTRUCTIONS: Using the scale below, please respond to the following evaluation statements. All responses should be recorded in the right-hand column of the FasTrax answer sheet, in the section marked "Evaluation." Be sure to fill in each corresponding answer circle completely using blue or black ink. Leave any remaining answer circles blank.

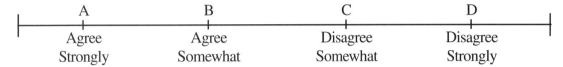

A	B	C	D
Agree Strongly	Agree Somewhat	Disagree Somewhat	Disagree Strongly

OBJECTIVES: Upon completion of this course, the learner will be able to

1. Explore ethical, legal, and cultural issues associated with mental health care and treatment.
2. Describe components for obtaining a relevant psychiatric history.
3. Describe common adult and child psychiatric disorders utilizing the *DSM-IV-TR* Guidelines.
4. Identify current treatment modalities and medications used for various mental health disorders.
5. Discuss a nursing plan of care and interventions for specific patient scenarios.
6. Identify appropriate nursing measures for promoting safety and maximizing function.

COURSE CONTENT

7. The course materials were presented in a well organized and clearly written manner.
8. The course content was presented in a fair, unbiased and balanced manner.
9. The course expanded my knowledge and enhanced my skills related to the subject matter.
10. I intend to apply the knowledge and skills I've learned to my nursing practice. (Select the appropriate response below.)
    A. Yes   B. Unsure   C. No   D. Not Applicable

ATTESTATION

11. By submitting this answer sheet, I certify that I have read the course materials and personally completed the final examination based on the material presented. Mark "A" for Agree and "B" for Disagree.

COURSE HOURS

12. Choose the response that best represents the total number of clock hours it took to complete this **30 hour** course.
    A. More than 32 hours B. 28–32 hours C. Less than 28 hours

Note: To provide additional feedback regarding this course, Western Schools services, or to suggest new course topics, use the space provided on the Important Information form found on the back of the FasTrax instruction sheet included with your course.

CONTENTS

FIGURES AND TABLES

PRETEST

1. Begin this course by taking the pretest. Circle the answers to the questions on this page, or write the answers on a separate sheet of paper. Do not log answers to the pretest questions on the FasTrax test sheet included with the course.

2. Compare your answers to the PRETEST KEY located at the end of the Pretest. The pretest key indicates the page where the content of that question is discussed. Make note of the questions you missed, so that you can focus on those areas as you complete the course.

3. Complete the course by reading the chapter and completing the exam questions at the end of the chapter. Answers to these exam questions should be logged on the FasTrax test sheet included with the course.

Note: Choose the one option that BEST answers each question.

1. In 1946 the United States passed the National Mental Health Act which resulted in the establishment of

    a. more state psychiatric institutions.
    b. the National Institute of Mental Health.
    c. guidelines for the testing of psychotropic drugs.
    d. Veteran's Administration mental health services.

2. Ethical principles are meant to

    a. guide the healthcare professional in decision-making.
    b. serve as rules for conduct in society.
    c. prevent errors in judgment.
    d. predict the behaviors of individuals.

3. The first element assessed in the Mental Status exam is

    a. eye contact.
    b. overall appearance.
    c. mood and affect.
    d. cognitive abilities.

4. A major focus of cognitive behavioral therapy is

    a. learning stress management strategies.
    b. challenging inaccurate beliefs.
    c. confronting issues from the past.
    d. teaching appropriate medication usage.

5. The percentage of persons in the United States diagnosed with schizophrenia is

    a. 1%.
    b. 5%.
    c. 20%.
    d. 40%.

6. Schizophrenia is caused by

    a. neurobiological alterations yet to be identified.
    b. impoverished home environments.
    c. mentally ill mothers with domineering personalities.
    d. chronic drug and alcohol abuse.

continued on next page

7. The percentage of individuals older than 65 years of age with a dementia disorder is

   a. 10% to 15%.

   b. 4% to 5%.

   c. 2% to 4%.

   d. 1%.

8. The chemical that causes the "hangover effect" of alcohol intoxication is

   a. acetaldehyde.

   b. ethanol.

   c. acetic acid.

   d. carbon dioxide.

9. Symptom sets associated with opioid withdrawal include

   a. hallucinations and paranoid delusions.

   b. neuron excitability and grand mal seizures.

   c. violent outbursts, followed by stupor.

   d. lacrimation, piloerection, muscle aches, and rhinorrhea.

10. Prevalence rates for major depression in women are

    a. 1%.

    b. 5%.

    c. 10%.

    d. 40%.

11. *DSM-IV-TR* criteria for diagnosing major depression must include

    a. a depressed mood or a loss of interest or pleasure in activities.

    b. weight increases or decreases.

    c. suicidal thoughts or behaviors.

    d. irritability or grouchiness.

12. Symptoms of mania associated with a bipolar I disorder must include

    a. delusions and hallucinations.

    b. an abnormal and elevated, expansive, or irritable mood.

    c. spending sprees and promiscuity.

    d. poor judgment, insight, or awareness of symptoms.

13. Diagnosing bipolar II disorder may take as long as

    a. 2 years.

    b. 5 years.

    c. 8 years.

    d. 12 years.

14. Generalized anxiety disorder is characterized by

    a. excessive worry about a variety of events or activities.

    b. specific fears of certain situations.

    c. hypervigilance and flashbacks.

    d. repetitive thoughts and actions.

15. Eating disorders often onset in

    a. early childhood.

    b. middle to late adolescence.

    c. college years.

    d. adulthood.

16. Narcolepsy is associated with

    a. excessive amphetamine abuse.

    b. problems with primary insomnia.

    c. a disturbance in REM sleep architecture.

    d. sleep apnea concerns.

17. Of women who are killed annually in the United States, the percentage that is secondary to domestic violence is

    a. 1% to 3%.

    b. 5% to 10%.

    c. 10% to 20%.

    d. 30% to 50%.

18. Psychological first aid is

    a. relaxation training used during a crisis.

    b. the same as cognitive behavioral therapy.

    c. used to comfort and provide immediate support for disaster victims.

    d. designed to only be used by psychologists.

19. Attention deficit hyperactivity disorder occurs in males at a rate that is

    a. 3 to 4 times higher than in females.

    b. twice as high as in females.

    c. the same as in females.

    d. half as much as in females.

20. The prevalence of Tourette's disorder is

    a. 1 in 1,000 children.

    b. 4 in 1,000 children.

    c. 1 in 10,000 children.

    d. 4 in 10,000 children.

PRETEST KEY

1.	B	chapter 1	6.	A	chapter 5	11.	A	chapter 9	16.	C	chapter 12
2.	A	chapter 2	7.	C	chapter 6	12.	B	chapter 10	17.	D	chapter 13
3.	B	chapter 3	8.	A	chapter 7	13.	D	chapter 10	18.	C	chapter 14
4.	B	chapter 4	9.	D	chapter 8	14.	A	chapter 11	19.	A	chapter 15
5.	A	chapter 5	10.	C	chapter 9	15.	B	chapter 12	20.	D	chapter 16

INTRODUCTION

In the 1948 book *Psychiatry in Nursing,* (Headlee & Corey), the psychiatric nurse is described as requiring an "entirely different set of values, new ways of thinking, new attitudes, and new techniques" (p. 210). The authors go on to say "making satisfactory contacts with human beings constitutes psychiatric nursing." Little has changed in the past 50 years regarding this basic humanistic approach. However, what has changed dramatically is the nurse's ability to practice with increasing autonomy in providing care for clients and to be perceived as an important member of the multidisciplinary healthcare team.

One of the purposes of this educational offering is to teach nurses about psychiatric disorders, various treatment modalities, therapeutic communication skills, medications, and cultural variances in the way mental illness is perceived and treated in adults and children.

Psychiatric nursing utilizes a continuum of care model. Clients with psychiatric disorders are no longer found exclusively within the hospital setting. Every year, new medications are launched with improved efficacy and fewer side effects. Acute psychiatric hospital stays are becoming shorter, with many hospital stays lasting only 3 to 5 days (historically, clients were hospitalized for the duration of their illnesses – often up to 3 months in an acute care hospital before transferring to a long-term care facility). The separation of mental health care from medical and surgical care has become an artificial distinction. Nurses who believe that they will have no need for ongoing education in psychiatric disorders or their treatment may find themselves to be at a distinct disadvantage, as indi-

viduals with psychiatric diagnoses are encountered in all treatment areas.

It is the goal of this course to assist nurses in updating their mental health skills and knowledge of current psychiatric treatments. Nurses must recognize and be able to care for clients in inpatient, residential, outpatient, or home settings as well as in numerous medical settings, such as nursing homes and primary practice offices. The concept of "least restrictive environment" has had a significant impact on the way psychiatric nursing is practiced. Key to nursing care is the therapeutic nurse-client relationship (which can be loosely defined as a genuine desire to help the client coupled with the practice of effective communication techniques and the demonstration of respect for the independence of the client). Communication is much more open and bi-directional now, necessitating a contract between clients and nurses in which clients are better informed regarding their conditions and participate more fully in planning their care.

In 1973 the American Nurses Association developed standards of practice to provide a framework for psychiatric nursing practice. This evolved in 1995 to the American Psychiatric Nurses Association's position paper, "Psychiatric-Mental Health Nursing Practice" (available at www.apna.org/i4a/pages/index.cfm?pageid=3343). These practice guidelines allow for the standardization of nursing care in all mental health care settings. Since 1988, the American Nurses Credentialing Center has provided nurses with an opportunity to obtain specialty certification as generalists or clinical specialists in psychiatric and mental health nursing through a certification examination (generalist or undergraduate level) or through a combination of clinical supervision, professional recommendations, and an examination (clinical specialist or graduate level).

This course will examine broad categories of psychiatric disorders utilizing the guidelines of the *Diagnostic and Statistical Manual of Mental Disorders,* 4th ed., Text Revision (*DSM-IV-TR*), (American Psychiatric Association, 2000). Adult and child disorders are reviewed, with attention placed on the more commonly encountered diagnoses. Practical applications are emphasized. In most chapters, a case study will be presented that will include study questions. The reader will also be provided with sample nursing care plans, which include significant nursing diagnoses plus appropriate objectives and interventions. Information on current treatment modalities and medications also will be provided. Chapter objectives and pretest and posttest questions will be used to measure the level of understanding of the reader.

This course is designed for the practicing registered nurse (RN) or licensed practical or vocational nurse (LPN or LVN). A basic understanding of medical terminology, abbreviations, and fundamental nursing care is assumed. Non-psychiatric nurses who are practicing in an advanced role (e.g., nurse practitioners) may find the sections on diagnosing health problems and medication options to be of particular interest. New to this edition is the inclusion of information on advanced practice psychiatric nursing and prescribing medications. This information is included to enhance learning for the reader, to stimulate thought, and (hopefully) to encourage nurses to consider returning to school for a master's or higher degree.

CHAPTER 1

HISTORY OF MENTAL HEALTH CARE

CHAPTER OBJECTIVE

At the end of this chapter, the reader will be able to discuss the epidemiology and history of mental health care, the diagnosing of psychiatric disorders, and some protective factors that may reduce negative outcomes caused by a psychiatric illness.

LEARNING OBJECTIVES

At the completion of this chapter, the reader will be able to

1. discuss epidemiological data in prevalence rates of psychiatric disorders, based on information gathered by the National Institute of Mental Health and the U.S. Census.

2. identify key trends in mental health care over the past century.

3. describe the *DSM-IV-TR* guidelines and how they are utilized in diagnosing psychiatric disorders.

4. describe predictors of a positive outcome in improving functional levels.

INTRODUCTION

The National Institute of Mental Health (NIMH) estimates that 26.2% of American adults experience a diagnosable psychiatric disorder at some point in their lives, with 6% experiencing a serious and disabling condition such as schizophrenia (National Institute of Mental Health [NIMH], 2008).

The most recent U.S. Census Bureau report (completed in 2000, reported March 2003) identified approximately 12.4 million Americans, or 4.8% of the population, as receiving disability benefits for a mental or emotional disorder. A disability is defined as difficulty in performing functional tasks or daily living activities. Poverty rates for the disabled were 25%, as compared to 15.7% of non-disabled persons (U.S. Census Bureau, 2003).

Co-morbidity is defined as the presence of two or more disease states at the same time. For persons diagnosed with a psychiatric illness, up to 45% have co-morbid conditions. To illustrate this better, nearly half of the children with attention deficit hyperactivity disorder (ADHD) will also have oppositional-defiant disorder, bipolar mood disorder, or learning disabilities. Some adults and children have numerous, overlapping conditions (see Figure 1-1).

This chapter presents some of the incidence and prevalence rates for several major psychiatric illnesses, including depression, anxiety, bipolar disorder, anorexia nervosa, alcoholism, ADHD and schizophrenia. The history of mental health care and treatment will be reviewed, covering the period known as "moral therapy" (late 1700s to early 1800s) to the present neurobiological approach. The manner in which psychiatric illnesses are diagnosed is provided, with a discussion on the emerging

FIGURE 1-1: CO-MORBIDITY OF PSYCHIATRIC DISORDERS

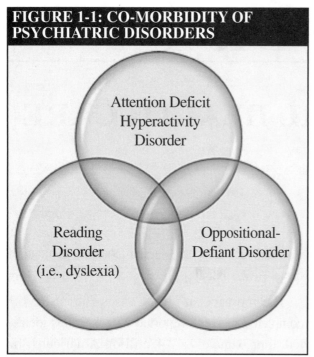

field of genetic studies since the completion of human genome mapping in 2003. Finally, social, familial, and individual characteristics that may reduce or prevent the development of mental illness or psychiatric disturbance will be reviewed.

EPIDEMIOLOGY

Nineteen million Americans are diagnosed with anxiety disorders each year in the United States. Rates are twice as high in women as compared to men. Approximately 2.3 million American adults are diagnosed annually with a bipolar mood disorder, which constitutes 8% to 10% of the total population of adults. In children and adolescents, approximately 4.1% are diagnosed with ADHD. In a typical American classroom, with an average of 25 students, at least one will meet the clinical criteria for ADHD, which is 2 to 3 times higher in boys than in girls. The reverse is true in eating disorders where only 5% to 15% of clients with an eating disorder are male. The rate of anorexia nervosa in young women is about 3.7% and the rate of bulimia nervosa is about 1.1%. Suicide is the third leading cause of death in 15- to 24-year-old individuals (NIMH, 2009). Approximately 5.8% of men and

9.5% of women worldwide experience a depressive episode at some point in their life (World Health Organization [WHO], 2007).

HISTORY OF MENTAL HEALTH CARE

During the middle-ages, persons with mental illness, or "the insane," were believed to be possessed by demons. Until the late 1700s, persons with mental illness were perceived as little better than wild animals; banishment and confinement were common practices. Although families were occasionally provided some assistance by the community, in most cases those with psychiatric disorders were left to wander and fend for themselves. Until 1770, a small fee was charged to visitors of St. Mary of Bethlehem Hospital (Bedlam) in England to view the patients. Treatments were torturous in nature and included forced feedings, purging, bleeding, and whippings (Keltner, Schwecke, & Bostrom, 2007, p. 3).

Philippe Pinel became superintendent of two separate institutions, one for men and one for women in France in 1793. While there, he noted the deplorable conditions and brutality of the attendants. He unchained clients and brought them out into the sunshine, instituting what became known as "moral therapy" (Weiner, 2008a, p. 308). In 1796, William Tuke in England founded a private facility, The York Retreat, which would ensure moral treatment, based on Quaker teachings. He saw his facility as a refuge, a place of asylum or safety. (Weiner, 2008b, p. 282) In the United States, Boston schoolteacher Dorothea Dix was instrumental in helping to open 32 state hospitals advocating warmth, food, and protection for residents. A movement toward seeing persons with mental illness as human beings with rights to dignity had begun with the new century (Keltner et al., 2007, p. 4).

The second major shift in the way mental illness was perceived occurred about 80 years later during the age of "scientific reason" (Decker, 2008, p. 587). Sigmund Freud began talking about the influence of early childhood experiences in shaping the psyche. Freud's work stimulated many others to follow (Carl Jung, Alfred Adler, and others), providing models of care that are still used today. Emil Kraepelin was the first to describe, classify, and label distinct mental disorders. Other theorists emerged making major contributions in the fields of behaviorism (Watson, Pavlov), somatic treatment (psychosurgery, electroconvulsive therapy, insulin shock), and biology. During this period, individuals with psychiatric disorders could finally receive medical care along with rehabilitative treatment (Decker, 2008).

In 1946, the United States passed the National Mental Health Act, which served to establish the NIMH. This Act was stimulated by the poor mental health of many returning World War II soldiers. The NIMH provides funding for research into the causes of mental illnesses and tuition for education in four core mental health disciplines: psychiatry, psychology, nursing, and social work (www.nimh.nih.gov). In the 1950s, rapid progress was made with the discovery of psychotropic medications. Chlorpromazine (Thorazine®) was the first such agent, and Lithium and imipramine (Tofranil®) were identified a few years later. Prior to chlorpromazine, various concoctions were used to calm clients. These often contained dangerous combinations of alcohol, barbiturates, or opiates. Chlorpromazine was different because the actual symptoms of the illnesses remitted in many clients. Lithium was accidentally discovered to reduce rapid and severe mood swings in clients during the study of its usefulness in epilepsy. It rapidly became a state-of-the-art medication for bipolar illness. Imipramine, a tricyclic antidepressant, was the first medication with treatment efficacy for clinical depression. It has since demonstrated usefulness in the treatment of anxiety and ADHD as well. Monoamine oxidase inhibitors followed tricyclic antidepressants in the treatment

of depression. With the availability of effective medications, a gradual shift in perspective among the public occurred. Clients were increasingly perceived as suffering from chemical imbalances or other, as yet unknown, physical defects that, hopefully, could be corrected through medical treatment.

The Community Mental Health Centers (CMHC) Act of 1963 initiated a trend to remove patients from psychiatric hospitals and return them to their home communities. This deinstitutionalization benchmark period began when state hospitals had reached their peak census populations in 1955. After the CMHC Act, federal legislation provided an income for persons with mental illness by providing definitions for disability and financial aid. This aid is now called Supplemental Security Income (SSI) and Social Security Disability Income (SSDI). Public law discontinued these benefits to individuals suffering exclusively from a drug or alcohol addiction in 1997. Finally, changes in involuntary commitment laws made it more difficult for individuals to be hospitalized unless there were specific criteria met that indicated the person was a danger to himself or herself or unable to provide for basic needs of food, shelter, and self-care. These changes were difficult for communities to accept, primarily because of their fear of persons with mentally illness, but also because of concerns regarding a potential increase in homelessness and crime. Community-based, regional centers were developed with a primary purpose of providing care for deinstitutionalized individuals and managing some of these public concerns. Today, hundreds of community mental health care centers are located throughout the United States, divided regionally. Each of these centers is charged with the task of assisting adults and children with chronic psychiatric, behavioral, or addictive disorders in maintaining their functions within the communities in which they reside.

THE DIFFICULTY OF DIAGNOSING AND THE *DSM-IV-TR*

Identifying and diagnosing a psychiatric disorder has always been a difficult task. Unlike most physical health disorders, blood tests cannot reveal a psychiatric illness and are primarily useful in ruling out other diagnoses. X-rays, computerized tomography (CT) scans, and magnetic resonance imaging (MRI) are only useful in identifying vascular or structural changes in the brain. Recently, positron emission tomography (PET) scans have been studied as a means of identifying some individuals with brain-based disorders. Early research with PET scans looks promising, with changes demonstrated in both the level of brain activity and physical structure in individuals with schizophrenia; however, the clinical value of this testing is currently indeterminate. Indirect measures have been practiced for years, notably 24-hour urine collections to evaluate serotonin breakdown in the form of 5HT excretion and the dexamethasone suppression test to indicate depression syndromes, but these are unreliable and difficult to administer. Additionally, clinicians have varied in their descriptions of psychiatric disorders and historically there has been a lack of common language for the psychiatric care provider.

Recently, research into genetics and deoxyribonucleic acid (DNA). DNA contains the biological instructions that make each species unique. The complete set of DNA in an organism is referred to as its genome. The Human Genome Project, completed in April 2003, served to map the human genome for the first time ever. This had led to a surge of research in health care, specifically in trying to identify genes that are associated with different diseases, looking for familial inheritance factors and key triggers. In December 2008 the NIMH awarded 19 million dollars to the University of Southern California to look for genetic markers for schizophrenia and bipolar disorder. The NIMH also awarded 9.8 million dollars in research funding to John Hopkins University to look at environment-triggered genetic changes in schizophrenia. This "epigenetic" research may help to explain why one identical twin may develop the illness, whereas the other twin does not, even thouogh identical twins share identical DNA (NIMH, 2008).

Kraepelin was one of the first clinicians to develop a set of criteria that could be used in differentiating various symptoms of psychiatric disorders and placing them into some type of categorization. In the United States, the need to collect statistical information resulted in early definitions of mental illnesses. Idiocy/insanity was the terminology utilized in the 1840 census. By 1880, seven categories were identified: mania, melancholia, monomania, paresis, dementia, dipsomania, and epilepsy. In 1917, the Committee on Statistics of the American Medico-Psychological Association (later renamed the American Psychiatric Association) developed a plan for the Census Bureau to gather uniform statistics by identifying nationally acceptable nomenclature to label mental disorders. Following World War II, the U.S. Army and Veteran's Administration expanded on these diagnostic categories to better incorporate the types of problems experienced by veterans. About the same time, the World Health Organization (WHO) published the sixth edition of the *International Classification of Diseases* (ICD-6). A variation of the ICD-6 was published in 1952 by the American Psychiatric Association and was the first edition of the *Diagnostic and Statistical Manual of Mental Disorders* (DSM-I). Revisions and new additions have occurred every 5 to 10 years to the present date. In 1994, the *DSM-IV* was published as the preeminent classification system for diagnosing and describing psychiatric disorders. More than 1,000 people, in 15 task groups, conducted a 3-stage empirical process that included comprehensive reviews of the published literature, reexamination of existing data sets, and extensive field trials that collected information on the reliability and characteristics of each criteria set. As the information in the text runs the risk of becoming increasingly outdated with each passing year and each new research study, a text revision was undertaken in 2000. No substantive changes in the criteria sets were made; neither were there any additions of new disorders or subtypes.

Since 2000, the American Psychiatric Association's *DSM-IV-TR* has been the primary educational and resource tool for evaluating and categorizing psychiatric disorders. The *ICD-10* was published by the WHO in 1992 and is fully coordinated with the *DSM-IV-TR* in codes and terms used. In the *DSM-IV-TR*, mental disorder is defined as a:

> *"clinically significant behavioral or psychological syndrome or pattern that occurs in an individual and that is associated with present distress (e.g., a painful symptom) or disability (i.e., impairment in one or more important areas of functioning) or with a significantly increased risk of suffering death, pain, disability, or an important loss of freedom,"* (American Psychiatric Association, 2000).

The manual goes on to say "that in order to be identified as a 'mental disorder,' the syndrome or pattern cannot be an expectable or culturally sanctioned response to an event such as bereavement seen after a death." Mental disorders are psychological or biological in nature and cannot be socially deviant behaviors or conflicts between the individual and society. (American Psychiatric Association, 2000, p. xxxi)

The *DSM-IV-TR* is limited by its use of catgorical classifications. Individuals vary in their symptoms and many do not fit neatly into one specific category. The diagnostic criteria provided should be utilized by trained clinicians and serve as a guideline to assist in making sound clinical decisions. Diagnosing does not imply etiology; therefore, using the *DSM-IV-TR* to predict dangerousness or future behavior is inappropriate. The disorders covered in this text will utilize criteria and definitions provided in the *DSM-IV-TR*.

Efforts were made to incorporate cultural awareness into the *DSM-IV-TR* because of the extent of diverse populations seen in today's healthcare settings. A clinician must have an awareness of culturally appropriate behaviors to avoid mislabeling a particular behavior as symptomatic of a mental disorder. The *DSM-IV-TR* contains information to aid mental health professionals in making culturally sensitive evaluations, including: 1) a discussion of cultural variations within clinical presentations; 2) a description of culture-bound syndromes; 3) an outline for cultural formulation to assist the clinician in systematically evaluating the impact of the client's cultural context.

Lastly, the *DSM-IV-TR* is organized in a five-axis format. Axis I consists of primary psychiatric disorders, which are diagnosed by comparing patient symptoms to a set of standardized criteria. In most cases, the client must meet a minimum number of criteria (e.g., four out of six) in order to receive a specific diagnosis. Within Axis I, a client may have one or many diagnoses. Axis II diagnoses are limited to personality disorders and mental retardation. Axis III refers to all medical conditions that may impact on the psychiatric condition. Axis IV is the clinician's assessment of the type and level of stress the client experiences in his or her social environment that may worsen or ameliorate the psychiatric disorder. Finally, Axis V is a standardized Global Assessment of Functioning (GAF) Scale numbering 1 to 100 that the clinician utilizes to assign a numerical rating on how well the client copes with his or her diagnoses, illnesses, and life stressors noted in Axes I to IV. This number is a useful tool for assessing outcomes as well as evaluating the degree of psychiatric impairment and safety risk. Table 1-1 demonstrates the use of the *DSM-IV-TR* multiaxial structure in conceptualizing an adult client's diagnoses. Table 1-2 applies the multiaxial *DSM-IV-TR* structure to a child client.

TABLE 1-1: MULTIAXIAL DIAGNOSES FOR AN ADULT CLIENT

Axis I	Schizophrenia, paranoid type Polysubstance dependence
Axis II	Mild mental retardation
Axis III	Type II diabetes mellitus Morbid obesity Hypertension
Axis IV	Moderate – problems with finances, lack of primary supports
Axis V	Current GAF:48

TABLE 1-2: MULTIAXIAL DIAGNOSES FOR A CHILD CLIENT

Axis I	Posttraumatic stress disorder Reactive attachment disorder Phonological disorder
Axis II	No diagnosis
Axis III	Mild asthma
Axis IV	Severe – foster home placement (3rd in 2 years), school failure
Axis V	Current GAF:50

PREDICTORS OF A POSITIVE OUTCOME

Positive outcomes consist of an increase in the overall functional level of the individual while minimizing detrimental symptoms and excessive resource utilization (cost). Keep in mind that what is perceived as desirable in an adult client, may appear to be different than that for a young child; however, some basic similarities clearly exist. For example, adults are expected to be able to participate in and contribute to society in productive ways, such as paid employment, volunteer work, or caring for a family. When an adult experiences a severe and disabling condition, this role performance is threatened; whereas, children only have expectations that they will participate in learning experiences through education and that they are fully involved members of their families and future members of society. Both populations benefit from healthy peer interactions and social relationships at a level considered developmentally appropriate. Clearly, a reduction in physical impairments and risk factors for serious physical and mental illnesses is another standard by which one can measure good health. Chronic mental illness impacts on all aspects of an individual's life. Current research focuses on strategies to alleviate symptoms and provide safe and effective interventions for individuals. Mental health care providers are challenged with the task of examining their clients' functional levels and problem areas, and working with them to identify interventions that will promote a maximum level of independence, good health, and happiness.

Negative outcomes cost society a great deal – not only in money spent on hospitalizations or incarcerations, but also in the loss of productive contributions that individuals may be capable of making in their lifetimes. In a meta-analysis of 26 studies (4490 participants) done by Marshall et al., there was a significant correlation between duration of psychotic symptoms and a poor positive outcome in patients (Marshall et al., 2005).

Protective factors are conditions that can increase resistance to disease or negative outcomes. They may be externally based (social, economic, familial, or environmental) or they may be individual attributes. Individual protective factors include such things as good self-esteem, positive thinking, good problem-solving abilities, good stress management, positive social skills, literacy, and feelings of mastery or control over one's environment. Social protective factors include social responsibility and tolerance, access to supports and community networks, empowerment, ethnic minority integration, and social participation. Conversely, risk factors include a sense of isolation, racial strife, poverty, war, and unemployment. Familial protective factors include good parenting, positive attachment and early bonding, and early cognitive (brain) stimulation. Even improvements in basic need access, such as better nutrition and safe housing, have been associated with prevention of mental disorders (WHO, 2004).

Treatment providers can intervene in a number of ways to maintain stability and reduce the risk of relapse. One such way is by encouraging clients to participate in self-help groups, especially when drugs or alcohol are involved. This consistently has been shown to positively impact on psychiatric stability. Advocacy and support through organizations, such as the National Alliance for the Mentally Ill (NAMI) or Children and Adults with Attention Deficit Disorder (CHADD), is recommended for family members and clients alike.

Psychiatric nurses can have a significant impact in mental health care promotion and disease prevention through educating clients and their families, encouraging self-help and advocacy programs, providing case management, monitoring medication administration and efficacy, and providing direct care. Psychiatric nurses are in a unique position in the multidisciplinary healthcare team of viewing "whole" clients and their support systems and being able to facilitate care planning in a manner designed to restore clients to optimal levels of functioning, for each client's own well-being and to the benefit of society in general.

THE ADVANCED PRACTICE PSYCHIATRIC NURSE

The first master's degree program in psychiatric nursing was implemented at Rutgers University in New Jersey under the direction of nurse Hildegard Peplau, author of the landmark 1952 text *Interpersonal Relations in Nursing*. Her program eventually graduated hundreds of clinical nurse specialists who went into clinical, leadership, and teaching roles in their communities.

The American Psychiatric Nurses Association statement on advanced practice nursing states that the advanced practice nurse is a:

"licensed registered nurse (RN) who is educationally prepared at a master's level, at a minimum, and is distinguished by a depth of knowledge of theory and practice, supervised clinical practice, and competence in advanced clinical nursing skills. The psychiatric-mental health advanced practice registered nurse has the ability to autonomously apply knowledge, skills, and experience to complex mental health problems."

(American Psychiatric Nurses Association [APNA], 1995)

Advanced practice nurses may be nurse practitioners (NP), clinical nurse specialists (CNS), nurse midwives, or nurse anesthetists. The general term APRN (advanced practice registered nurse) can refer to any of these, although usually only NPs and CNSs are found in the psychiatric specialty area. There are also nurse therapists, who are nurses who have a master's or doctoral degree in another discipline, such as psychology or counseling. APRNs may be qualified to sit for certifying exams by the American Nurse Credentialing Center (ANCC). The psychiatric CNS and NP certification requires extensive clinical supervision, graduation from an accredited master's degree program, and passing a board-certifying examination. After certification, the nurse must recertify every 5 years, with a combination of continuing education and other scholarly pursuits in the specialty, such as teaching or writing.

A psychiatric APRN may practice in a variety of settings, including offices, hospitals, clinics, schools, and nursing homes. Graduate education will include coursework and some experiences in providing individual and family therapy, managing group therapy, and prescribing medications. A nurse practitioner focuses chiefly on clinical (direct patient care), management, and leadership activities, often in an outpatient office or clinic setting. Clinical nurse specialists are taught to practice in a variety of roles, including direct care, program development, leadership and management, education, consultation, and research.

Some APRNs elect to apply for prescriptive privileges. Prescriptive privileging is now available throughout the country; however, regulations vary from state to state. Some states require a close collaborative arrangement with a physician and will only allow the APRN to prescribe if pre-established protocols are used, whereas other states have no collaborative or supervisory regulations and the APRN may prescribe independently. Some states will allow the APRN to prescribe controlled substances, whereas others will not. Interestingly, the more urban the population, the more restrictions there seem to be. In very remote areas such as Alaska, APRNs have very little supervisory restrictions. This is perhaps due to the paucity of licensed mental health providers in medically-underserved, healthcare professional shortage areas. The nurse is responsible for knowing the license regulations that exist in his or her state.

Most insurance companies will now reimburse the APRN for the direct care of clients. Medicaid rules vary by state. Medicare reimburses at 85% of the physician-approved rate, unless the physician is on-site, in which case they will reimburse the same as the physician. Most third-party insurance providers set contractual reimbursement rates. Grant-funded programs such as the Federally Qualified Health Clinic program sponsored by the Health and Human Resource Administration are designed to have a majority of the care provided by an APRN.

SUMMARY

Psychiatric and mental health issues are a major problem in the United States as well as worldwide. Persons with psychiatric disabilities have a higher incidence of poverty than do persons without those disabilities. Prevalence rates for mental health problems range from 4% to 10%, with higher rates in comorbid (two or more disorders) situations. The treatment of persons with mental illness has likewise varied over time, based on the perception of the cause of the disorder. The age of moral therapy in the late 1790s was followed by the age of scientific reasoning and the advent of psychotropic medications. Today, a major focus and emphasis of research is on genetic studies and the interaction between genes and the environment. The *DSM-IV-TR* multiaxial assessment is the primary diagnostic tool used in psychiatry and psychology because, currently, there are no reliable medical tests or X-rays for mental illnesses. Lastly, characteristics exist within the individual, the family, and the environment that may contribute to more serious illnesses or that may reduce the impact of the disorder when it occurs. This is particularly evident in the identification and treatment of posttraumatic stress disorders.

EXAM QUESTIONS

CHAPTER 1
Questions 1-6

Note: Choose the one option that BEST answers each question.

1. The percentage of women worldwide who will experience a depressive episode in their lifetime is approximately

   a. 9%.
   b. 18%.
   c. 27%.
   d. 36%.

2. The major shift in the perception of mental illness as a medical disorder is known as the age of

   a. religious exorcisms.
   b. shunning.
   c. home-based care.
   d. scientific reason.

3. The *DSM-IV-TR*

   a. does not address cultural variations.
   b. contains information to aid in making culturally-sensitive evaluations.
   c. is only relevant to diagnosing U.S. citizens.
   d. is a culturally-biased tool.

4. The *DSM-IV-TR* utilizes a five-axis format. Axis-IV represents

   a. the degree of social stress experienced by the client.
   b. the primary psychiatric diagnosis.
   c. the client's medical diagnosis.
   d. personality and basic character traits.

5. Role performance expectations that are important in childhood include

   a. maintaining a household and caring for siblings.
   b. volunteering for community organizations.
   c. participating in the national economy through paid employment.
   d. participating in the learning experience through education.

6. Which of the following is considered a protective factor in preventing mental illness?

   a. A sense of isolation
   b. Good healthcare insurance
   c. Good problem solving abilities
   d. Challenges to one's self esteem

CHAPTER 2

ETHICS, LAW, AND CULTURAL VARIATIONS

CHAPTER OBJECTIVE

At the end of this chapter the reader will be able to discuss some of the ethical, legal, and cultural issues associated with mental health care and treatment.

LEARNING OBJECTIVES

At the completion of this chapter, the reader will be able to

1. discuss the role of ethics in mental health care.

2. differentiate between voluntary and involuntary clients.

3. verbalize the importance of maintaining confidentiality and when it may be necessary to break confidentiality.

4. examine cultural differences as related to mental health care in minority populations in the United States.

INTRODUCTION

A review of mental health care and treatment would not be complete without a discussion of some of the ethical and legal issues surrounding care of the individual with a psychiatric illness. History has shown us many ways in which people with mental illness or emotional distress were abused and mistreated. The American Psychological Association has

worked diligently to provide ethical guidelines for client care, which will be presented in this chapter. Because of these past maltreatments, legal actions were taken in 1971 to ensure that clients who have psychiatric illnesses are not deprived of their basic rights to life, liberty, and the pursuit of happiness. For example, a person may not be hospitalized against his or her will simply because the presence of psychiatric symptoms; there must be some evidence of grave disability or of a danger to self or to others. This chapter will discuss in some depth these legal protections and some of the history upon which they are based. Despite legal protections and ethical obligations, many people still experience problems in accessing good healthcare because of social issues, such as poverty or homelessness, and ethnic discrimination. Some variations in care, based on cultural differences, will be presented as well as demographics relevant to the mental health of these populations.

ETHICAL PRINCIPLES AND BEHAVIORS

Ethics refer to the beliefs about right and wrong in a person and the standards of right or wrong in a society. Ethical standards may or may not be consistent with societal norms or laws. Nurses need to have a thorough understanding of general ethical principles in order to make reasonable, fair, and sound judgments in providing care. Ethical principles cause us to look at how we act in relationships and how we live with one another. Nurses who choose to work in the specialty of mental health care will encounter ethical questions on nearly a daily basis. Issues, such as confidentiality, patient protection, therapeutic relationships, clinical competency, and mental health research, are particularly complicated. To better guide the nurse in making ethical choices, an understanding of general principles will be useful.

The American Nurses Association (ANA) has developed a Code of Ethics for nurses, which are intended to serve as a framework for use in analyzing situations and making ethical decisions in the provision of nursing care. The ANA Code may not be copied or reproduced for the purposes of this book, but it may be viewed at no charge on the ANA Web site (www.nursingworld.org). The ANA Code divides ethical issues into nine provisions, based on general ethical principles:

- Provision 1 provides guidelines and directions for treating patients with dignity and respect (1.1) and encouraging self-determination (1.4). It also discusses relationships with clients (1.2) and colleagues (1.5) as well as the nature of health problems (1.3).

- Provision 2 states that the nurse's primary commitment is to the patient, whether an individual, family, or group (2.1). It covers conflicts of interest (2.2), collaboration (2.3), and professional boundaries (2.4).

- Provision 3 deals with protecting the privacy (3.1), confidentiality (3.2), and research participation (3.3) of patients. Ensuring nursing standards of practice (3.4), addressing impaired practice (3.6), and acting on questionable practices (3.5) all serve to protect patient safety and security.

- Provision 4 is concerned with accepting responsibility for patient care (4.1), being accountable for nursing judgment and action (4.2), and taking responsibility for nursing judgment and action (4.3). Delegating nursing care to others is discussed in provision 4.4.

- Provision 5 covers moral self-respect (5.1), professional growth and competence (5.2), wholeness of character of the nurse (5.3), and the preservation of integrity (5.4), which refers to being honest with the patient and oneself.

- Provision 6 is concerned with the influence of the environment on moral values (6.1) and the influence of the environment on ethical obligations (6.2). Each nurse's responsibility for the health care environment is discussed in provision 6.3.

- Provision 7 discusses the advancement of nursing practice through active involvement in the field and in healthcare policy (7.1), in developing and maintaining professional standards (7.2), and through knowledge development and dissemination to other nurses (7.3).

- Provision 8 addresses the promotion of community, national, and international efforts to meet health needs and concerns (8.1) and responsibilities to the public (8.2).

- Provision 9 reviews how the profession of nursing is expected to articulate nursing values (9.1) and carry out its collective responsibility through professional associations (9.2). Intraprofessional integrity (9.3) and social reform (9.4) are discussed here (Americaan Nurses Association, 2005).

General ethical principles fall into five broad categories. The American Psychological Association's Ethics Office discusses these on their Web site (www.apa.org/ethics). These principles are meant to be guidelines to help the healthcare provider in decision-making.

1. *Beneficence and Nonmaleficence* – Healthcare providers must have the desire to be professional and help the client and, in doing so, to do no harm. The nurse should guard against using undue influence to pressure a client into desired actions. Medication compliance is a good example of where decisions are frequently made that present ethical dilemmas. The healthcare provider must weigh the pros and cons of administering antipsychotic medications against a client's will, in order to address the greater good of ameliorating the psychotic condition or protecting society. Involuntary treatment may be necessary to benefit the client and to prevent future harm.

2. *Fidelity and Responsibility* – Healthcare providers have a duty to be honest and trustworthy with their clients. The inherent power in the relationship lies with the caregiver. Clients are asked to be trusting and to believe that others have their best interests in mind. This ascribes a high degree of responsibility on the healthcare provider to tell the truth and to be accountable for professional behaviors. Ethical issues often arise regarding clinical research and informed consent.

3. *Integrity* – Healthcare providers must be professional and maintain a high level of clinical expertise. Nurses practicing in psychiatric settings should obtain continuing education in the mental health specialty and maintain a certain level of competency. Healthcare providers must also guard against establishing personal or sexual relationships with clients. In most settings, psychiatric staff members are not permitted to engage in any commerce (buying or selling) with clients for an extended period of time to avoid the appearance of impropriety or accusations that the staff member is taking advantage of the dependent nature of the staff-client relationship.

4. *Justice* – Healthcare providers must recognize that all persons are entitled to equal treatment and quality of care, even in the mental health realm. It can be particularly difficult to provide emotional support and counseling equally to both the family harmed by an intoxicated driver and to the driver himself. Healthcare providers should strive to be nonjudgmental and fair to all clients, regardless of age, gender, race, sexual orientation, diagnosis, or any other differentiating characteristic.

5. *Respect* – Healthcare providers need to respect the dignity and worth of all people and the rights of individuals to confidentiality, privacy, and freedom of choice. The psychiatric nurse should also respect religious and cultural differences and strive to avoid ethnocentrism. Clients experiencing an acute exacerbation of a psychiatric disorder may behave oddly or inappropriately at times. The nurse needs to refrain from laughing or otherwise demeaning the client and protect the client as much as possible from a loss of dignity (American Psychological Association, 2002).

When faced with a difficult decision, it is useful to have a framework for decision-making to guide the healthcare provider. First, it is important to gather all of the facts of a situation: What is the dilemma? Who will be affected? What are possible outcomes? For each course of action, what may be the result? Are there legal issues at stake? After making a thorough examination of the relevant information, one can next consider alternative actions from various moral perspectives.

The Virtue Perspective

- Identifies moral values as what are inherently positive character traits

- Includes honesty, faithfulness, integrity, compassion, truthfulness, and courage

- Decisions are based on what is *the right thing to do*

The Utilitarian Perspective

- Weighs the effects of actions against the consequence there will be to society; may sacrifice rights of the individual for the greater good

- Decisions are based on what is *best for the majority*

The Rights Perspective

- Focuses on the rights of the individual (civil, political) and respects the dignity of the person

- Includes issues of "right to free speech," "right to liberty," and "right to privacy"

- Decisions are based on what *protects basic rights*

The Fairness (or Justice) Perspective

- States that all must be treated equally and consistently, unless there is moral justification for treating some differently (some "deserve" it more)

- Involves moral justification, which may be based on needs, merit, or faults

- Decisions are based on *treating based on moral justifications*

The Common Good Perspective

- Describes that the good of the individual is bound to the common good of the community; the community has shared values and goals

- Decisions are based on *the advancement of the community*

The nurse is then faced with making a decision. Decisions do not have to be made alone – in fact, involving the multidisciplinary mental health care team (usually comprised of nursing, medicine, social work, rehabilitation, and psychology) can provide a safety net for the nurse and ensure that personal biases are eliminated.

As a final step, those involved need to reflect on the decision made, actions, and subsequent results. What, if anything, should have been done differently? Were the basic principles of beneficence, fidelity, integrity, justice, and respect maintained? Were goals accomplished? How will these actions influence the client's future care?

Additionally, one should consider the issue of ethical relativism. Ethical relativism deals with the differences in ethical beliefs relative to one's societal norms. An action deemed appropriate or right in one culture, may be very unacceptable in another. Some ethicists claim that there is no universal moral standard – all ethics are culture bound and moral standards can only be determined within a specific society – whereas others believe that fundamental principles exist in all cultures and are inherent in all human beings. Consider the act of infanticide. American culture treats the killing of infants equal to the killing of any person, whereas other cultures have practiced infanticide when obvious birth defects are present or starvation of other children is at risk. Relativism is also evident on a historical basis. Hundreds of years ago, intermarriage with first cousins and even siblings (royalty) was encouraged to maintain the family bloodlines. Today it is unacceptable in most parts of the world.

LEGAL CONSIDERATIONS: VOLUNTARY VERSUS INVOLUNTARY CLIENTS

In Section 1 of the 14th Amendment of the U.S. Constitution, it states that

All persons born or naturalized in the United States, and subject to the jurisdiction thereof, are citizens of the United States and of the state wherein they reside. No state shall…deprive any person of life, liberty, or property, without due process of law; nor deny to any person within its jurisdiction the equal protection of the laws.

The issue of liberty has been tested repeatedly in settings where United States citizens have been held against their will, including in psychiatric institutions.

Keltner et al. (2007, pp. 53-54) do an excellent job of providing an overview of landmark legal decisions related to individuals with psychiatric disorders. They identify 10 rulings that have historically made a marked impact on the legal rights of the identified clients and on affected other parties. A summary of each of these legal decisions follows.

1. 1843 – The *M'Naghten rule* first identified a legal defense of "not guilty by reason of insanity" by stating that persons who do not understand the nature of their actions cannot be held legally responsible for those actions.

2. 1965 – In *Griswold v. Connecticut,* the U.S. Supreme Court first recognized that an individual has a "right of personal privacy" under the Constitution of the United States.

3. 1966 – *Rouse v. Cameron* was a case in which the courts found that a person committed to an institution must be actively receiving treatment and not merely warehoused.

4. 1968 – *Whitree v. State of New York* was a case in which a client who had been institutionalized for 14 years successfully sued the state of New York claiming that if he had received adequate treatment he could have been discharged after only 2 years.

5. 1968 – In *Meier v. Ross General Hospital,* a physician was found liable for the death of his hospitalized client who committed suicide while under his care. The client had a previous suicide attempt prior to the hospital stay. The physician was liable for failing in his "duty to warn" of the threat of suicide in this client.

6. 1972 – In *Wyatt v. Stickney,* the entire mental health care system of Alabama was sued for an inadequate treatment program. The court ruled that each institution within the mental health care system must: a) stop using clients for hospital labor needs, b) ensure a humane environment, c) maintain minimum staffing levels, d) establish human rights committees, and e) provide the least restrictive environment possible for the client.

7. 1976 – In the well-known case of *Tarasoff v. The Regents of the University of California,* the parents of Tatiana Tarasoff sued the university following the 1969 death of their daughter at the hands of Prosenjit Poddar. Poddar had told his therapist that he planned to kill Tarasoff when she returned from summer break. Although the therapist had contacted the police, they released Poddar because he appeared rational. The court found that the therapist had a "duty to warn of threats of harm to others" and was negligent in not notifying Tarasoff of the threats that had been made against her.

8. 1979 – Clients at Boston State Hospital sought the "right to refuse treatment" in *Rogers v. Okin.* Based on the 1965 decision regarding the "right of personal privacy," the court found that the hospital could not force nonviolent clients to take medication against their will. This ruling also included the directive that clients or their guardians must give informed consent before medications could be given.

9. 1983 – In *Rennie v. Klein,* a client claimed his rights were violated by the hospital when he was forced to take psychotropic medications. The ruling again addressed the "right to refuse treatment" and the "right to privacy," and furthered the necessity of obtaining informed consent.

10. 1972 – *Jackson v. Indiana,* and 1992 — *Foucha v. Louisiana* demonstrated that the nature of a (ongoing) psychiatric commitment must "bear some reasonable relation to the purpose for which the individual is committed" (Foucha v. Louisiana, 1992). When Jackson and Foucha were first hospitalized, they were

deemed to be mentally ill and dangerous. The ruling recognized that individuals who are no longer mentally ill do not require hospitalization, and that individuals are not required to prove themselves to be no longer dangerous.

THE BAKER ACT

In 1971, the legislature of Florida adopted the Florida Mental Health Act, also known as the *Baker Act*, thus dramatically revising and updating almost 100 years of mental health involuntary commitment practice. The Baker Act was named after Maxine Baker, the former state representative from Miami who sponsored the act after serving as chairperson of the House Committee on Mental Health. The overall purpose of the Baker Act was to systematically address the limitations on liberty placed upon an individual with a psychiatric disorder. The Baker Act has since been revised, with its most recent reform occurring in 1996 to further reinforce, among other things, protection for voluntarily admitted clients, clients being released from state treatment facilities, informed consent and guardian advocacy, and expanded notice requirements (State of Florida Department of Children and Families Mental Health Program Office, 2002).

The Baker Act is broad in its coverage. It ensures that individuals are treated humanely and fairly and includes the rights to send and receive mail and telephone calls, to keep one's own possessions and clothing, and the right to register and vote in public elections. It guarantees clients the right to have visitors when requested and covers the right to receive appropriate treatment or to refuse treatment. The use of restraints, seclusion, isolation, and other management techniques are closely monitored and complaint resolution is required. The Baker Act ensures that clients have the right to ask the court to review the cause and legality of any detention or unjust denial of a right, privilege, or

authorized procedure. Additionally, the client has the right to participate in treatment and discharge planning and to seek out a practitioner of his or her choice. In any instance where these rights are denied, the healthcare providers must be able to thoroughly document the rationale for the denial and notify the client, preferably in writing. The healthcare provider may never restrict telephone calls to the client's attorney.

As a consequence of the Baker Act, an admission to a psychiatric facility differs from an admission to a medical facility in that there must be a clear (not implied) legal status of the client. Preferentially, all hospitalized clients are admitted voluntarily and have agreed, in writing, to receiving inpatient care. Prior to admission, the client must be informed of the reason for admission, purpose of the proposed treatment, the approximate length of care, and side effects that may be incurred as a result of treatment. Adults must be deemed mentally competent to give their consent or an involuntary commitment needs to be obtained (discussed later in this section). A minor child can only be admitted to a psychiatric facility upon the application and signature of a legal guardian. Occasionally, a voluntarily admitted client will decide to leave the hospital against medical or clinical advice. The attending physician must determine whether the client's thoughts or behaviors will constitute a danger to himself or to others, or whether the client is so gravely ill that he will be unable to provide for basic needs of food, shelter, clothing, and protection from the elements. If the determination is made that the client is not safe to leave the facility, then involuntary commitment proceedings are initiated. This decision must be made within 24 hours of the client's request to be discharged.

Particular care must be taken when hospitalizing an adult client with a dementia disorder, or one who has a healthcare surrogate or proxy, to a psychiatric facility. Prior to the admission, these clients must be assessed as to their ability to provide informed consent for the admission. If there is a question as to the competency of the client, it may be preferable to refuse a voluntary admission and obtain a court order for an involuntary examination. A competency hearing may also be necessary.

Clients can be evaluated on an involuntary basis when they refuse voluntary treatment or if they are not competent to consent to voluntary treatment. Without care or treatment, clients are likely to suffer from neglect. This can result in a real and present threat to the client, with a substantial likelihood that serious bodily harm may be caused to the client or others in the near future. Involuntary admission laws may vary somewhat from state to state. An involuntary examination can be requested, or petitioned, by any concerned party; however, it is usually done by a family member. It can be initiated by any one of the following: A court can enter an ex parte order based upon sworn testimony; a law enforcement officer can take the client into custody and deliver him or her to a treatment facility; or a physician, clinical psychologist, psychiatric nurse, or clinical social worker can execute a certificate stating that the client has been examined within the past 48 hours and found to meet the criteria for involuntary admission, after which a court will issue an order to admit the client involuntarily to the nearest accepting treatment facility. After an involuntary admission has been initiated, the receiving facility has 72 working hours (does not include weekends or legal holidays) to examine the client and determine whether psychiatric treatment is required. At the end of the 72 hours, the client must be released (to outpatient care; if charged with a crime, then to the appropriate police department), sign a voluntary admission application, or the attending physician must petition the court for involuntary placement. In some cases, the attending physician may be able to renew the 72-hour detention order if admission to a secure psychiatric facility has not yet been obtained (i.e., the client has been held in the emergency department pending an inpatient placement).

An involuntary placement may be ordered by the court when there is clear and convincing evidence that the client has a mental illness and has refused voluntary treatment (or is unable to decide) and, without the placement, a real and present threat of substantial harm to the clients' well-being exists; or, without the placement, there is a substantial likelihood that the client will inflict self-harm, or harm others, and all available less-restrictive treatment alternatives have been deemed inappropriate. The court then states the length of time that the client will be under an involuntary placement order. At the end of this time, the healthcare team must decide whether to pursue continued involuntary placement.

Psychiatric nurses should become familiar with their individual state laws that govern the specifics of voluntary and involuntary psychiatric admissions as well as the procedures followed by specific healthcare facilities. It is not unusual to find variations on the interpretation of the Baker Act from state to state or in different regions of the country.

CONFIDENTIALITY AND THE BILL OF RIGHTS

In 1998, President Clinton appointed the Advisory Commission on Consumer Protection and Quality in the Health Care Industry. The Commission, co-chaired by Donna Shalala, secretary of the Department of Health and Human Services, issued its final report, which included a Consumer Bill of Rights and Responsibilities (see Table 2-1). Of particular interest to psychiatric nurses is the section on confidentiality of health information. Psychiatric clients are expressly protected in the confidentiality of their records; information may not be shared with any third-party, without the express written consent of the client or his or her legal guardian. Consent to release infor-

TABLE 2-1: CONSUMER BILL OF RIGHTS AND RESPONSIBILITIES

I. *Information Disclosure* – You have the right to receive accurate and easily understood information about your health plan, healthcare professionals, and healthcare facilities. If you speak another language, have a physical or mental disability, or just don't understand something, assistance will be provided so you can make informed healthcare decisions.

II. *Choice of Providers and Plans* – You have the right to a choice of healthcare providers that is sufficient to provide you with access to appropriate high-quality healthcare.

III. *Access to Emergency Services* – If you have severe pain, an injury, or sudden illness that convinces you that your health is in serious jeopardy, you have the right to receive screening and stabilization emergency services whenever and wherever needed, without prior authorization or financial penalty.

IV. *Participation in Treatment Decisions* – You have the right to know all of your treatment options and to participate in decisions about your care. Parents, guardians, family members, or other individuals that you designate can represent you if you cannot make your own decisions.

V. *Respect and Nondiscrimination* – You have the right to considerate, respectful, and nondiscriminatory care from your doctors, health plan representatives, and other healthcare providers.

VI. *Confidentiality of Health Information* – You have the right to talk in confidence with healthcare providers and to have your healthcare information protected. You also have the right to review and copy your own medical record and request that your physician amend your record if it is not accurate, relevant, or complete.

VII. *Complaints and Appeals* – You have the right to a fair, fast, and objective review of any complaint you have against your health plan, doctors, hospitals or other healthcare personnel. This includes complaints about waiting times, operating hours, the conduct of healthcare personnel, and the adequacy of healthcare facilities.

(Presidents Advisory Commission on Consumer Protection and Quality in the Health Care Industry, 1997).

mation can be withdrawn at any time by the client. Few exceptions to this exist. Confidentiality may be violated only in the situations:

1. The client has made a direct threat against another person, and the healthcare provider has a clear duty to warn the endangered individual.

2. The client has reported actual or suspected abuse (including molestation) or neglect of a minor child. The healthcare provider has an obligation to report this to the appropriate Child Protective Services division of the state's Office of Family and Children.

3. The healthcare provider can discuss the information provided in a commitment document with the relevant physician, officer of the court, and petitioner(s) of the commitment.

4. When an insanity defense is utilized to defend against a criminal charge, the entire clinical record becomes public.

5. A judge may order documents (clinical records) to be turned over to the court for examination. A subpoena to appear in court does not constitute a judge's order to release information; it merely mandates the appearance of the subpoenaed individual.

Violation of the confidentiality of a client with a psychiatric illness in situations other than those outlined here may subject the nurse to legal action as well as licensure censure. Most agencies have an acceptable form that identifies to whom information can be released, date that the release is valid, and particular types of information that can be shared. The Health Insurance Portability and Accountability Act (HIPAA) was enacted in 1996 and went into effect in 2003. This act is designed to protect the client's health information more securely and it encourages the use of electronic health records, data submission, and documentation.

CULTURAL DIVERSITY ISSUES

Culture influences various aspects of mental health, including the recognition and expression of psychiatric symptoms, coping styles, community supports, and the willingness to seek treatment. Culture-bound syndromes are recurrent, locality-specific patterns of aberrant behavior that are not linked to a specific *DSM-IV-TR* diagnostic category. Most of these are limited to specific ethnic populations and are, in essence, diagnostic categories used to identify, discuss, and treat specific problem behaviors or symptoms within that culture. Appendix A examines some culture-bound syndromes identified in the *DSM-IV-TR,* along with characteristic traits of each syndrome.

In 1999, the U.S. Department of Health and Human Services, Office of the Surgeon General, collected data on the mental health of various cultures and ethnic populations in the United States. Four primary ethnicities were studied: African Americans, Asian American/Pacific Islanders, Latinos/Hispanic Americans, and Native American Indians/Alaska Natives. A supplement to the Surgeon General's report entitled, "Mental Health: Culture, Race and Ethnicity" was written in 2001 to provide a better framework for understanding cultural and racial differences, but also to reinforce what was found in the original data regarding the effect stigma and shame has on many Americans in their pursuit (or lack of) mental health treatment. The U.S. Census Bureau provided updated information in its 2005 to 2007 American Community Survey that described characteristics of populations in the country. Table 2-2 presents a summary of some of the differences identified in these populations, as compared to the general population of all U.S. citizens. Mental health problems including depression, PTSD and alcoholism have long been associated with social problems of poverty, homelessness, poor education, and incarceration.

TABLE 2-2: SOCIAL DEMOGRAPHICS OF CULTURAL MINORITIES IN THE UNITED STATES

	Total U.S. Population	White/ Caucasian	Black/ African-American	Latino/ Hispanic American	Asian American	Native Hawaiian/ Pacific Islander	American Indian/ Alaskan	Two or more Races	Some other Race
% of all U.S. citizens	100	74	12.4	14.7	4.3	4.7	0.8	2.1	6.2
% living at or below 100% of poverty	13.3	10.5	25.3	21.5	11	16.7	25.8	17.3	22
% with a high school education or above	84	86.5	79.3	59.9	85.4	83.9	75.7	86.4	57.6
% that are veterans	10.4	11.6	9.3	3.8	2.9	9.1	10	10.5	3

(U.S. Census Bureau, 2008)

Table 2-3 looks at the percentage of homeless and incarcerated individuals in minority populations and in those who are mentally ill or substance dependent. The number of homeless people in the United States is estimated to be between 6% and 10% of the total population (Substance Abuse and Mental Health Services Administration [SAMHSA], 1999).

African Americans constitute approximately 12% of the U.S. population. In the 1999 data, 25.3% lived below poverty guidelines. Mental health providers are predominately not African American, with only about 2% of psychiatrists and psychologists and 4% of social workers represented by the race. Few clinical trials have focused primarily on the African American population. Limited data suggests that mental health rates are the same for all ethnic groups, but there is alarming cause for concerns in diagnostic accuracy. African Americans are more likely than whites to be diagnosed with schizophrenia and less likely than whites to be diagnosed with or treated for depression. Additionally, African Americans are more likely to be treated in hospital settings and less likely to receive outpatient services. The Surgeon General's Report found that older African Americans (especially women) were found to enter post-hospital home care with higher levels of physical and cognitive impairments and to have caregivers with more limitations than did older whites. Older African American adults may also be reluctant to share information with non-African American healthcare providers because of historical experiences with racism and the belief that they will not be listened to or shown respect (SAMHSA, 1999).

The Latino/Hispanic American population is rapidly growing. If trends continue, Latino/Hispanics will comprise 25% of Americans by the year 2050. Mexican Americans constitute nearly two-thirds of the Hispanic population. Rates of mental health disorders are similar to non-Hispanic Whites, with some exceptions: Adult immigrants have lower rates of mental disorders than American-born Mexican Americans or Puerto Ricans; Latino youths experience more anxiety and delinquency problems, depression, and drug use than do non-Hispanic White youths; depression in older adults is closely correlated with physical illness; and suicide rates were about 50% that of non-Hispanic Whites (although suicide ideation and unsuccessful attempts were higher). There is a higher incidence of PTSD in Hispanic men that is associated with refugees exposed to civil wars in their home countries and to Vietnam War veterans. Substance abuse rates are slightly lower in Hispanic women and slightly higher in Hispanic men. Hispanics are approximately twice as likely as Whites to die from liver cirrhosis, which is possibly related to a higher incidence of hepatitis C. There are few Hispanic children in the child welfare system, but Latino men are four times more likely than Whites to be incarcerated at some point in their lifetime. The lack of Spanish-speaking mental health care providers has been a problem, causing fewer than 1 in 11 individuals with a psychiatric disorder to seek treatment. Misdiagnosing is common related to language barriers. Hispanic Americans are

TABLE 2-3: CHARACTERISTICS OF ADULT INCARCERATED MALES WHO WERE HOMELESS IN THE PRECEDING YEAR

White/ Caucasian	Black/ African American	Latino/ Hispanic	Other	Mentally Ill: all ethnicities	Drug abuse or dependency	Alcohol abuse or dependency	Trauma history (physical or sexual abuse)
41%	50%	16%	13%	75%	68%	55%	31%

(Greenberg & Rosenheck, 2008)

more likely to utilize folk remedies solely, or as a complement to traditional care, and some may consult folk healers for more traditional care. Older people and those who are ill are more likely to be cared for within the home community, partly due to the strength of family values (SAMHSA,1999).

Asian Americans/Pacific Islanders comprise just over 9% of the U.S. population. There are more than 43 different ethnic subgroups included in the Asian American/Pacific Islander category, with over 100 languages and dialects. About 35% of these individuals live in households where there is limited English proficiency. Mental health care needs have not been well studied in this group. Prevalence rates for depression are about 3% to 7% using traditional scales. Asian Americans tend to exhibit somatic (physical) symptoms of depression more frequently than emotional symptoms. Culture-bound syndromes may include neurasthenia, which is characterized by fatigue, weakness, poor concentration, memory loss, irritability, aches and pains, sleep disturbances, and Hwa-byung (Appendix A). The focus on physical symptoms can serve as a barrier to seeking mental health care. Older Asian Americans may not understand questions or the intent of a medical interview, and may answer, "Yes" to avoid confrontation. Suicide rates tend to be lower overall among minorities with the exceptions being Native Hawaiian adolescents, and older Asian American women (older than 65 years of age). Social isolation may be a factor in the higher suicide rates of older adults. Many Asian Americans and Pacific Islanders are heavily represented among refugee populations and, as such, are at higher risk for PTSD – in some studies as high as 70% for Southeast Asian refugees. Nearly 50% of this population has difficulty accessing mental health care services because of language barriers. Utilization of mental health care services is extremely low. Shame and stigma are believed to figure prominently in these low utilization rates. The use of complementary therapies (such as

herbal therapy) is higher than in the general population. Many Asian Americans have a decreased activity of the enzyme aldehyde dehydrogenase-2, a necessary component for the metabolism of alcohol. As a result, alcohol tolerance and dependency is very low (SAMHSA, 1999).

In the general population, less than 1% of the population is identified as being of American Indian or Alaska Native heritage. There are at least 561 different American Indian and Alaska Native tribes and over 200 indigenous languages. In 1996, 4500 children between 9 and 13 years of age were screened in the Great Smoky Mountains Study of Youth for psychiatric and substance use disorders. The study found that American Indian children were the same as White children in rates of psychiatric disorders, with lower rates of neurological tic disorders; however, 13-year-old American Indian and Alaska native children had higher rates of substance abuse than did White children in the study (Costello et al., 1996). According to the 1999 Surgeon General's data, suicide rates for American Indian and Alaska Natives are 1.5 times the national average. Alcohol and drug problems are higher than in other populations (up to 70% in Northern Plains Indians). Deaths from chronic liver disease and cirrhosis are about four times more prevalent among American Indian and Alaska Natives than in the general U.S. population. The Indian Health Service (IHS) is the federal agency responsible for providing healthcare to native populations. Only about 20% of Native American Indians report access to IHS clinics, which are located on reservations. Mental health treatment rates appear to be the same or similar to those of non-American Indian/Alaska Native Whites – about 32% of those with an identified disorder seek treatment. Among Cherokee children, only one in seven received professional treatment, and they were more likely than White children to be seen in the juvenile justice system. There is a limited availability of skilled and intermediate long-term care facilities on reservations. In 1999, there were only 15 such facilities among the nearly 300 reservations. Healthcare is more likely to be provided within the home community. American Indian and Alaska Native cultures tend to view illness as a natural part of the aging process; thus, healthcare may not be readily sought and there is a greater reliance on native remedies (SAMHSA, 1999).

SUMMARY

Society has known about psychiatric and mental/behavioral disorders for centuries; however, the ethical and humane treatment of persons experiencing these problems is a relatively new phenomenon. Only in the past century have the legal rights of individuals with mental illness been addressed, through the enactment of the Baker Act in Florida in 1971 that ensured basic rights, such as the right to receive mail and phone calls, see visitors (or refuse them), and to refuse medical treatment. For clients who refuse treatment, doctors and psychologists must now petition the courts to enforce treatment, including medications, of psychiatric clients who do not want care. Very strict guidelines exist as to the criteria required for court intervention, although these may vary somewhat from state to state. Confidentiality is closely protected, and the Consumer Bill of Rights and Responsibilities (adopted in 2003) further provides individuals with the right to participate in their care and keep their medical records secure. Mental health providers are faced daily with ethical dilemmas and issues in weighing the costs versus benefits of treatment, the need to treat all clients equally, and the need to be honest and forthright with clients and families about their care. General ethical principles help to guide in decision making, and nursing organizations have put out more specific guidelines for the practice of nursing care. Psychiatric disorders are prevalent across all populations, regardless of ethnicity, although discrimination and racism adversely affect health status as well as the willingness to seek treatment because of stigma and shame. Stigmas about mental disorders and their treatments are as great, or even greater, in minority populations as in the general U.S. population, and mistrust of mental health care services has been a major deterrent to treatment.

EXAM QUESTIONS

CHAPTER 2
Questions 7-12

Note: Choose the one option that BEST answers each question.

7. Ethical decisions ideally should be made by a

    a. physician.

    b. nurse.

    c. family.

    d. multidisciplinary team.

8. The Baker Act of 1971 guarantees the right to

    a. smoke in designated hospital rooms.

    b. send and receive mail.

    c. take weekend long passes.

    d. commit suicide if terminally ill.

9. An involuntary hospital admission is most likely to be necessary with a

    a. person who is hallucinating but is not making threats to harm himself or herself or others.

    b. person who is confused and talking about alien invasions, is sleeping on the streets, and is dehydrated and malnourished.

    c. person who is intoxicated and angry with the staff of the emergency department of a hospital.

    d. teenager who writes a letter to his girlfriend telling her that he wants to run away with her.

10. One criterion for an involuntary hospital admission is

    a. refusal to take medications.

    b. illegal acts such as burglary.

    c. alcohol intoxication.

    d. a suicide attempt or threat.

11. Confidentiality of an individual receiving psychiatric treatment can only be violated without the client's consent when the

    a. police have a warrant to arrest the individual.

    b. client reports physical or sexual abuse of a child.

    c. client's spouse is calling for information.

    d. client's employer needs to know how long the client will be in treatment.

12. The ethnic group studied in the 1999 Surgeon General's Report that is expected to comprise 25% of the U.S. population by the year 2050 is

    a. African American.

    b. Latino/Hispanic American.

    c. Asian American/Pacific Islander.

    d. American Indian/Alaska Native.

CHAPTER 3

ASSESSING THE CLIENT WITH A PSYCHIATRIC DISORDER

CHAPTER OBJECTIVE

At the end of this chapter, the reader will be able to describe components of a relevant history of a client with a psychiatric disorder and an effective nursing care plan.

LEARNING OBJECTIVES

At the end of this chapter, the reader will be able to

1. perform a mental status examination.

2. identify possible defense mechanisms that may impact on care.

3. identify key elements of information that need to be obtained in a mental health history.

4. write a nursing care plan with appropriate nursing diagnoses, long-term treatment goals, short-term objectives, and interventions.

INTRODUCTION

Individuals experiencing psychiatric and mental health or emotional problems are more difficult to evaluate than are those with physical health issues. In medicine, laboratory and diagnostic tests can identify the presence or absence of specific disease states, such as a complete blood count for anemia, X-rays to reveal fractures, CT scans to identify masses and tumors, and physical evaluations to pin-point such conditions as abnormal heart sounds or fluid in the lungs. As discussed in Chapter 1, there are no medical tests that will definitively and consistently diagnose a psychiatric or mental health problem. As a result, the history and presenting symptoms of the client are of utmost importance.

In this chapter, the evaluation of a client with psychiatric symptoms will be presented, utilizing a systematic approach. The mental status exam will be discussed in detail, and examples will be given of some of the striking alterations in thought processes and content that can occur. Unknown or unexamined psychological processes that may interfere with, or are counterproductive to, a client's ability to participate in his or her care will be presented. These defense mechanisms are often unknown by the client and, once identified, may form the foundation for the therapeutic interventions discussed in Chapter 4. For practicing clinicians, key elements of information to be obtained in a mental health assessment and the application of the nursing process are reviewed. A sample care plan is provided. Finally, components of a standard psychiatric evaluation are presented for the advanced practice nurse clinician.

MENTAL STATUS EXAMS

Mental Status Exams are a structured means of examining the mental and emotional state of a client with a psychiatric disorder to better lead to an appropriate diagnosis. They can also point the clinician toward significant problem areas to be targeted in a care plan. Mental status exams are an essential tool for evaluating safety for both the client and the caregivers. Exams may follow many different formats, and most healthcare facilities have a form already in place. All exams include the same basic elements: an examination of the client's behaviors, thoughts, and moods.

Appearance

Overall appearance is the first element assessed in a mental status exam. How is the client groomed? Is his or her clothing or person soiled? Is there an odor present? Is the client wearing clothing that is appropriate to the weather and environment? It is important to take housing and financial means into consideration, as a client who is homeless or indigent may have less access to stylish clothing or hygiene items than one who lives in a middle-class, suburban setting.

Behavior

The client's behavior during the interview should be noted. Is the client cooperative and maintaining good eye contact or does the client present as evasive, guarded, or hostile? Is the client calm and sitting quietly or pacing and restless? Does the client appear to be attending to stimuli within his own mind, such as picking at the air or talking to empty space? Does the client have any motor tics or other unusual motor movements, which may be indicative of medication side effects, or is the client using any unusual gesturing.

Mood and Affect

Mood and affect are assessed together. In general, a client's mood reflects overall emotional state. Mood is fairly consistent, whereas affect is the current emotional presentation and may be situation-dependent or may change rapidly. A dysphoric mood indicates the client is persistently depressed, lethargic, apathetic, or down. It is usually accompanied by a depressed affect, but the affect may also be described as anxious or irritable. A euphoric mood is an elevated emotional state that may be associated with an affect that is giddy, cheerful, or excessively bright. A labile affect is one that is rapidly changing and unpredictable – the client may be cheerful, then suddenly becomes enraged with little provocation or may burst into tears unexpectedly. Dysphoric moods are often associated with depression, whereas euphoric moods may be associated with mania. Substance abuse affects the client's mood in many ways, depending on the degree of intoxication, substance used, and any withdrawal symptoms. Clients may also be described as having an affect that is flat or blunted. Some medications can interfere with the physical expression of an emotion through blunting, the emotions or impacting negatively on the facial muscles. A client who is slow to respond emotionally, or responds at a degree less than expected, may be referred to as blunted. A client who demonstrates no emotional response at all may be considered as having a flat affect.

Thought Processes

Thought processes refer to the way thoughts are organized and structured. Normally, thoughts are logical, sequential, and easily understood by others (in the absence of a known speech or communication disorder). Clients with disorganized thoughts may seem to have nonsensical speech. They may have difficulty in performing simple activities, such as bathing or eating, without assistance, even in the absence of a physical impairment. Clients may mix up or confuse medications when a structured system (such as a weekly pill dispenser) is not available. Thoughts also may be rapid, racing, or slowed. Poverty-of-thoughts occurs when the client has a paucity of ideas or content of thoughts – questions are answered with one or two words, and clients may be unable to expand or utilize imagination. Thoughts can be abstract or concrete. The common proverb, "A rolling stone gathers no moss," will be perceived by an abstract-thinking person as a metaphor for life and interpreted as such; whereas a concrete-thinking person may interpret it as "When you roll rocks, they don't get moss on them." Tangential thoughts are seen when a client loses the central thread of a conversation. The clinician will note that one idea leads to another, which then leads to a third idea, and so forth. "I came here in an ambulance, the driver was a man. I was married to a man once. I had a beautiful wedding. My sister makes flower arrangements for weddings. I hate my sister!" is an example of a tangential thought process. The term flight-of-ideas may also be used to describe a client's thought processes: "I came here in an ambulance. I wish I had more money! Did you see that TV show on Pekinese dogs the other night?" When a client is experiencing flight-of-ideas, thoughts are somewhat random and have little association with one another. Word-salad is another phenomenon seen when assessing a client's thought processes. In a word-salad, there are no logical connections, and the thoughts are jumbled, "I don't. Here, he said. My house. Mouse. Spouse." The previous statement also gives an example of clang associations – or using words because they have similar sounds and not because of the actual meanings of the words. Lastly, a client may use neologisms, or words that don't exist in the English language. Words such as "frugelzip" or "rappeliciosity" will have a meaning that is clear only to the client.

Thought Content

Thought content refers to what the client is thinking about. Initially, it is helpful to assess for preoccupations or obsessions on real-life events, such as finances, employment, or relationships. An intrusive thought is an idea that comes unbidden and occurs when the client has difficulty thinking about anything else. Ruminative thoughts are thoughts that seem to be "stuck" in the client's mind, much like a cow that will "ruminate" by chewing repeatedly. An obsessive client will tend to have ruminative thoughts that may be unusual in nature, such as a desire to check the door repeatedly to ensure it is locked or the belief that germs may be everywhere. Often, obsessive thoughts will lead to compulsive behaviors – such as ritualized handwashing – in part as an attempt to ameliorate those thoughts and their accompanying anxiety.

Two particular thought content problems are of essential importance: hallucinations and delusions. Hallucinations are disordered sensory perceptions. Auditory, visual, olfactory, gustatory, or tactile symptoms may be present. Auditory hallucinations, such as hearing voices, occur most often in the presence of a primary psychiatric illness. Visual hallucinations are most commonly seen in psychiatric disorders and in delirium states, such as those caused by alcohol withdrawal or drug toxicity (including prescription medications). Olfactory and gustatory hallucinations are rare in psychiatric illnesses, but are quite common as prodromal symptoms of an impending seizure. Occasionally, a client with a psychiatric illness will report a tactile hallucination, such as "hands touching me," "bugs crawling on me;" however, these are more often associated with alcohol or drug withdrawal states. When working with a client experiencing hallucinations, it is important to remember that the brain actually perceives the reported sensation and, to the client, it is very real. Pointing out that the hallucination does not exist is usually fruitless and may jeopardize the development of a secure clinician-client relationship.

Delusions are false beliefs. The client experiencing a delusion is certain that something is true, when there is no substantiating evidence to prove these beliefs. Paranoid delusions are common in mental health clients. Paranoid clients are usually quite frightened, as they may believe they are being watched, monitored, or spied upon by others. They may report cars following them or mysterious phone calls late at night. Occasionally, a client with paranoia may fear being poisoned and refuse medications or food. Religious delusions are another common phenomena. Clients having a religious delusion may feel persecuted by demons or may be very excited about a special relationship with God or with angels. The healthcare provider needs to exert further care in obtaining a thorough history to determine a client's baseline religious beliefs, so as not to label a thought as delusional when it is a well-accepted belief within the client's social network. Somatic delusions are uncomfortable beliefs that there is something terribly wrong with one's body. Some clients may believe that their bowels are necrotic or dead or that their brain is missing. Other delusions may exist, ranging from a belief that aliens are broadcasting signals, to one's loved ones have been replaced by clones. It is always essential to determine the feeling states that are produced by the client's delusional thoughts. Paranoid thoughts will drive fear and fight-or-flight responses. The client may set up protective traps around the home to prevent others from entering. Religious delusions may be pleasant and make the client feel special, or they may be so persecutory that the client becomes depressed and suicidal. Somatic delusions can lead to excess visits to family practitioners and emergency departments and result in the label of "hypochondriac" for the client.

"Ideas of reference" are thought content that occurs when the client believes that events in the environment have a personal connection to the self. Clients may report that television news broadcasters are giving them messages or that ambulance sirens mean that something bad is about to happen. These beliefs can be so strong that the client has a great deal of discomfort with any form of public news or media, for fear of hidden meanings or messages. Sometimes, ideas of reference are associated with grandiosity, or the belief that one is especially important or powerful; an elderly home-maker who suddenly believes herself to be the next Marilyn Monroe may be experiencing grandiosity. Grandiose clients attempt to convince others of their importance and may present as rude or arrogant to the casual observer.

Memory and Cognition

Cognitive abilities are those elements of thinking that determine attention, concentration, perception, reasoning, intellect, and memory. They are generally thought of as higher functioning areas of thought. Attention span is particularly important in evaluating the mental status of children. An inability to attend to a task for an adequate length of time will impair learning. Decreased concentration levels and distractibility may be seen in clients with attentional problems as well as in clients who are depressed or impaired due to chemical substances. Perception and reasoning can be evaluated by asking the client to perform simple multi-step tasks, such as "write a sentence using your name in it" or "count backward from 100 by 3's." An evaluation of intellectual capability is often quite detailed and lengthy, involving psychological testing. Intellect is measured in intellectual quotient, or IQ, scores. An IQ score below 70 is considered below normal, 55 to 69 indicates a mild degree of mental retardation, 40 to 54 a moderate degree, 25 to 39 a severe degree, and less than 25 is considered profound. Intellect can sometimes be estimated by asking the client about years of schooling and special education needs as a child; however, this is unreliable due to the variability of educational and cultural environments.

An assessment of memory consists of three basic parts: immediate recall, short-term memory, and long-term memory. A simple test of recall is to give the client three items to remember, such as apple, car, and house, and then 5 minutes later ask the client to state those items. Immediate recall can be quickly determined by asking what a client consumed for breakfast. Short-term memory is recall of one to several days. Questions regarding family members' names or place of residence helps to assess short-term memory. Long-term memory is recall from several days to a lifetime. Asking clients where they grew up, what their parents' names were, or where they went to school readily provides this information. Memory assessments are important to help in differentiating a thought disorder from a dementia disorder. Clients with a primary psychiatric disturbance may be delusional in their beliefs, but extremely accurate in memory and recital of facts and dates. A client with early dementia will generally lose some short-term memory first, progressing to the loss of immediate recall, then finally to long-term memory loss. Clients with dementia may initially present with delusional beliefs as well. "Orientation" is a word commonly utilized in healthcare settings. "Oriented x 3" usually means that clients know who they are, where they are at the present time, and the approximate time, date, and day. A disoriented person may be suffering from a dementia disorder, drug or alcohol intoxication or withdrawal (including prescribed medications or drug interactions), or a number of physical health problems.

Insight and Motivation

When clients appear to have good understanding of their illnesses and the steps necessary to treat or manage their disorders, they are said to have good insight. The determination of a client's level of insight is often associated with treatment compliance. Presumably, understanding leads to compliance. Occasionally clinicians will encounter clients who have good insight into their illnesses, and have been well educated, but continue to demonstrate noncompliance with recommended treatments. This apparent lack of motivation may be related to factors other than education. Clinicians should ask these clients about possible barriers to treatment, such as poor finances or a lack of health insurance. The stigma of having a psychiatric diagnosis may lead the client to feel ashamed or angry. Anger may be causing the client

to intentionally deny and refuse adequate treatment. Hidden motivations, such as the defense mechanisms described in the following section, may be having a significant impact on the client.

Judgment

The choices that clients make in their healthcare treatments are a reflection of their judgment. The diabetic client who continues to eat sugary desserts is demonstrating poor judgment, as is the alcoholic client who continues to go to nightclubs. The client who recognizes that an increase in paranoia is a sign of decompensation and seeks out emergency treatment is demonstrating good judgment. Judgment and insight are linked, but are not always positively correlated. Assessing and understanding a client's ability to make good or poor choices is invaluable in planning care.

Safety

Finally, an evaluation of safety is important in any mental status assessment. The essential areas to examine include safety to the self and safety to others. The clinician should determine if a client has been intentionally or unintentionally harming himself or herself recently, or has any thoughts or urges to do so.

Clients experiencing extreme emotional pain may self-mutilate by cutting or burning their arms, legs, or trunk. Although this is not considered suicidal behavior, it is high-risk in that infection and scarring may result and the client is obviously in distress. When suicidal thoughts are noted, inpatient treatment should be considered. Assessing suicide risk consists of asking the client about means to harm oneself and the availability of those means. A hunter who thinks about shooting himself is at much higher risk than the office worker who doesn't own a gun. Determining the lethality of the means available is also essential. Overdosing on prescription cardiac agents or tricyclic antidepressants is far more dangerous than overdosing on selective serotonin reuptake inhibitors. Many adolescent clients cause serious liver damage every year by overdosing on relatively small amounts of acetaminophen, which is easily accessible to a minor. Another important assessment tool is to determine if the client has developed a suicide plan. A well-developed suicide plan with means at hand may necessitate forcing an involuntary hospital stay, whereas an impulsive episode of self-mutilating may be best treated by an intensive outpatient program and family supervision.

The clinician should also determine the degree of risk to others involved. There are two distinct areas in which clients with a psychiatric disorder lose their rights to confidentiality: a direct threat to harm or kill another person and the report of child abuse, neglect, or molestation. "Duty to warn" is the term that refers to the duty carried by the healthcare provider to notify another individual when a threat has been made against that individual's life. The clinician must use all means necessary to reasonably contact the individual, including notifying the police. In most healthcare settings, there are policies to be followed to ensure the report is made accurately and documented appropriately. If a client tells the clinician about the knowledge of the abuse, molestation, or neglect of a minor child, the clinician is obligated to report this to the local child protective services. Not reporting suspected abuse or neglect constitutes a major ethical problem and may jeopardize the clinician's license and employment. Again, most healthcare facilities have policies in place to coordinate these types of reports. Ultimately, the clinician is responsible for seeing that the report has been made.

PSYCHIATRIC DEFENSE MECHANISMS

Sigmund Freud, the "grandfather" of psychotherapy, believed that most psychiatric disturbances arise out of childhood experiences and the way human beings respond to their environment and are based on unconscious drives or motivations.

Freudian therapy, developed in 1936 and referred to as psychoanalysis, attempts to bring the unconscious into consciousness to allow individuals to work through past issues and develop insight into present behaviors. Although some of his theories seem unusual or even laughable to the clinician today, perhaps the most practical application of Freud's teaching is the idea of defense mechanisms. These are behaviors that an individual adopts in order to deal with stressors. Defense mechanisms can be beneficial and protective for the client, or counterproductive and maladaptive. Table 3-1 provides an overview of commonly accepted defense mechanisms; a brief discussion of some of these follows.

The phrase "he's in denial," is often heard in a hospital setting. This is a reflection of the defense mechanism of denial, which basically says that a person finds himself or herself unable to believe some type of news or information or act on that information in a helpful manner. This may be due to unconscious forces that override the person's rational thoughts; changing a behavior is more difficult and anxiety-provoking than continuing the behavior. For example, a man with lung cancer may continue to smoke because quitting smoking may mean acknowledging a life-threatening illness or a woman with alcoholism may continue to drink to avoid facing her dysfunctional marriage. Denial provides protection by allowing the psyche to slowly grasp traumatic events (e.g., death of a loved one), but it becomes maladaptive when the person can't move on. Understanding denial as a psychological process makes sense when trying to understand why a client is not compliant with his or her care.

Repression and suppression as defense mechanisms are commonly confused with one another. In repression, a person cannot voluntarily recall a traumatic event, such as a rape or terrorist attack. Only through therapy, and sometimes hypnosis, can the memories start to painfully resurface; when they do, the event will be as acutely distressful as if it had just happened. In suppression, a person chooses to ignore or forget painful events; however, when queried, he or she is able to instantly recall them. This can be very productive for the clinician in an emergency situation, when he or she is able to

TABLE 3-1: DEFENSE MECHANISMS

Defense Mechanism	Definition	Example
Repression	Involuntarily forgetting painful events	A woman who was sexually abused as a child cannot remember that it occurred.
Suppression	Voluntarily refusing to remember events	An emergency room nurse refuses to think about the child who is dying from an auto accident.
Denial	Refusing to admit certain things to one's self	An alcoholic man refuses to believe that he has a problem, in spite of evidence otherwise.
Rationalization	Trying to prove one's feelings are justifiable	A student insists that poor academic advice is the reason he cannot graduate on time.
Intellectualization	Using logic without feelings	A father analyzes why his son is depressed, without expressing any emotions of concern.
Identification	Attempting to model the self after an admired other	An adolescent tries to look and dress like his favorite musician to feel stronger and more in control.
Displacement	Discharging pent-up feelings (usually anger) on another	A child who is yelled at by her parents goes outside and kicks the dog.
Projection	Blaming someone else for one's thoughts or feelings	A jealous man states his wife is at fault for his hitting her.
Dissociation	Unconsciously separating painful feelings and thoughts from awareness	A rape victim "goes numb" and feels like she is floating outside of her body.
Regression	Return to an earlier developmental level	A 7-year-old child starts talking like a baby after the birth of a sibling.
Compensation	Covering up for a weakness by overemphasizing another trait	A skinny, nonathletic kid becomes a chess champion.
Reaction formation	Acting exactly opposite to an unconscious desire or drive	A man acts homophobic when he secretly believes he is gay.
Introjection	Taking on values, qualities, and traits of others	A 12-year-old girl acts like her teacher when the teacher is out of the room.
Sublimation	Channeling unacceptable drives into acceptable outlets	An angry woman joins a martial arts club and takes lessons.
Conversion	Converting psychiatric conflict into physical symptoms	A lonely, elderly woman develops vague aches and pains all over.
Undoing	Trying to counteract or make up for something	A man who yells at his boss sends her flowers the next day to "make up."

temporarily push aside personal feelings and reactions to deal with the crisis at hand.

Some people encounter the defense mechanism of displacement nearly every day. When you are having a bad day and you take it out on your spouse or children, then you have displaced your feelings away from the intended object (your job, boss, etc.) and onto an innocent and unsuspecting other. Displacement can be the defense mechanism behind seemingly unprecipitated anger outbursts such as road rage.

Rationalizing is the attempt to explain away situations, while not taking responsibilities for one's own actions. A senator who is arrested for taking gifts or money from lobbyists may try to rationalize this behavior by saying, "Everyone in Washington does it," or "That's the way you get business done."

An adolescent who tries to emulate a respected authority figure is using identification. Identifying with others and trying to be like them is adaptive and useful when the role model is a positive influence (e.g., father, mother, minister), but can be very maladaptive when the role model is a negative influence (e.g., gang leader, rock star with drug problems).

The following case study provides an example of a man with domestic violence issues. It applies his use of defense mechanisms to explain his behaviors and to provide a framework as to why they continue.

CASE STUDY: DEFENSE MECHANISMS IN DOMESTIC VIOLENCE

Samuel is a 36-year-old man who has been married for 8 years. He was raised in a divorced home, and his father was an alcoholic who left his mother for a younger woman. His mother remarried three times, and two of her husbands were violent and abusive to her in front of the children. Samuel is the middle child of 5. Samuel's marriage went well during the first 3 years; however, after the birth of their third child, his wife decided to quit work and be a homemaker. Samuel works in construction, and his work is hard and erratic. Samuel and his wife have a lot of financial stressors and may lose their home. Nearly everyday throughout the past year, Samuel has been staying late after work to "have a drink with the boys." When he gets home, his wife is often upset and she berates him for not being a good provider or helping her more with the kids and chores. He has started to blow up with her and, for the first time, has started hitting her. The next day he says he can't remember doing it, but says that it's her fault anyway for nagging him so much and not helping out financially.

Questions

1. What are the defense mechanisms that Samuel is demonstrating?

2. How does Samuel's upbringing likely impact on his current behaviors?

3. What role does alcohol play in this situation?

Discussion

Samuel is utilizing the defense mechanisms of denial (not dealing directly with his financial stressors), displacement (taking his feelings of anger out physically on his wife), rationalization (saying he wouldn't behave this way if she didn't nag him so much), and suppression (states he can't remember what he does). Samuel's childhood exposure to domestic violence predisposes him to resort to this behavior when he is under undue stress. He has likely identified with his father and/or stepfathers and has tried to emulate them in some ways. Alcohol serves to disinhibit a person, which can lead him to commit acts that would typically be unacceptable. Additionally, alcohol may contribute to some memory impairments of the events that occurred.

THE NURSING PROCESS AND CLINICAL REASONING

The nursing process is a systematic way of approaching the nursing care of an individual who is experiencing a disruption in health status – whether physical or psychiatric. The nursing process consists of assessment and diagnosis, care planning, carrying out selected interventions, and evaluating the outcome or effectiveness of those interventions. Clinical reasoning takes this a step further by incorporating evidence-based practice to encourage the nurse to think systematically about a real or potential problem and to make decisions based on facts and moral and ethical actions (as opposed to feelings or intuition).

The first crucial step in the nursing process is to obtain a thorough history of the client, incorporating elements of current and past health problems, social issues impacting health, and cultural or spiritual beliefs that may support or interfere with prescribed healthcare treatments. The nursing history should be obtained in an environment conducive to effective communication between the clinician and the client. Family members and significant others may or may not be present, or they may be present for a portion of the time and then be asked to step out to maintain the client's sense of confidentiality. Interviews should be done in a private conference room or client's room (if inpatient or residential), rather than in a public area where others may overhear. If personal safety is a concern, the clinician may request another staff member to be present. Distracting elements, such as television or radio, should be removed. If the clinician determines that the client is too ill to be able to provide accurate information or that the interview process itself will be detrimental to the client's health, then information should be obtained from other reliable sources, such as family members, social workers, therapists, and primary physicians. Documentation of the source of information is important, particularly when the client is unable to provide an accurate history.

Most healthcare facilities have an existing form to guide the clinician in data collection. Appendix B provides an example of a form that incorporates key elements of the nursing history. Whatever format is utilized, the information obtained should readily lead to the development of a problem list, which may be fairly extensive. At this point, the clinician needs to utilize the skill of prioritizing to determine which problems can realistically be addressed, given the time and resources available.

After essential real or potential problems have been identified (usually not more than four to six problems, depending on the severity of the disorder), the clinician should be prepared to write nursing diagnoses to address the problem. Nursing diagnoses are important in structuring the care provided for the client in the most efficient and appropriate manner possible. They also serve as a common language between healthcare providers to better facilitate communication. The North American Nursing Diagnosis Association (NANDA) International is an organization that has developed a list of commonly used nursing diagnoses. By utilizing NANDA diagnoses, the clinician can better identify existing or potential problems, contributing factors, and the behavioral expression or symptoms of the disorder. Identifying contributing factors and behavioral symptoms can directly lead to the development of short- and long-term goals to measure the success of treatment.

DEVELOPING A NURSING CARE PLAN

Long-term goals are useful in helping the client to determine what the overall desired outcome of care will be. Long-term goals are generally expressed in broad or general terms and can represent months or years of treatment. For example, in a depressed client, a long-term goal might be, "The client will have complete symptom remission for a period of one year." It may be helpful to discuss some of the contributing factors identified in the nursing diagnosis with the client, in order to better understand what elements may interfere with the success of a long-term goal. In the example given, contributing factors could include a lack of prescription medication or healthcare insurance, which prevents the client from receiving therapy or regular medication treatment. Long-term and short-term goals are expressed in terms of what the client will be able to achieve.

Short-term goals, often called objectives, are outcome measures that can realistically be achieved during the current course of treatment. These can usually be met within hours, days, or a few weeks. Objectives need to be behavioral in nature. They should be written in such a way as to allow them to be easily measured by the clinician. Verbs, such as "demonstrates," "verbalizes," and "lists," are more appropriate than "knows," "has," or "is" in writing objectives. It is important that the objectives be developed in collaboration with the client so that there is an understanding of what the clinician and other healthcare providers identify as primary needs. In this way, the client becomes an active part of the healthcare team. Each nursing diagnosis will lead to at least one objective; however, more commonly, two to four goals or objectives are identified for each diagnosis. Each objective should lead logically to several nursing interventions that are specifically designed to address that objective.

Nursing interventions should be expressed in terms of what the clinician, or other healthcare providers, will do to help the client meet the objectives and, ultimately, the long-term goals. A statement such as, "The client will go to A.A. meetings every day," is inappropriate because it is not focused on the healthcare provider. An appropriate intervention would read, "Staff will provide transportation to A.A. meetings on a daily basis." Another common error in writing nursing interven-

tions is that they are often too generalized and vague. Saying a clinician will "Reorient the client to reality" does not specify how the client will be reoriented, what techniques or tools are needed, or what role each specific healthcare provider will carry out in the reorientation process. It is more useful for the clinician to select a smaller number of very specific objectives and nursing interventions that can be understood and attained, rather than to write a "laundry list" of objectives and interventions that can not realistically be utilized by the healthcare staff.

The final phase of the nursing process consists of reflecting on the goals and objectives written and determining whether the interventions were effective. This evaluation of care should be systematic and address each of the objectives identified. When objectives are written in very specific, behavioral measures, then it is a simple matter to assess goal attainment. If an objective is, "The client will demonstrate how to measure and self-administer his insulin accurately every time," then the clinician can easily determine if this objective is met at 100%, 50%, or not at all. The final task is to determine what prevented the client from meeting the objectives. Perhaps they were not developed in collaboration with the client. In this case, there were likely unidentified barriers that prevented the objectives from being met. It may be that the objectives set were too vague or could not be met in the time available. Interventions may not have been clear, carried out, or associated with the care goals. The initial problem identification, prioritization, and nursing diagnosis may not have accurately reflected which problems were primary. A thorough examination of goal attainment will lead the clinician to revise the care plan to more effectively target the problems identified. Table 3-2 provides an outline of the nursing process and its components.

TABLE 3-2: THE NURSING PROCESS	
Assessment	Mental status exams
	Nursing histories
	Review of systems
	Medical histories
	Medication review
	Psychosocial issues
	Drug and alcohol issues
	Community support networks
	Spiritual beliefs and sources of strength
	Personal strengths (predictors of a positive outcome)
Problem identification	List of problems found in assessments
	Prioritize the problems: most urgent to least urgent
Planning care	Select the most relevant or immediate problems
	Develop performance measures ("client will"):
	Short-term objectives (to meet)
	Long-term goals
	Identify nursing interventions ("nurse will")
Implementing care	Carry out planned interventions
Evaluating effectiveness	Assess whether short-term objectives were met
	Assess whether interventions were useful or not
	Decide how to alter planning of care

NURSING CARE PLAN CASE EXAMPLE

*S*ally is a 25-year-old single woman with a history of numerous psychiatric inpatient stays for a diagnosis of bipolar disorder. The clinician is interviewing her in a hospital room where she was admitted for an acute manic episode. The dialogue between the nurse and the client will be utilized to demonstrate the application of the nursing process in writing a nursing care plan:

Nurse: *"I understand you've been having some trouble sleeping?"*

Sally: *"I haven't slept in 3 or 4 days. But I don't need sleep! Don't you see? I have been rebirthed in the spirit of our lady, Athena, the goddess of light and dark. She has given me the ability to see far-reaching into the future!*

Would you like me to tell you about your true love? Love is grand. Love is dandy. Love is like candy. Sandy beaches and moonlight. True light. Blue light is shining on me. There! Do you see!?"

Nurse: *"Let's focus on what we can do to help you get some rest. When this happened to you last fall, you were able to get some relief with sleeping medication."*

Sally: *"Medicine. Schmedicine. I don't need any of that drug stuff. The stars will take me away, sailing away and I'll never sleep again. (Starts to cry.) Oh, can't I ever be like everyone else? Why does this keep happening? If only I could get some rest."*

Nurse: *"Remember when you were here before. It only lasted a little while, then you got better.*

And you will get better again. The first step is to get you settled down. Later, I'm going to get you a cup of warm milk and some extra blankets. Then I'll set up the relaxation tape we keep here in the foyer outside your room. I'll give you a sleeping pill and play the relaxation tape. I'll bet you'll drift right off and feel much better tomorrow."

Sally: *"I don't know if it will help…but…okay. I'll try anything. You'll be here won't you? To make sure I'm okay? I'm always scared in the hospital."*

Nurse: *"I work until 11:30 p.m. I'll check on you before I go home. Then the night nurse will check on you throughout the night."*

Problem Listing

- Inadequate sleep
- Labile moods
- Mild grandiosity
- Anxiety over being in the hospital

Primary Nursing Diagnosis

Sleep disturbance (insomnia) due to the acute exacerbation of a manic episode as demonstrated by three nights with no sleep and a highly labile mood.

Long-term Treatment Goal

Client will master techniques for self-management of sleep within 2 weeks.

Short-term Objectives

1. Client will verbalize techniques for getting a good night's sleep.
2. Client will ask for the as needed medications that are available.
3. Client will participate in learning activities to self-manage sleep patterns.

Interventions

1. Staff will administer a bedtime sedative at 10:00 p.m. and document results.

2. Staff will offer warm milk and extra blankets at bedtime.
3. Staff will turn down lights and keep noise to a minimum.
4. Staff will teach the client deep breathing and relaxation techniques, utilizing relaxation cassette tapes or soft music.
5. Staff will utilize a nonconfrontational, supportive approach with the client to support a sense of security and safety.

The final stage of the nursing process, evaluating the effectiveness of interventions and the completion of objectives, is done on a daily basis. In the example given above, the client slept only 4 hours after the interventions. The nurse documented the objectives as partially met and continued the care plan with no alterations.

ADVANCED PRACTICE NURSING: THE PSYCHIATRIC EVALUATION

Advanced practice nurses, like psychiatrists, may perform psychiatric evaluations of clients, although forensic evaluations are usually only done by a psychiatrist or psychologist because of the stringent requirements for insanity and competence required by the legal system. Most licensing or credentialing organizations have certain minimal criteria that must be included in a psychiatric evaluation. These are:

1. *Identifying information* – client's name, age, gender, sometimes race or ethnicity (if relevant), place of residence, and other information that helps to identify him or her to the reader.

2. *Chief complaint* – what the client or significant other states is the primary reason for the evaluation.

3. *History of present illness* – what are the detailed events that led up to this event and evaluation? Presenting symptoms are usually found here, although they may be in a separate and independent section as well.

4. *Psychiatric history* – past psychiatric or mental health treatments, including hospitalizations. It is helpful to include past medication trials and effectiveness (and who prescribed them). May also include past sexual or physical abuse exposure; however, that may be included as a part of a social history. May also include chemical dependency history (drugs, alcohol) and past treatment or lack thereof.

5. *Family psychiatric history* – the goal of this section is to discuss pertinent family history that may impact the client or have some genetic inheritance factor. The family history should identify psychiatric disorders found in first and second degree relatives, including parents, siblings, grandparents, aunts, and uncles.

6. *Social history* – for adults, this will include employment, marriages, children, current living situation, healthcare insurance and, possibly, a family-of-origin (childhood) review. For children and adolescents, family description is essential, including place in the family, whether parents are together or divorced, stepparents, siblings, place in the sibling line-up, and so forth. Also, school performance and academic functioning must be included for children and adolescents.

7. *Medical history* – should include all pertinent healthcare concerns, current health problems, medication use, primary care provider when known, all past surgeries or health crises, allergies, recent and relevant lab work done, and so forth. For children and adolescents, may also include birth and developmental information if there is not a separate section on developmental history.

8. *Mental status assessment or exam* – a mental status assessment that covers the basics of appearance, behavior, thought processes and content, mood and affect, memory, insight, motivation, and safety concerns, such as the risk of danger to self or others, should be included.

9. *Summary of data and diagnoses* – an overall statement of the pertinent problems identified and the preliminary psychiatric diagnoses made based on the *DSM-IV-TR* multiaxial structure.

10. *Plan of care* – a preliminary plan of treatment that may include therapy, outside referrals, and medications. Should include follow-up plans with the APRN.

11. *Patient education* – any patient education provided at the time, particularly in regard to plan of care and to medications.

SUMMARY

This chapter has provided a means of assessing a person who presents with a psychiatric or mental health disturbance. Mental status examinations are done in every psychiatric setting, regardless of the client's age, and are one of the primary sources of information needed to help in making a psychiatric diagnosis. Mental status examinations also serve to provide a common language for mental health care practitioners, allowing for better communication between providers. Defense mechanisms are conscious or unconscious drives that help us to explain a person's behaviors and to identify adaptive and maladaptive coping strategies that can be encouraged or remediated as a course of treatment. Some defense mechanisms are more common that others, but all can have their place in protecting the human psyche in times of great stress. It is only when they are overused or the individual is "stuck" in a pattern of behavior that is harmful to himself or to others, that they can become dysfunctional.

Nurses working in all settings follow a systematic approach to planning patient care that is called the nursing process. This process allows for effective problem identification and planning of care while focusing on priority issues. The nursing care plan incorporates the nursing process and applies it to real life patient care situations. Advanced practice nurses are able to perform more detailed psychiatric evaluations that lead to *DSM-IV-TR* diagnoses and treatment plans, which may include medications.

EXAM QUESTIONS

CHAPTER 3
Questions 13-18

Note: Choose the one option that BEST answers each question.

13. Sam is a 19-year-old client who presents with the following statement, "I had to come in here! There was a man stalking me outside of my apartment. I stayed up all night watching and I kept seeing shadows. I'm sure the government is in on it! Can you help me to prove there's a conspiracy against me?" This statement represents

    a. religious preoccupations.

    b. flight-of-ideas.

    c. paranoid delusions.

    d. auditory hallucinations.

14. When evaluating safety in a mental status assessment, the statement that best reflects a high risk for a suicide attempt is

    a. "Next week my kids are coming to visit and I am so stressed that I want to just escape from it all."

    b. "I don't see a future for myself. I've been thinking a lot lately about dying and how peaceful it would be to take my heart pills and go to sleep forever."

    c. "I wish I had a knife! I get so tensed up that I just want to stab something!"

    d. "Everyone hates me. My parents and my friends think I'm dumb. I just wish I were dead!"

15. A man who has a bad day at the office and comes home shouting at his wife and kids is demonstrating the defense mechanism of

    a. identification.

    b. rationalization.

    c. displacement.

    d. reaction formation.

16. It is very common for pre-adolescent girls to want to dress like and emulate female pop stars (e.g., Madonna in the 1980s, Hannah Montana in 2008). This defense mechanism is an example of

    a. identification.

    b. rationalization.

    c. denial.

    d. suppression.

17. A nursing action conducive to obtaining a thorough and accurate nursing history would be

    a. keeping the TV and radio turned off and distraction to a minimum.

    b. obtaining information only from secondary sources and records.

    c. interviewing the client at the nurse's station for safety.

    d. focusing only on psychiatric symptomatology.

continued on next page

18. Jack is a 45-year-old man who presents in the emergency department confused and staggering. He has had numerous past admissions for alcohol detoxification, which was complicated by withdrawal seizures and liver failure. The nursing diagnosis most appropriate for his first 24 hours of care is

    a. ineffective denial related to guilt as evidenced by refusing to accept treatment voluntarily.

    b. ineffective family coping related to destructive family patterns as evidenced by inappropriate anger demonstrations.

    c. risk for injury related to changes in mental status and a history of seizures as evidenced by confusion and a staggering gait.

    d. impaired social interactions related to emotional lability as evidenced by tearfulness and isolation on admission.

CHAPTER 4

THERAPEUTIC INTERVENTIONS

CHAPTER OBJECTIVE

At the end of this chapter, the reader will be able to discuss various therapeutic interventions, including which interventions are appropriate in select situations.

LEARNING OBJECTIVES

At the end of this chapter, the reader will be able to

1. apply active listening techniques to interactions with clients.

2. differentiate cognitive-behavioral therapy, family therapy, and group therapy in promoting individual client change.

3. discuss the importance of community support groups in aiding recovery.

4. review various types of somatic, alternative, and complementary therapies.

INTRODUCTION

Assessing the client, performing mental status assessments, identifying priority problems, developing goals and objectives, and writing nursing care plans is the initial part of systematic client care. The next step is the provision of relevant and appropriate interventions. Nursing interventions for healthcare problems include comfort measures such as the provision of a quiet, warm environment; educational measures such as teaching the client about his or her medication or disease process; and technical interventions, such as starting an IV or managing telemetry in a cardiac patient. In this chapter, techniques are presented that are used commonly in a psychiatric or mental health setting. Interpersonal communication skills that are applicable to all healthcare providers, regardless of specialty area, are discussed. An evidence-based style of individual therapy, called *cognitive-behavioral therapy* is presented with examples to illustrate the concept. Environmental, or *milieu* therapy found in inpatient settings is reviewed. This is followed by a discussion of group dynamics and group therapy techniques, based on the work of Irvin Yalom, and the concept of psychoeducational groups, more often facilitated by nurses. The use of group therapy to impact individual change will be illustrated. The importance of community-based support groups to aide in recovery and provide resources for clients as well as family members is well recognized and will be discussed.

The word "somatic" occurs frequently in psychiatric and psychological teachings. Somatic comes from the root word "soma," roughly meaning "of the body." A review of somatic (physiological) interventions including the use of magnets, electroconvulsive therapy, and vagus nerve stimulation, is presented. A brief discussion of medications is included; however, detailed medication information is presented, throughout the text in appropriate chapters. Finally, alternative (or complementary) interventions are presented, including massage, acupuncture, hypnosis, mindfulness meditation, and over-the-counter herbal preparations.

INTERPERSONAL COMMUNICATIONS

In 1953, Harry Stack Sullivan developed a model for therapy based on the interpersonal relationship. His model considered psychiatric disturbances to be a disruption in the relationship between the individual and others. Therapy consisted of correcting the relationship defects to relieve anxiety and tension, resulting in more mature, adult relationships. In order to do this, Sullivan incorporated the therapist as a tool, by using sessions to present reality and validate or confront the client's beliefs. The therapist might make such statements as, "You say you aren't angry, but I see you clenching your fists and hear you raising your voice." Interpersonal communication skills are taught to nursing students today, based on the early beliefs of Sullivan. These techniques emphasize active listening and allowing the client to lead the content of the interaction, as opposed to an agenda led, question and answer format (Keltner et al., 2007, p. 41). A sampling of therapeutic and non-therapeutic communication techniques is provided in Table 4-1.

Hildegard Peplau applied Sullivan's teaching to nursing practice in 1963. Peplau viewed the nurse-patient relationship as representative of the patient's relationship with other important people in his or her life (husband, wife, mother, father, etc.). By analyzing the dynamic between the self and the patient, nurses can draw inferences about how clients interact with others and help clients to develop insight into these behaviors in order to promote change. Furthermore, Peplau applied Sullivan's views on anxiety as a driving force

behind behaviors and related these to nursing practice and a patient's ability to perceive and learn. For example, mild anxiety promotes learning; whereas, severe or panic levels of anxiety prevent learning and distort perceptions (Keltner et al., 2007, p. 43). Practicing the therapeutic communication techniques provided in Table 4-1 and applying them to interactions with clients (whether in psychiatry or not) will go far in assisting the nurse to develop helpful and empathic relationships with his or her clients.

COGNITIVE-BEHAVIORAL THERAPY

Cognitive behavioral therapy (CBT) has gained in both popularity and implementation in the past few years. Aaron Beck (1967) and Albert Ellis (1973) first focused on the relationship between a client's perceptions about events and the resultant feelings and behaviors. This cycle of thoughts that triggers feelings and behaviors is demonstrated in the following example:

Imagine you are driving down the interstate at 65 miles per hour. You look into your rear view mirror and see the flashing lights of a state trooper. Knowing that you are a little over the speed limit, you are certain he is pulling you over to give you a ticket. You think of the two glasses of wine you just had with dinner. "What if my blood alcohol level is too high? I can't be arrested! I would lose my job! They'll take away my nursing license! You feel your palms get sweaty and your heart start to race. Barely able to contain your panic, you swerve quickly into the right-hand lane, without signaling, and cut off a car coming up behind you. The car honks, you get onto the shoulder, and finally stop. In dread, you look out the window for the trooper. He continues past you down the highway.

In this example, the driver's thoughts of breaking the law by speeding and getting arrested for drunk driving cause the driver to feel anxious and panic,

TABLE 4-1: THERAPEUTIC AND NON-THERAPEUTIC COMMUNICATION TECHNIQUES	
Therapeutic	**Example**
Open-ended question	"How are you feeling?"
Offering self	"I'll sit here with you for a while."
Giving general leads	"Go on…you were saying."
Silence	(sitting quietly)
Active listening	Leaning forward, making eye contact, attentive
Restating	"So what you're saying is…"
Clarification	"I don't quite understand. Could you explain…"
Making observations	"I notice that you shake when you say that."
Reflecting feelings	"You seem sad."
Encouraging comparisons	"How did you handle this situation before?"
Interpreting	"It sounds like what you mean is…"
Non-therapeutic	**Example**
Close-ended question	"Did you do this?"
Challenging	"Why did you do this?"
Arguing	"No. That's not true."
Not listening	Body turned away, poor eye contact
Changing the subject	(client states he is sad) "Where do you work?"
Being superficial	"I'm sure things will turn out just fine!"
Being sarcastic	"Just what do you mean by that, huh?"
Using clichés	"All's well that ends well"
Being flippant	"I wouldn't worry about it"
Showing disapproval	"That was a bad thing to do"
Ignoring the client	"Did anyone read the paper today?"
Making false promises	"I'll make the doctor listen to you!"

which results in erratic behavior and nearly causes an accident. Now consider this example:

Imagine yourself driving down the interstate. You look into your mirror and see the flashing lights of a state trooper. You know you're a little over the speed limit, but so is everyone around you. You think of the two glasses of wine you had with dinner, but you did eat a large portion and you don't feel drowsy – besides, that was an hour ago. You deduce that there must be an accident further down the road. You signal a right turn, check your mirrors, and carefully pull over onto the shoulder. After the trooper passes, you continue on your journey.

Cognitive behavioral therapy is based on the supposition that behaviors are a result of distorted thinking about situations. These distortions can take the shape of catastrophizing, which is thinking that the worst that can possibly happen will happen; perceiving threats where none exist; thinking only of negative outcomes; or making sweeping generalizations. In anxiety disorders, fear is the driving force for these distorted thoughts. Cognitive restructuring is used to help the client examine his beliefs in more detail and to break down the resultant feelings and behaviors into A (antecedent), B (behavior), and C (consequence). Exposure is a CBT technique that provokes the client's anxiety over a feared idea or object in a controlled, supportive environment. For example, a person afraid of heights might be asked to stand on a foot-stool for 5 minutes in the clinician's office. Gradual exposure to the situation allows the clients to systematically desensitize to the stressor. Flooding exposes the client to the stressful object or idea all at once and may produce panic symptoms. Skills training may also be employed in CBT; it specifically trains the individual based on his or her needs. Cognitive behavioral techniques are useful when treating a client with depression, anxiety, or PTSD. Helping the client to identify beliefs (true or false) about situations will enable the client to challenge the beliefs that are detrimental to recovery (Fleming & O'Brien, 2008, pp. 343-345).

FAMILY THERAPY

Individuals with psychiatric, mental health, or behavioral problems do not usually live in a vacuum. Children and adolescents are still living in a family unit, even if in foster care or residential treatment, although the nature of "family" may differ in these situations. Adults may live alone or with others, be married or single, and live with or without children of their own. Even adults that live alone often have significant family relationships with parents, children, or others. The idea of "family" is identified by the client, but usually involves other persons with whom the client interacts on nearly a daily basis and in whom the client has significant emotional investment; therefore, a same-sex partner arrangement would constitute "family," whereas a roommate would not.

Family therapy is based on the idea that although there is an identified patient, problems may arise out of dysfunctions within the family system. Treating the client apart from his or her family will not correct these system problems and

relapse is likely. The most commonly practiced form of family therapy is systems therapy.

In systems therapy, the individuals making up a family are thought to be in balance with one another. Change in one part of the system upsets that balance and invokes a necessary change in other places. For example, a wife and mother who is being emotionally and physically abused takes steps through counseling to stop the abuse, thus altering the power structure within the family. In turn, her abuser (in this case her husband) becomes more controlling to try to re-establish previous roles, and he may become more violent. This serves to override her resolve and ends with her returning to her previous role. Family therapy would require the husband and wife to both participate in treatment, exposing and exploring these unconscious behaviors and trying to ascribe meaning to them (perhaps he is fearful she will outgrow him and he will grow old alone if she is allowed to change). The children would also be involved in therapy to allow them to see that change is possible and to break any emergent dysfunctional patterns that they are developing, such as battering behaviors in the boys and victim behaviors in the girls. In this way, family therapy seeks to re-align balance and power within the family unit, allowing each individual member to become emotionally healthy and well developed.

Family therapy is complex, and master's or doctorally prepared clinicians should be utilized for this type of intense treatment. The American Academy of Marriage and Family Therapists provides certification for family therapists to ensure a high quality and standard of care.

GROUP DYNAMICS

Irvin Yalom, MD, has been highly influential in the development of group therapy. Dr. Yalom postulated that when individuals are grouped together, certain characteristics of the individuals will emerge that are reflective of family-of-origin and childhood issues. By using groups of people, these negative or destructive childhood events can be reworked and reframed, leading to healthier adult coping responses. Additionally, groups themselves develop identities and go through phases. His first publication, *The Theory and Practice of Group Psychotherapy* in 1970 became the textbook for all serious psychotherapists and nurses interested in group therapy. Dr. Yalom is still publishing; in fact, *The Theory and Practice of Group Psychotherapy* is in its 5th edition (2005) co-authored with M. Leszcz. Dr. Yalom is currently a Professor Emeritus at the Stanford University School of Medicine.

By working in a group setting, clients can receive feedback from others in a unique manner, different from that encountered in individual therapy. Group members may be able to perceive responses in one another that the group leader is blinded to, and they are adept at pointing out inconsistencies and maladaptive reactions to one another. Group members also offer a built-in support mechanism – a well-functioning group usually has members who all have something in common. Thus, a universality or "we are all in this together" camaraderie develops, which serves to encourage trust and move the group into productivity. Individual group members grow and develop self-awareness through the relationships and feedback from those around them.

Groups go through readily identifiable stages. This seems to be true for all groups of human beings, even those without therapy intent (e.g., reality television shows such as "Survivor"). The first developmental stage of a group is the honeymoon, or pre-affiliation, stage. At this time, group members are polite to one another and somewhat superficial. The tasks of the group at this time are to get to know one another better and to begin to develop trust in one another and in the group leader. Experiential activities that require the group to plan and work together to accomplish an important task

may accelerate this stage. The second stage of development of a group is the conflict, or power phase. During this stage, members develop disagreements with one another and challenge one another and the group leader. This stage serves to establish working rules, mores, norms, and standards and to set the tone for how conflict will be managed. Established and inherent group leaders also emerge. In the third, or working, phase of a group, activities become more directly focused on problem solving. Very powerful personal changes can occur during this stage in a therapy-oriented group. An insightful group leader uses this stage of the group to accomplish tasks and forward progress of the group's overall goals. The final stage of group process is the termination of the group. Again, psychological issues can emerge, as members have to deal with loss, grief and, sometimes, a sense of abandonment. Members may attempt to delay termination by exchanging phone numbers and making promises to contact one another.

The best size for a therapy group is usually 5 to 15 members (with 8 to 10 as ideal). If larger, some members may be ignored or can avoid participation. If smaller, the group can turn into a series of individual therapy sessions with the group leader, while everyone else watches. Training in facilitating therapy groups is standard in graduate programs for advanced practice nurses, psychiatric and psychological master's programs, and clinical doctoral programs.

PSYCHOEDUCATIONAL GROUPS

Nurses are often found facilitating psychoeducational groups in mental health settings. These groups are a hybrid of a classroom or teaching environment and a supportive, therapeutic environment. There is always a defined group leader and a specific content or topic to be discussed. Topics are frequently based on developing skills important to daily living and maximizing the quality of life. Some topic examples include medication education, coping with stress, understanding one's illness, leisure pursuits, reducing cigarette smoking, and relapse prevention. There is some emphasis on group member interaction and participation, but there is also an emphasis on learning new behaviors. Hands-on activities may be provided and sometimes, homework assignments are made. Other non-nurse personnel may conduct psychoeducational groups; however, nurses are in a unique position of crossing the bridge between physical and mental health, based on their education, training, and holistic approaches. Psychoeducational groups may be larger than strictly therapeutic groups, although more than 25 members can be difficult to manage.

MILIEU THERAPY

Milieu therapy is the therapeutic use of the environment as a tool in treatment. The underlying idea is that all persons are affected by their physical, social, and emotional surroundings. If one alters that environment, then change will be effected within the individual. Effects of the environment can easily be understood by thinking about some common events in our own lives: Going to a party evokes a sense of festivity, joy, and excitement; going to a funeral causes us to feel somber, quiet, and sad; when walking into a hushed and quiet library, a person may feel the need to whisper and walk softly; and a starkly painted, tiled hospital room may lead us to feel fearful, anonymous, or disengaged. Even schools reflect environmental or milieu manipulation and effects (consider a Montessori-style school, as compared to a stricter military school). Therapeutic environments all have the following characteristics:

1. The client is protected from injury from self or others.

2. The client's physical needs are met.

3. Programming is structured and routines are encouraged.

4. Staff members remain relatively consistent.

5. Emphasis is placed on social interaction among clients and staff.

6. Decision-making authority is clearly defined.

7. The client is respected as an individual and is encouraged to express his or her opinions.

8. The client is afforded opportunities for freedom of choice.

9. The environment provides opportunity for testing new behaviors (Taylor, 2008).

Inpatient psychiatric settings and residential settings are the most common places that milieu therapy is consciously thought about and orchestrated by staff. A client who is disorganized, paranoid, or agitated responds better to an environment that is calm, well structured, and predictable, with staff persons who are pleasant in nature, but directive and firm.

COMMUNITY SUPPORT GROUPS

Many support groups exist to help individuals who are experiencing specific problems. In one Internet search, 38 different mental health associated groups were identified. One of the most common of these, the Alcoholic Anonymous group will be discussed in a later chapter. Groups exist for gambling addiction, rape and sexual abuse support, bipolar disorder, depression, grief and bereavement, suicide, attention-deficit disorder, Tourette's disorder, and many more. Support groups differ from therapy groups in several important ways: Support groups are a network of members with similar traits or characteristics; support groups are leaderless – they may have a nominated leader but that person is also a victim, client, group member; support groups are not managed by a therapist; support groups are free (some may have annual dues but no one is charged for participating); support groups may meet less frequently than therapy groups, but for a longer period of time (years to indefinitely); and support groups are usually self-sustaining. If members lose interest, can't find a place to meet, or membership wanes, then the group may end.

The National Alliance on Mental Illness (NAMI) is the nation's largest grassroots support organization for families and persons affected by mental illness. Established in 1979, NAMI is a powerful lobbying force in Washington, with affiliates in every state and more than 1100 communities across the country. NAMI provides support, including sponsoring support groups, education, and advocacy for families and clients with psychiatric illnesses. Fighting against the stigma associated with mental illnesses is a key project of NAMI.

SOMATIC (PHYSIOLOGICAL) INTERVENTIONS

Medications are utilized in nearly every psychiatric condition. Even such conditions as mental retardation and developmental disabilities can have co-morbidity with moodswings, irritability, depression, or psychosis, for which medication is prescribed. For the purposes of this text, medications will be classified into seven broad categories: antidepressants, anti-anxiety agents (also called anxiolytics), antipsychotics and their "partners" anticholinergics (used to reverse some side effects), mood stabilizers, sedative-hypnotics, medications for attention-deficit disorder, and miscellaneous medications designed to reduce or prevent alcohol or drug dependence, including nicotine. Many medications are used off-label to treat psychiatric complaints or conditions. The U.S. Food and Drug Administration (FDA) defines "off-label" use as the use of a prescription medication for any purpose that it has not expressly approved. Every medication approved by the FDA is approved for a specific

diagnosis, for a specific age group or population, and in a specific dose range. If a medication is given to someone outside of the approved age range, in a higher (or lower) dosage than approved, or for any disorder other than that studied and approved, then it is said to be off-label. Off-label use does not mean illegal or even inappropriate; prescribing clinicians safely and effectively use many medications off-label every day. Medication usage will be addressed throughout the remainder of this text in the corresponding chapters.

Electro-convulsive Therapy (ECT) was introduced in the 1930s to treat a broad range of psychiatric disturbances. Today, its use has been refined considerably and it is primarily only used to treat severe and persistent, treatment-resistant depression. Medications and therapy should be tried before ECT is given. ECT has an effectiveness rate of about 60% to 70% in depression (SAMHSA, 1999). To perform ECT, the client is given a short-acting sedative, followed by a muscle relaxant agent. The muscle relaxant prevents tonic-clonic jerking of the body, caused by seizure activity that, historically, was the cause of physical injuries to the client. After the client is asleep, electrodes are placed on the sides of his or her head and an electrical stimulus that is sufficient to trigger a seizure is given. Ideally, the seizure activity lasts about 15-seconds. Breathing is supported during the procedure. ECT is repeated two to three times a week for 3 to 4 weeks and is often done as an outpatient. There are no absolute contraindications to ECT; however, caution should be used in pregnancy or in patients with cardiac conditions. Side effects of ECT include memory loss and some confusion for events right before and after the procedure. Some people complain of long-term memory and cognitive problems. Also, complications related to the use of anesthetics (allergy, respiratory suppression) can occur.

Transcranial magnetic stimulation (TMS) therapy is a non-invasive treatment for depression. The client is exposed to electrical energy that is passed through a coil of wires to produce a powerful magnetic field. Magnetic waves pass through the brain and skull painlessly and the client remains awake for the procedure. It is most effective when administered for 40 minutes daily, for 4 to 6 weeks. The FDA approved TMS for depression treatment in the fall of 2008. It is thought to work by stimulating nerve cells to produce the neurotransmitters that relieve depression. Side effects of TMS are nearly nonexistent, with only complaints of mild headaches reported. TMS cannot be used if the client has implanted or permanent metal in the skull or brain.

Approved in 2005, vagus nerve stimulator (VNS) therapy is an adjunctive, long-term treatment for adult clients with serious and persistent depression. Most of these individuals have failed on four or more antidepressants. A VNS implant is a small, battery-powered device, similar to a cardiac pacemaker, that is surgically implanted subcutaneously under the skin of the upper left or right chest. Internally, a wire runs from the device to the vagus nerve, which then carries electrical impulses to the brain. These impulses are emitted every few minutes. The device is thought to work by electrically stimulating the production of neurotransmitters that are associated with depression treatment. The side effects of vagus nerve stimulation include a tickle in the throat (may trigger a cough reflex), mild hoarseness or other voice changes and rarely, difficulty swallowing, shortness of breath, neck pain, and a prickling sensation in the skin. VNS therapy has also been used since 1977 to treat severe epilepsy.

ALTERNATE OR COMPLEMENTARY TREATMENT MODALITIES

Massage is the manipulation of the body's soft tissues to promote circulation and relaxation. Used for over 4000 years, it is one of the most natural and risk-free ways to treat stress, reduce anxiety, and improve sleep. There are numerous types of massage techniques; a brief search of the Internet found 26 different types, varying from light touch to deep muscle work and from specific to generalized body parts. "Bodywork" incorporates therapeutic massage and other touch techniques, often with the intent of healing a specific problem, such as insomnia or poor digestion. Reflexology, also called *zone therapy,* is the application of massage or pressure to the hands and feet to alleviate distress in different parts of the body. The theory is that all of the body is represented in areas in the hands and feet, and that stimulating these trigger points can eliminate distress.

According to traditional Chinese medical theory, acupuncture points are situated along meridians in the body, along with vital energy flow. This energy flow, called Qi, gets disrupted by illness or distress. Acupuncturists insert tiny, filiform needles along the meridians to stimulate and readjust the energy flow. Practitioners diagnose which systems in the body are affected, based on inspection, auscultation, olfactory senses, palpation, and taking a limited history of symptoms. Side effects to the treatment are generally mild and may include slight headaches, nausea, or pain in certain areas.

Hypnosis is a technique that induces a deep relaxation and calm, trance-like state of mind. The client's focus of awareness becomes so restricted that external noise and distractions are no longer present in the conscious mind. Hypnotherapy is practiced by highly trained clinicians, often psychologists, to achieve certain therapeutic goals with the client, such as recovering memories lost through the defense mechanism of repression, learning to be less anxious when faced with typically anxiety-provoking situations, or reducing an undesirable behavior such as smoking. Hypnotherapy requires a client who is relaxed and receptive to the procedure. A client who is under hypnosis cannot be made to violate his or her own ethics or beliefs.

Mindfulness is a concentrated awareness of thoughts and feelings through the use of meditation. Mindfulness has been studied as a means of reducing chronic pain, improving immune system responsiveness, relieving stress and anxiety, and promoting wound healing.

Herbals and nutritional supplements have gained a lot of interest in the past few years, as people search for home remedies to reduce the cost of obtaining healthcare. Many people feel that herbal remedies are more natural, and thus, healthier and safer overall. The FDA considers herbal supplements, vitamins, and other nutritional supplements as food sources and, as such, does not regulate their usage. This can result in wide variances in the amount of active ingredient that may be available in a certain product; some products have even been found to contain no active ingredients when subjected to laboratory evaluation.

A few herbal supplements have found their way into mental health care. Please note: This discussion is theoretical and is not fully supported by scientific research – the reader should consider this as informational only. Children or pregnant or nursing women should never take any of these products without medical consultation. Table 4-2 is a summary of the following discussion on herbal remedies.

St. John's Wort (*Hypericum perforatum*) is derived from the St. John's Wort plant. It is primarily used to treat depression. St. John's Wort is thought to affect serotonin and monoamine oxidase inhibitors in the brain, similar to antidepressants. In fact, there are case reports of drug-to-drug interactions in clients who used St. John's Wort while taking

antidepressants, resulting in emergency room visits for serotonin syndrome or mania. St. John's Wort should not be taken in combination with prescription antidepressants.

Valerian (*Valerian officinalis*) root is powdered and taken in a capsule. It is believed to help in alleviating anxiety and treating insomnia. Valerian is also believed to work on the GABA (gamma-aminobutyric acid) system to produce its effects. Folklore tells us that valerian is the root word for "Valium" (diazepam), a potent benzodiazepine that has been on the market for over 30 years. Valerian should not be taken with other central nervous system depressants, as it can potentiate their effects (especially anesthetics, barbiturates, and benzodiazepines). Side effects include headaches, uneasiness, dizziness and, sometimes, excitability.

Kava-kava (*Piper methysticum*) is a South Pacific oceanic herb with sedative, analgesic, and mild euphoria properties. Kava-kava may act on GABA in a manner similar to benzodiazepines, and it does have drug-to-drug interaction effects with those products. Long-term use of kava-kava has been associated with liver problems in at least 36 people. Despite this, kava-kava is still widely available for over-the-counter or Internet purchase, without restriction. Other side effects of kava-kava can include stomach disturbances, dizziness, and a temporary yellowing of the skin. A person with liver impairment or one who is a heavy alcohol user should never use kava-kava. Long-term use may also result in a serious skin scaling condition.

Ginseng (*Panax ginseng*) is a stimulating herb that can produce energy similar to caffeine, which results in improved endurance and reduced fatigue. Jitteriness and nervousness can be side effects of ginseng, as can insomnia, hypertension, restlessness and, possibly, mania.

Ephedra (*Ephedra sinica*) is a Chinese herb, from which the herbal remedy Ma Huang has been extracted. Ephedra is a potent central nervous system stimulant. It increases energy, reduces

TABLE 4-2: COMMON HERBAL REMEDIES IN MENTAL HEALTH CARE

Name of Herb	Common Usage	Possible Side Effects	Precautions	Comments
St. Johns Wort	Depression	Allergic reactions	Can interact with antidepressants	Has resulted in Serotonin Syndrome, Mania reactions
Valerian	Insomnia, anxiety	Dizziness, headaches, excitability	Can potentiate other central nervous depressants	Do not take wtih CNS depressants including alcohol
Kava-kava	Anxiety, sedation	GI upset, dizziness, yellow or scaly skin	36 cases of liver problems associated with its use	Can potentiate other central nervous depressants including alcohol
Ginseng	Improves endurance, reduces fatigue	Irritability, excitability, nervousness	Can potentiate other CNS stimulants such as caffeine	Has induced hypertension and mania
Ephedra	Reduces fatigue, increases energy	Irritability, excitability, nervousness	Has been implicated in 34 deaths when used in Diet Tea. No longer available	Found in herb Ma Huang; similar to OTC product pseudoephedrine
Ginkgo Biloba	Improves memory, circulation	Nausea, GI upset, headaches, skin allergies	Anti-coagulant effects	Should not be used in combination with blood thinners
Mint or Chamomile Teas	Calming, mildly sedating, anitspasmodic (mint)	Allergic reactions	None	Safe for most populations

appetite, and is thought to improve mood. In 2004, its availability in the United States was restricted because of deaths associated with its use in a diet tea (up to 34 by 1997). Ephedra can also induce symptoms of psychosis and mania, similar to amphetamines. The synthetic product used in cold and sinus formulations, pseudoephedrine (commonly known as Sudafed), has some of the same stimulant properties. Sudafed© is one of the ingredients in the illegal manufacturing of methamphetamine; thus, access to Sudafed© is also monitored.

Ginkgo biloba (*Ginkgo biloba*) has gained popularity in theoretically improving blood flow to the brain to promote alertness, mental sharpness and memory; to treat fatigue and stress; and to improve endurance. Ginkgo biloba appears to be a powerful antioxidant, reducing free radicals in the body that cause cellular death. Ginkgo biloba can interfere with blood clotting and reduce platelet action, leading to increases in bleeding times. It may interfere with anticoagulant therapy and should not be taken by clients with circulatory problems who are taking such medications as Coumadin©, Plavix©, or aspirin. Side effects of ginkgo biloba include headaches, nausea, vomiting, stomach upset and, occasionally, skin allergies (Vermani, Milosevic, Smith, & Katzman, 2005).

Mint teas and chamomile tea are gentle and some find them calming. Mint is a mild antispasmodic in the stomach. Both of these are safe for children to drink.

Data on vitamin and mineral supplementation has not generally supported much in the field of mental health. Iron deficiency is associated with fatigue and also with some behavioral disorders in children. A one-a-day multivitamin supplement for adults and a chewable daily supplement for children (taken at bedtime) are advisable. Omega-3 fatty acids (fish oil, flax seed oil) have shown some positive benefits in treating behavioral problems such as attention-deficit disorder and such psychiatric problems as bipolar disorder and depression; however, data is inconsistent. Fat-soluble vitamins A, D, and K can be dangerous in high doses. Vitamin K is a good antioxidant and has become more popular as an adjunct treatment for the prevention of neuromuscular side effects associated with antipsychotic medications. It is usually dosed at 400 International Units once or twice a day. Water-soluble vitamins C and B complex must be consumed nearly every day for good health. B-complex vitamins are associated with energy and good moods, may help to reduce premenstrual symptoms, and are generally safe in a person with normal kidney function. One form of folic acid (a B vitamin) is now available in prescription strength. This product, Deplin©, is still considered a nutritional supplement but it has demonstrated effectiveness in enhancing the treatment of depression.

ADVANCED PRACTICE NURSING: THE NURSE AS THERAPIST

Graduate programs that prepare the clinical nurse specialist or nurse practitioner in psychiatric and mental health nursing all include some component of education and experience in providing individual, group, and family therapy. The usual process is an intensive didactic training, with practicum experiences in these areas. Additionally, graduate programs now include pharmacology and psychopharmacology to meet the requirements for prescribing privileges. APRNs have the opportunity to provide counseling and medication management for their clients – something that is not available to master's level clinicians in other disciplines (although, in some states, clinical psychologists are able to prescribe medications as well). APRNs have quite a bit of autonomy in making decisions on providing therapy and medications, based on their education and experience.

CASE STUDY: THERAPEUTIC INTERVENTIONS

Donald is a 45-year-old man employed as a financial manager by a fairly large bank. Due to economic downturns, there have not been as many accounts available and competition between brokers on the job has become fierce. Donald presented to his primary care provider's office complaining of episodes of shortness of breath, sweating, anxiety, and the strong feeling that he was about to die. An electrocardiogram and stress test were performed, which were both normal. Similarly, laboratory testing was also normal. These symptoms had started out occurring once or twice a week, but within a few months they were happening daily and he began to be afraid of leaving his home for fear of another attack. His attendance at work became poor, and he was told that he might lose his job as a result. This caused problems between he and his wife, and she started talking about leaving him to move back in with her parents. Donald was put on alprazolam (Xanax®) by his primary care provider, which helped a little bit, and he was referred to the local mental health center for treatment. Once there, he met with a therapist for a fuller assessment of his symptoms and was diagnosed with panic disorder with agoraphobia. He was then referred to the psychiatric nurse practitioner for a medication evaluation and treatment. She advised that he start taking sertraline (Zoloft®) 100 mg daily and that he use the Xanax® only as needed, to avoid dependency and tolerance.

Questions

1. What type of therapy would be most beneficial for Donald?

2. Are there any ancillary services that could be helpful?

3. What are other recommendations that you might make to Donald or his wife?

Discussion

Panic attacks and panic disorder are very treatable and respond well to medications and therapy: Cognitive-behavioral therapy is indicated to help this client learn to identify anxiety-provoking triggers and reframe how he thinks about these events; and relaxation training would be helpful in teaching Donald a means of reducing the anxiety once it occurs. The types of relaxation training that would be particularly helpful include guided imagery and mindfulness meditation. Another recommendation for Donald would be to include daily, regular exercise in his routine (aerobic or weight-lifting) because exercising can have a significantly positive effect on panic disorder treatment. He and his wife may want to have some marital therapy sessions with his treatment provider to work on improving their communication. They may also want to join the support group NAMI to learn more about psychiatric disorders and the rights of individuals who have such disorders. Finally, mental and behavioral health problems are considered medical problems and are protected under the federal Family and Medical Leave Act guidelines. Donald's nurse practitioner can provide him with a work statement and absence excuse that should help to protect his employment status and prevent him from losing his job, while he is under her care.

SUMMARY

Developing an effective plan of care with a client requires a systematic approach. After problems are identified and prioritized and goals are established, therapeutic interventions can be implemented to meet these goals and objectives. Individual-based interventions may be based on active listening skills, which encourage clients to open up and expand on subjective concerns in a nonjudgmental environment, or they may be more formally structured, as seen with cognitive-behavioral therapy. Individual therapy may not be effective in the long-term unless family dynamics are taken into consideration. Some clients benefit greatly from adding family therapy to their care plan but it should be provided by a qualified clinician. Manipulation and management of the environment for the client to promote change is known as milieu therapy. It is most often found in the hospital or residential setting. Group therapy is a powerful mechanism for change. In this chapter, two kinds of groups were discussed: therapeutic groups based on the works of Yalom and psychoeducational groups that are a hybrid of teaching and active listening and are commonly facilitated by nurses. Community support groups exist to provide clients and families with an understanding network of others who are experiencing the same or similar problems. Support groups are client-led, usually long-term, low cost, and are less focused on therapeutic changes than they are on education and providing resources for the members. Some support groups are very politically active and have resulted in policy changes in the treatment of persons with mental illnesses. NAMI is one such active group. The chapter concludes with a discussion of somatic therapies, including ECT, VNS implants, and magnets, and a review of alternative or complementary interventions that are relatively common. Many people are self-medicating with herbal home remedies. It is important for the clinician to have a basic understanding of these preparations and their possible mental health effects to be able to counsel clients about side effects, drug-to-drug interactions, and potential dangerous effects. The case study provided an example of how multiple treatment modalities can be combined to develop an effective plan of care for a client with a psychiatric illness.

EXAM QUESTIONS

CHAPTER 4
Questions 19-25

Note: Choose the one option that BEST answers each question.

19. "How does that make you feel?" is an example of what communication technique?

    a. Non-therapeutic, close-ended question

    b. Non-therapeutic, challenging

    c. Therapeutic, open-ended question

    d. Therapeutic, offering self

20. "Are you sad?" is an example of what communication technique?

    a. Non-therapeutic, close-ended question

    b. Non-therapeutic, challenging

    c. Therapeutic, open-ended question

    d. Therapeutic, offering self

21. Cognitive behavioral therapy techniques offer distinct advantages to clients because

    a. insurance companies reimburse at a better rate.

    b. clients are taught to challenge beliefs that are detrimental to recovery.

    c. childhood traumas are thoroughly explored.

    d. of the use of positive and negative reinforcers.

22. Psychoeducational groups

    a. are effective ways to educate clients to develop life skills.

    b. should always be done by psychologists.

    c. require a high degree of training.

    d. effect change by altering balances of power in the family system.

23. Community support groups are useful because they provide

    a. individual and group therapy.

    b. an opportunity to gain employment.

    c. connections to community political leaders.

    d. a network of peers experiencing similar problems.

24. ECT is utilized primarily to treat

    a. schizophrenia.

    b. treatment-resistant depression.

    c. severe aggression and agitation.

    d. epilepsy.

25. The problem with using over-the-counter herbal remedies is that they

    a. don't work.

    b. are dangerous.

    c. are too expensive.

    d. have not been tested or approved by the FDA.

CHAPTER 5

SCHIZOPHRENIA AND RELATED DISORDERS

CHAPTER OBJECTIVE

At the end of this chapter the reader will be able to identify symptoms of a thought disorder and the appropriate nursing care and medication treatment.

LEARNING OBJECTIVES

At the end of this chapter, the reader will be able to

1. describe the symptoms of schizophrenia.

2. differentiate schizophrenia from other psychotic disorders.

3. discuss antipsychotic medications and their side effects.

INTRODUCTION

Schizophrenia was recognized as far back as there are written records, with thought disturbances typical in schizophrenia described in ancient Egyptian writings. The word schizophrenia is derived from the Greek roots "schizo" (split) and "phrene" (mind), leading to a common misconception that schizophrenia is the same as multiple personality disorder (now called dissociative identity disorder). In 1887, Dr. Emile Krapelin was the first person to classify psychiatric disorders into categories (see Chapter 1), initially calling the disease of schizophrenia "dementia praecox." The Swiss psychiatrist Eugen Bleuler coined the term "schizophrenia" in 1911, noting that the disease has significant differences from dementia, can onset later in life, and is characterized by both positive and negative symptoms.

In this chapter, the etiology, development, and diagnostic criteria of schizophrenia will be presented. Related disorders, with hallucinations, delusions, or gross disorganization of thoughts (psychosis) as primary symptoms, will be discussed in comparison with schizophrenia. Antipsychotic medications are presented, following a brief discussion of chemicals in the brain known as neurotransmitters. Antipsychotic medications are divided into two groups: traditional medications first utilized in the early 1950's and new generation medications approved after 1980. Side effects of these medications are reviewed in some detail, with particular attention to the metabolic syndrome – hyperglycemia, dyslipidemia, hypertension and obesity – that predisposes an individual to the development of diabetes and cardiac disease. Nursing care of the client with schizophrenia is discussed, and a case study, accompanied by a comprehensive nursing care plan for the client with schizophrenia, is provided.

SCHIZOPHRENIA: ETIOLOGY AND DEVELOPMENT

Schizophrenia is a severe psychiatric disorder that is chronic and can be very disabling to the individual. The incidence of schizophrenia in the population is about 1% and affects both genders approximately the same. The average age of onset varies slightly with the majority of men becoming ill between 20 and 25 years of age or 30 and 35 years of age. Women tend to experience a disease onset approximately 5 years later than men. After 45 years of age, the ratio of women to men in newly diagnosed cases becomes 2 to 1. Schizophrenia is believed to be a brain-based medical disorder with distinct, yet unknown, neurobiological causes.

Although schizophrenia has been noted to have familial tendencies (first-degree relatives have a risk for the disorder at a rate of 10 times the general population), more than 60% of persons with schizophrenia have no family history of the disorder and the concordance rate for monozygotic (identical) twins is only 50%. This would imply that nongenetic factors are also important in the development of the disease (Nasrallah & Smeltzer, 2002).

To diagnose schizophrenia, the individual must have an occurrence of symptoms that lasts for 6 months and include at least 1 month of clear positive or negative symptom groups (American Psychiatric Association, 2000). Positive symptoms may include hallucinations of any type, delusional beliefs, grossly disorganized behavior or speech, or catatonic behaviors. Negative symptoms are more difficult to identify and reflect a loss of normal functioning. Three major negative symptom characteristics are associated with most clients with schizophrenia. These include affective flattening, alogia, and avolition. Affective flattening refers to an apparent lack of emotional responsivity in the client. The client may demonstrate poor eye contact, few facial gestures, and reduced body contact.

The client may be able to briefly smile or laugh, but the intensity and duration of the emotional response are impaired. Alogia, also referred to as poverty-of-speech, is exhibited by brief replies to questions and a lack of elaboration or colorful details in speech content. The client may answer questions with only one or two words, then lapse into silence. Alogia is associated with a diminished range and content of thoughts, reflected in the decrease in speech. Lastly, avolition is exhibited by a decreased ability to initiate or maintain activities. Clients may appear to be staring off into space for long periods of time and may require frequent reminders to participate in daily activities. Together, negative symptoms have a profound impact on social relationships, employment, continued education, self-care abilities, and other life endeavors. Medication treatment of schizophrenia consists of antipsychotic agents.

To diagnose schizophrenia, six criteria are provided by the *DSM-IV-TR*.

1. *Characteristic symptoms:* Two or more of the following must be present, each for most of a 1-month period:
   a. Delusions
   b. Hallucinations
   c. Disorganized speech
   d. Grossly disorganized or catatonic behavior
   e. Negative symptoms (affective flattening, alogia, or avolition)

2. *Social and occupational dysfunction:* One or more major areas of functioning (work, relationships) or self-care are markedly below the level expected for the individual (child) or the level achieved previously (adult).

3. *Duration:* Continuous symptoms persist for at least 6 months, with at least 1 month of criterion-1 symptoms.

4. *Schizoaffective and mood disorder exclusion:* No major depressive, manic, or mixed-mood episodes have occurred concurrently with the criterion-1 symptoms (or mood symptoms are brief).

5. *Substance and general medical condition exclusion:* Drugs, alcohol, or medical conditions cannot be associated with the symptoms.

6. *Relationship to a pervasive developmental disorder:* In the presence of a history of autism or pervasive developmental disorder, prominent symptoms of delusions or hallucinations must be present for at least 1 month.

Schizophrenia is further differentiated in the *DSM-IV-TR* into five subtypes: paranoid, disorganized, catatonic, undifferentiated, and residual. Each of these subtypes is identified based on the symptom clusters that are experienced by the client. A brief description of these subtypes follows.

Paranoid schizophrenia is expressed by an overall good organization of thought processes that is accompanied by delusions that may be persecutory, grandiose, jealous, religious, or somatic. Delusions usually center on a specific theme and may be very intricate and detailed. Hallucinations may also be present. Associated mood states may be fear, anger, suspiciousness, irritability, mistrust, anxiety, arrogance, or aloofness. The combination of persecutory delusions with anger can predispose the client to violence or suicidal tendencies. There is little cognitive impairment and clients, though resistant to treatment, may respond well to antipsychotic agents. Occupational functioning and self-care abilities are impacted to a lesser degree with this subtype than with the other four.

Clients with disorganized schizophrenia have great difficulty in managing their affairs and living independently. Speech, thoughts, and behavior may all be disorganized, and the client may demonstrate a flat or inappropriate affect. Hallucinations and delusions, when present, may be scattered and aren't as clearly thematic in nature as in paranoid schizophrenia. Clients who are acutely ill may be unable to complete a sentence, express a simple idea, or perform basic self-care activities, such as bathing and dressing. Associated features may include odd or bizarre grimacing or behavioral mannerisms.

The essential feature of catatonic schizophrenia is an extreme psychomotor slowing or retardation that may cause stupor, immobility, mutism, echolalia (echoing others' words or phrases), echopraxia (imitating the behavior of others), negativism, or agitated activity that is non-goal oriented and purposeless. Catalepsy (also called *waxy flexibility*) is an unusual symptom that allows the healthcare provider to pose an immobile client, much like a department store manikin, and the client will hold his position for a long period of time. During an acute phase, the client requires a great deal of nursing care to prevent self-harm, malnutrition, dehydration, and injury. Hallucinations are difficult to assess and the client may seem to be devoid of emotions or affect.

A client with undifferentiated schizophrenia has symptoms that meet the criterion-1 category, but do not meet the criteria to be classified as paranoid, disorganized, or catatonic. Occasionally, this diagnosis is used when the clinical picture is variable.

Residual schizophrenia is diagnosed when a client has had at least one episode of the disorder, but the current presentation is without significant positive symptoms. Associated positive symptoms may be present (odd mannerisms or gesturing) and there is continued evidence of negative symptoms. Any delusions or hallucinations are minimal, and there is no associated change in affect. Residual schizophrenia may be brief and occur between acute episodes, or it may become a long-term, baseline presentation.

SCHIZOAFFECTIVE DISORDER

Schizoaffective disorder is a neurobiological (brain-based) disorder in which there is a clear episode of clinical depression, mania, or mixed depressive and manic symptoms, concurrent with criterion-1 symptoms of schizophrenia. The symptoms cannot be due to the effect of substances (e.g., amphetamines) or a medical condition. The mood symptoms must be present for a prominent period of time. This time period requires clinical judgment, but can be no less than 1 full week in the case of mania or mixed mania/depression or 2 weeks in the case of depression. Prominent hallucinations or delusions must also be present during the course of the illness (which differentiates this disorder from a primary major depression or bipolar illness). Two subtypes of schizoaffective disorder are identified: bipolar type and depressed type. Medication treatment of a schizoaffective disorder may include antipsychotics, antidepressants, and mood stabilizers.

OTHER PSYCHOTIC DISORDERS

Other, less common, disorders related to thought processes and thought content are presented in the *DSM-IV-TR*. A brief description of each follows.

1. *Schizophreniform disorder* – the client meets the first three criteria for schizophrenia, but the duration of the disorder is less than 6 months. Impaired social or occupational functioning is not required.

2. *Delusional disorder* – the client has one or more irrational or inaccurate beliefs that persists for at least 1 month. Hallucinations may be associated with the delusion; however, behavior and psychosocial functioning are not impaired. Several subtypes exist: erotomanic (the belief that another person is in love with the individ-

ual), grandiose (the belief that one has a great, but unrecognized, talent, insight, or discovery or that one has a special relationship with someone famous), jealous (the belief that a spouse or lover is unfaithful), persecutory (the belief that one is being conspired against), somatic (the belief that something is gravely wrong with one's body), mixed (seen when no one theme emerges), or unspecified (when the delusional belief cannot be readily determined).

3. *Brief psychotic disorder* – sudden onset of at least one of the criterion-1 symptoms, with no known etiology (e.g., substances or illness), lasting from 1 day to 1 month, with full return to a premorbid state. This disorder may be seen after a traumatic psychosocial stressor occurs.

4. *Shared psychotic disorder* – formerly called folie á deux, a delusion develops in an individual who is closely involved with another person who is experiencing a psychotic disorder with prominent delusions.

5. *Psychotic disorder due to a general medical condition* – diagnosed when an individual develops criterion-1 symptoms that can be clearly linked to a medical event, such as a head injury, dementia, or a metabolic disturbance.

6. *Substance-induced psychotic disorder* – diagnosed when an individual develops criterion-1 symptoms that are associated with either the use or the withdrawal of a substance, such as alcohol, illegal drugs, prescription medications, or a variety of other offending agents.

7. *Psychotic disorder not otherwise specified* – diagnosis used when the etiology of the psychosis is unclear or a full diagnostic workup has not yet been completed (inadequate information).

ANTIPSYCHOTIC MEDICATIONS

Medications have been used in psychiatric disorders since they were first available. Early mental health treatment consisted primarily of chemical restraints on behaviors. Various concoctions were used – all containing blends of opiates, alcohol, or other sedating chemicals. The first generation of medications specifically targeted to reduce the symptoms of schizophrenia was developed in the early 1950s with chlorpromazine (Thorazine®), a phenothiazine agent with pronounced antihistamine properties. Several others soon followed, and by 1975 there were more than 10 first-generation antipsychotics available. Although efficacious for the positive symptoms of schizophrenia and psychotic disorders, the traditional agents are all high in side effects and do little to ameliorate the negative symptoms. Table 5-1 presents an overview of the traditional antipsychotic agents, along with a comparison of their potency levels and side effect profiles. Of these products, haloperidol (Haldol®) and fluphenazine

(Prolixin®) are available in long-acting, decanoate injections that are given intramuscularly every 4 weeks or 2 to 3 weeks respectively.

The primary mechanism of action of the traditional antipsychotic agents is postsynaptic dopamine receptor antagonism – that is, the medication binds with the dopamine receptors in the neurons of the brain, thus reducing (or blocking) the transmission of the neurotransmitter dopamine through the brain. Dopamine blockade from these agents is nonspecific, which has contributed to numerous unwanted neurological effects. The most severe of these side effects are medication-induced pseudoparkinsonism, secondary to dopamine blockade in the extrapyramidal tract of the brain (commonly referred to as extrapyramidal syndrome), and tardive dyskinesia, whose etiology is unclear. Symptoms of extrapyramidal syndrome include tremors of the skeletal muscles (most commonly noticed in the upper extremities), a blunting or stiffening of the facial muscles that results in a mask-like facial expression, slowed gait (bradykinesia), shuffling gait, stiffening of the skeletal

TABLE 5-1: TRADITIONAL ANTIPSYCHOTIC MEDICATIONS IN COMMON USAGE									
Generic Name	Trade Name	Relative Potency	EPS Risk	TD Risk	Ortho B/P Risk	Sedation	Weight Gain	Anticholinergic Properties	Comments
Chlorpromazine	Thorazine®	+	++	++	+++	++	+++	+++	1st antipsychotic developed
Thioridazine	Mellaril®	+	+	+	+++	+++	+++	+++	QTc prolongation problematic
Fluphenazine	Prolixin®	+++	+++	+++	+	+	+	++	Available in long-acting decanoate injection
Perphenazine	Trilafon®	++	++	++	+++	++	+	++	Available combined w/amitriptyline (Triavil®)
Trifluoperazine	Stelazine®	+++	+++	+++	++	+	+	++	
Thiothixene	Navane®	+++	+++	+++	+	++	++	++	
Haloperidol	Haldol®	+++	+++	++	+	+	++	++	Available in long-acting decanoate injection
Loxapine	Loxitane®	++	++	++	++	++	+	+	
Molindone	Moban®	++	++	++	+	+	+	+	
Pimozide	Orap®	+++	+++	++	++	++	+	+++	QTc prolongation a concern. Primary use is in Tourette's syndrome.

+++ High   ++ Moderate   + Low
EPS: Extrapyramidal syndrome   TD: Tardive dykinesia   Ortho B/P: Orthostatic blood pressure

muscles, a purposeless sense of restlessness and, occasionally, a sudden muscle dystonia or unremitting contraction, often noted in the muscles of the neck, shoulders, or eyes. Extrapyramidal syndrome symptoms often can be partially or completely relieved by the addition of anticholinergic medications (see Table 5-2). Tardive dyskinesia is a central nervous system (CNS) disorder more likely to occur after prolonged exposure to traditional antipsychotics. Tardive dyskinesia is characterized by abnormal, choreiform movements of the muscles, resulting is repetitive, often slow or writhing, body movements. Tardive dyskinesia does not respond to anticholinergic medications and it rarely remits spontaneously. There is no current treatment for tardive dyskinesia, although switching to one of the newer antipsychotic agents may be useful. Some recent research has suggested that antioxidants, such as vitamin E, may reduce some of the symptoms. When utilized, vitamin E should be administered at 800 to 1,200 international units daily.

Other CNS side effects may include an elevation in prolactin levels in the brain, resulting in dysmenorrhea, reduced libido, breast enlargement, or false breast milk (galactorrhea); inappropriate antidiuretic hormone, resulting in water toxicity (also called polygenic polydipsia); seizures (rarely); thermoregulatory abnormalities, resulting in hyperthermia or hypothermia; and neuroleptic malignant syndrome, a poorly understood syndrome in which body temperature rises rapidly and skeletal muscle breakdown occurs. Without emergency treatment, neuroleptic malignant syndrome can be life threatening.

Non-CNS side effects are also prominent with traditional antipsychotics. Antihistamine-like properties cause drowsiness and an increased appetite (and weight gain). Cardiovascular effects can occur and are evidenced by orthostatic hypotension, tachycardia (rapid heartbeat), and prolongation of the Q-Tc interval in electrical conduction through the heart, which can trigger a sudden cardiac arrest associated with a ventricular fibrillation known as torsades de pointes. Thioridazine (Mellaril®) now carries a black-box warning due to its potential for Q-Tc prolongation. Anticholinergic properties of traditional antipsychotics can cause dry mouth, constipation, and urinary retention. Some blood dyscrasias can occur with traditional antipsychotics. Ocular disorders have emerged in clients taking traditional antipsychotics: an increase in retinal pigmentation has been seen as well as an increase in cataract development. Agents used to treat extrapyramidal syndrome may also cause ocular disturbances – primarily, blurred vision, dry eyes, and acute glaucoma symptoms. Gastrointestinal problems include dry mouth, constipation, elevated liver enzymes, and paralytic ileus. Finally, photosensitivity reactions can

TABLE 5-2: MEDICATIONS USED TO TREAT EXTRAPYRAMIDAL SYNDROME EFFECTS ASSOCIATED WITH ANTIPSYCHOTICS

Generic Name	Trade Name	Classification	Comments
Benztropine	Cogentin®	Anticholinergic	Available in oral or intramuscular formulation
Trihexyphenidyl	Artane®	Anticholinergic	Some clients report decreased dry mouth
Amantadine	Symmetrel®	Dopamine agonist	Antiviral activities as well as EPS treatment
Bromocriptine	Parlodel®	Dopamine agonist	Inhibits prolactin release, used in NMS
Diphenhydramine	Benadryl®	Antihistamine	Often used in children and adolescents
Propranolol	Inderal®	Beta-adrenergic blocker	Primarily for tremors
Lorazepam	Ativan®	Benzodiazepine	Useful for restlessness, pacing

EPS: Extrapyramidal syndrome   NMS: Neuroleptic malignant syndrome occur, causing excess sunburn and rashes (Nasrallah & Smeltzer, 2002).

Altered glucose metabolism and an increased risk for diabetes are seen in clients taking antipsychotic agents. Usually this is an adult-onset, type II diabetes associated with obesity, but there have been reports of diabetic ketoacidosis, in the absence of significant weight gain, along with an increase in serum lipid levels and triglycerides. This has led to recommendations from the FDA that clients taking antipsychotic medications be evaluated at least annually for diabetes through laboratory testing.

Special consideration must be used when utilizing antipsychotic agents during pregnancy. There is no current evidence of teratogenicity (congenital abnormalities or birth defects), but the literature is sparse. A risk/benefit analysis should be done that considers the potential benefit to the expectant mother in terms of psychiatric stability and prenatal care and compares that to the risk of decompensated mental illness, including postpartum psychosis and danger to the infant. Breast-feeding is often discouraged because of the lack of information on the effects on the infant.

Certain ethnic populations may metabolize antipsychotic agents differently or at a slower rate than the general population. African American and Asian populations tend to have a genetic variant of the enzyme CYP2D6 – that causes slower drug metabolism and a higher incidence of extrapyramidal syndrome and tardive dyskinesia. Lower drug dosages may be indicated.

Tobacco induces cytochrome enzymes and can significantly increase the oxidation of some antipsychotics, reducing the serum concentrations and bioavailability of the drug. When a client chooses to stop smoking, serum medication levels may rise and cause an increase in side effects at the same dosage as previously taken.

New Generation Antipsychotics

After four decades, it became evident that newer medications were needed. Drug development started to focus on continued treatment efficacy; targeting the negative symptoms of avolition, alogia, and affective flattening; and attempting to reduce the noxious side effects of the traditional agents. The first of these newer agents was clozapine (Clozaril®). Clozapine was initially developed in 1959; however, the trends in medicating at the time dictated that psychotic remission was synonymous with extrapyramidal syndrome emergence. Because clozapine had no extrapyramidal syndrome side effects, it was initially thought to be a poor medication. Research continued and it was launched in Europe in 1972. The United States did not initially approve clozapine because of concerns about hypotension and increased seizure risk. Three years after its European launch, it became clear that there were several cases of agranulocytosis (low white blood cells) leading to death. It was removed from the market at that time but continued to be studied. Clozapine was reintroduced to the FDA for approval in the 1980s due to its marked superiority in treatment efficacy over traditional agents. In 1988, the FDA approved clozapine, only after other medications had been tried and failed, and with the caveat that all clients receiving the drug would have to have weekly white blood cell (WBC) count monitoring. A few years ago, this restriction was eased to allow clients on the medication successfully for at least 1 year to have less frequent blood draws. Currently, clients who are medicated with clozapine must have their WBC counts done weekly for the first 6 months of treatment, biweekly for the second 6 months of treatment, then monthly thereafter for life. Absolute neutrophil counts are even more specific for agranulocytosis and should be calculated with each WBC count. Even without extrapyramidal syndrome or tardive dyskinesia side effects, clozapine can cause hypotension, saliorrhea (excess salivation), sedation, weight gain (and increased risk for diabetes), and increased seizure risk. Additionally, the drug is metabolized quickly in the body and a client will rapidly decompensate after only a few missed doses. Rebound hypertension and tachycardia can occur with sudden withdrawal of clozapine.

After clozapine, several other new generation, atypical antipsychotics were introduced. These include risperidone (Risperdal®) in 1994, olanzapine (Zyprexa®) in 1996, quetiapine (Seroquel®) in 1997, ziprasidone (Geodon®) in 2001, aripiprazole (Abilify®) in 2002, paliperidone (Invega®) in 2006, and aliperidone (Fanapt®) and asenapine (Saphris®) in 2009. A distinguishing characteristic of the newer generation drugs is that, although they are still primarily dopamine antagonists, they also have serotonin reuptake blocking effects, which seem to be associated with improvement in the negative symptoms, including cognitive functioning in schizophrenia and other chronic, psychotic disorders (see Table 5-3). Atypical antipsychotics are also available in long-acting injectable forms. Risperdal-Consta is available in a long-acting intra-

TABLE 5-3: NEW GENERATION ANTIPSYCHOTIC MEDICATIONS

Generic Name	Trade Name	EPS Risk	TD Risk	Ortho B/P	Sedation Risk	Weight Gain	Anticholinergic Properties	Comments
Clozapine	Clozaril®	+	+	+++	+++	+++	++	* WBC/ANC monitoring required * Increased risk of seizures
Risperidone	Risperdal®	++	+	+	++	++	++	* Pronounced prolactin elevation in some clients * Approved for pediatric usage in autism * Available in biweekly injection and dissolvable tablet
Paliperidone	Invega®	++	+	+	+	+	+	* Oros™ delivery system for morning dosing *Available in monthly injection
Aliperidone	Fanapt®	++	+	+	+	+	+	*Potential drug interactions with Cytochrome P450, 2D6
Olanzapine	Zyprexa®	+	+	+	+++	+++	+	* Weight gain associated with metabolic syndrome *Zydis® is rapid-dissolving wafer formulation *Available in biweekly or monthly injection
Quetiapine	Seroquel®	+	+	++	+++	++	++	* Pronounced anti-anxiety effects *Sedation, weight gain, and triglyceride concerns
Asenapine	Saphris®	+	+	+	++	+	+	*Sublingual twice daily dosing. Less weight gain.
Ziprasidone	Geodon®	+	+	+	+	+	+	* Difficult to dose *No weight gain. May reduce lipids
Aripiprazole	Abilify®	++	+	+	+	+	+	*Approved for ages 13-17
+++ High ++ Moderate + Low EPS: Extrapyramidal syndrome								
TD: Tardive dyskinesia Ortho B/P: Orthostatic blood pressure WBC/ANC: White blood cell/absolute nutrophil count								

muscular injection given every 2 weeks. Invega Sustenna injectable is given monthly after initiation, and Zyprexa Relprevv can be given either biweekly or monthly. All of these products must be given intramuscularly. These are particularly helpful for clients who are noncompliant with oral medications. All of the new generation products, with the exception of clozapine, paliperidone, and aliperidone, are now also approved for the treatment of bipolar disorder, which will be discussed more fully in a later chapter.

In 2005, the FDA warned that data suggested an increased risk of death secondary to cerebrovascular accidents (strokes) in elderly persons with dementia who were taking new generation antipsychotics for agitation or hallucinations. This has resulted in the addition of an FDA black box warning for these products. Currently, more traditional antipsychotics are also being considered for this warning. Options are limited for treating elderly persons with dementia who are also hallucinating, delusional, or agitated. Healthcare providers must weigh the costs and benefits of treatment for each client individually, consulting with family members when possible.

METABOLIC SYNDROME

Metabolic syndrome is a term used to describe a group of physical health problems that predispose individuals to the development of diabetes mellitus and cardiovascular disease. This syndrome may help to explain why deaths in persons with schizophrenia occur on average up to 25 years earlier than in individuals without the disease. Symptoms of metabolic syndrome are illustrated in Table 5-4 along with their non-genetic contributory lifestyle factors. Metabolic syndrome, in particular weight gain and hyperglycemia, has become associated with new generation antipsychotics and there have been several law suits settled over this issue, although a cause-and-effect relationship has not

been demonstrated. However, due to the increase in case reports of diabetes onset and elevated lipid levels, the FDA recommends that clients on these medications have initial and annual laboratory monitoring for these diseases.

POST-INJECTION DELIRIUM/SEDATION SYNDROME

A new antipsychotic adverse reaction was identified in research trials for the long-acting injectable antipsychotic Zyprexa Relprevv®. In two studies totaling over 200 patients, 0.7% demonstrated a rapid onset of post-injection delirium/sedation syndrome (PDSS). Most cases of PDSS occurred within the first hour, with the majority occuring within the first few hours. Only 6% of cases occurred after 4 hours. PDSS is characterized by the occurrence of sedation, sometimes extreme, accompanied by confusion and delirium. All 37 cases seen in the initial trials largely recovered, including two clients who were prophylactically intubated after receiving benzodiazepines for agitation and aggression. The sedation seen was significant and lasted up to 72 hours (Eli Lilly & Company, 2010).

The mechanism of action as to why PDSS occurs is unclear. The manufacturer (Lilly, USA) theorizes that the medication olanzapine, which is bonded with pamoic acid in the form of pamoate crystals, manages to get into the vasculature system, causing an immediate break in the bond. This results in a large quantity of olanzapine being delivered immediately to the patient, which was intended to be delivered over a 2-week or 4-week period. In fact, the company advises any healthcare providers who detect PDSS, to tell the emergency medical responders and emergency department that the client is suffering from "a suspected overdose of olanzapine following a Zyprexa Relprevv® injection" (Eli Lilly & Company, 2010).

TABLE 5-4: METABOLIC SYNDROME AND RISK FACTORS	
Insulin-resistance	Fasting blood glucose >100 Hemoglobin > flex 6.5
Dyslipidemia	Total cholesterol >200 High-density lipoprotein cholesterol < flex 40 in men; < flex 50 in women Triglycerides >150
Hypertension	Blood pressure > 130/85
Obesity	Body mass index >28 Waist circumference > flex 40" in men Waist circumference > flex 35" in women
Contributory Risk Factors for Metabolic Syndrome	
Cigarette smoking, other tobacco product use	Vasoconstriction, poor oxygen transport, increased heart rate from nicotine (stimulant)
Sedentary lifestyle	Calorie expenditure not equal to calorie intake, loss of muscle tone, increased fat storage, osteoporosis
Diet high in animal fats, starches, sugar, soft drinks, fast foods	Increase load on pancreas to produce insulin; excess calorie intake in relation to expenditure, leading to stored fat
Poor primary health care	Lack of early identification of risk factors or disease; worsening disease, leading to chronic conditions and complications

Because of the unknown cause and the seriousness of PDSS, the FDA has approved the use of Zyprexa Relprevv® with certain restrictions. The first of these is that all prescribers, pharmacies, healthcare facilities, and patients using the product must be registered in a national database and renewed every 3 years. Second, every dose of Zyprexa Relprevv® given must be recorded in the database as well as any PDSS event. In addition, the patient receiving Zyprexa Relprevv® must be observed and monitored by trained staff for 3 hours after every dose and may not be released until he or she is accompanied home by a friend or family member.

Nurses who give Zyprexa Relprevv® must be trained in using the product and in recognizing PDSS. The medication itself can only be dispensed to the healthcare facility (not to the client) and it requires reconstitution prior to its administration. Lilly, USA is providing training to prescribers, nurses, and healthcare facilties at no charge to help manage this product (Eli Lilly & Company, 2010).

NURSING CARE OF THE CLIENT WITH SCHIZOPHRENIA AND RELATED DISORDERS

Psychiatric nursing roles center around many areas of holistic care. They include maintaining safety of the client and staff; assessing for mental and physical health alterations, including monitoring weight, blood pressure, and laboratory values; supporting basic needs for nutrition, hydration, sleep, warmth, elimination, and hygiene; and supporting and educating the client, family, and significant others about the disease process and appropriate treatments, which may include medication education and reducing metabolic syndrome risks.

Safety and risk assessment involve monitoring clients for any evidence of harmful behavior to self, and for any signs of increasing tension or agitation. Most healthcare facilities provide training for staff in crisis prevention, and how to de-escalate a situation. In an outpatient setting, the nurse should watch for clues that a client is becoming increasingly psychotic, manic, or depressed. Changes in mental status can be associated with emergent suicidal or violent thought, or severe disorganization, leading to an inability to provide basic self-care. Medication changes or hospitalization (voluntary or involuntary) may be necessary. Clients who are abusing alcohol or drugs in combination with an underlying psychiatric disorder are at particular risk for self-injury or harm to others.

Seclusion is the involuntary placement of a client in a safe, contained environment apart from other clients. Restraints are mechanical devices used to limit the client's mobility. Secluding and restraining persons with mental illness have been used for hundreds of years. Today, the client must present a clear and imminent danger to oneself or others in order to justify the use of seclusion or restraints because both procedures deprive the person of his or her rights to liberty as granted by the U.S. Constitution. It is inappropriate to seclude or restrain a client for the purposes of punishment. The nurse must chart the justification for the seclusion or restraint, the type of restraint used, alternative means that were tried before resorting to seclusion or restraint, the amount of time the client was in seclusion or restrainted, the objectives to be reached by utilizing seclusion or restraint, regular safety checks of the client, and the measures taken to ensure hydration, nutrition, and proper toileting for the client while in seclusion or restraint. As needed, or PRN, medication orders are never deemed to be appropriate. Each occurrence is treated as a separate and distinct event and must be documented as such. Seclusion and restraint are not appropriate for outpatient or residential settings caring for clients with psychiatric disorders. In many hospitals, physicians are required to assess the client within 30 to 60 minutes of the application of seclusion or restraints and strict protocols are observed.

Administering medications, teaching about the effects and side effects of those medications, assessing for medication efficacy, and monitoring for noncompliance are important nursing interventions. Antipsychotic medications come in oral and injectable intramuscular (IM) formulations. The nurse should document the medication given as well as any observations of the client during that time, paying particular attention to CNS side effects such as extrapyramidal syndrome and tardive dyskinesia. For as needed medications, the effectiveness and outcome should also be noted.

The psychiatric nurse fulfills a vital role in performing mental and physical health assessments. General knowledge of body systems and disease processes is essential. The nurse is often viewed as a resource by non-nursing and non-medical counseling and support staff. Identifying symptoms and placing symptom clusters into a framework helps the nurse to differentiate an acute psychiatric disturbance from a medical disease (e.g., presenting symptoms of anxiety and paranoid delusions may be triggered by a decreased oxygen level, secondary to congestive heart failure). The ability to prioritize and triage in emergency situations is essential. Developing care plans focusing on reducing the factors that contribute to metabolic syndrome may be an essential function of nurses working in mental health care settings.

Supporting clients in nutrition, hydration, elimination, hygiene, and other basic needs is especially important in the acute phase of a psychiatric decompensation. Clients who are disorganized or catatonic may experience fluid and electrolyte imbalances. Constipation can lead to intense discomfort and bowel perforations, necessitating surgery. Poor hygiene can result in skin lesions or parasites as well as social ostracization. Inadequate dental care can lead to cavities or infections of the mouth, jaw, and oral structures. Occasionally, a mouth infection becomes systemic and can cause septic shock. Assisting clients with basic care will help them preserve their dignity and integrity.

Education is a cornerstone of psychiatric nursing. Individuals with mental disorders are not sick in the traditional sense of the word; rather, they are experiencing an acute disruption in role performance and overall functioning. Assisting the client and family members or significant others in understanding psychiatric illnesses and their treatment promotes better treatment compliance and improves overall health. Teaching practical skills such as relaxation techniques provides clients with alternative coping strategies in times of increased stress. Learning to understand and recognize signs of decompensation, and seeking help early, decreases the length and intensity of acute illness episodes. Families with acutely ill loved ones often have difficulty in comprehending issues of personal freedom and the right to refuse treatment. The nurse can educate them about the legal process and support them when they are feeling helpless to intervene.

CASE STUDY: CLIENT WITH SCHIZOPHRENIA

Bob is a 46-year-old man diagnosed with schizophrenia, paranoid type. He first became ill at age 19. He came home from his freshman year of college to tell his parents that CIA agents had attempted to make contact with him using the computer lab in his dormitory. He has been hospitalized 6 times since then, with one state hospitalization lasting 18 months, after he assaulted his therapist (he accused the therapist of planting listening devices in his apartment). Bob has been put on the decanoate injectable form of the antipsychotic haloperidol (Haldol®), which he receives once a month at the mental health center. He takes Zyprexa® at bedtime to enhance the activity of the haloperidol. The nurse notes that Bob is rocking back and forth, rubbing his fingertips together, blinking rapidly, and smacking his lips. He is also taking the anticholinergic medication benztropine (Cogentin®) to control his tremors and muscle stiffness.

Bob is seen in the outpatient clinic office by the nurse. He weighs 278 lb at a height of 5'11". His blood pressure is 168/110, heart rate is 96, and respiratory rate is 24. He is unemployed, does not have any friends, and does not leave his home most days. Bob tells the nurse that he drinks two pots of coffee and smokes two packs of cigarettes daily. He is complaining about difficulty going to sleep before 4:00 a.m. and says he is unable to waken before 1:00 p.m. the following day. Bob also reports ongoing auditory hallucinations that are derogatory in nature. The voices tell him, "You are worthless. They're coming to get you! They'll lock you up again! Watch out!"

Questions

1. What are the positive symptoms of Bob's illness?

2. What are the extrapyramidal side effects of Bob's medication? What are the signs of tardive dyskinesia?

3. Which behaviors are likely to cause this client to develop significant health problems in the next few years?

Discussion

Bob's positive symptoms are his paranoid delusions of being watched or spied on by others. These symptoms are most amenable to antipsychotic medications. He is experiencing extrapyramidal side effects (tremors, muscle stiffness) and tardive dyskinesia (rocking, blinking rapidly, smacking his lips, rubbing fingertips together) because of these medications. Bob's greatest risks to his health in the next few years are his cardiac risk factors: obesity, smoking hypertension, and excessive caffeine intake.

NURSING CARE PLAN: CLIENT WITH SCHIZOPHRENIA

Problem Listing

- Poor nutrition – overweight
- Elevated blood pressure
- Shortness of breath
- Sleep cycle disturbance
- Caffeine abuse/dependence
- Nicotine dependence
- Auditory/derogatory hallucinations
- Probable tardive dyskinesia
- Lack of employment or structured daytime activities.

Nursing Diagnoses

1. Imbalanced nutrition: more than body requirements related to excessive intake of food, as evidenced by weight of 278 lb at 5'11".

2. Ineffective health maintenance related to knowledge deficit, as evidenced by blood pressure reading of 168/110.

3. Sleep pattern disorder related to excess intake of caffeine late at night, as evidenced by a pattern of sleeping from 4:00 a.m. to 1:00 p.m.

4. Disturbed sensory perceptions: auditory hallucinations related to disease process, as evidenced by patient report of "hearing voices."

5. Health behavior: risk prone related to excessive cigarette smoking, with risk for respiratory and cardiac disease.

6. Impaired physical mobility related to antipsychotic medication treatment, as evidenced by symptoms of tardive dyskinesia.

7. Impaired self-esteem related to derogatory hallucinations, as evidenced by lack of social contacts, social isolation, and unemployment.

Long-term Goal

Client will have improved physical and mental health status, with a decreased risk for diabetes, cardiac, and respiratory diseases leading to a return to an active and productive life.

Short-term Objectives

1. Client will reach a goal weight of 200 lb by the end of 1 year.

2. Client will demonstrate blood pressure readings consistently lower than 130/85.

3. Client will go to sleep by 11:00 p.m. nightly.

4. Client will demonstrate compliance with antipsychotic medications.

5. Client will decrease nicotine use by 50% in 6 months, and will stop smoking in 1 year.

6. Client will walk 30 minutes at least 5 times a week and go to the YMCA weekly with the life-skills training group program.

7. Client will participate in Clubhouse and vocational rehabilitation activities.

Nursing Interventions

1. a. Educate the client about the importance of good nutrition for health.

   b. Facilitate a dietary consult.

   c. Assist the client in identifying ways to build activity into the daily routine.

   d. Weigh the client weekly to monthly to assess progress.

   e. Educate the client in completing a daily food diary to track intake.

   f. Meet with the client weekly to assess progress.

2. a. Check blood pressure with each monthly injection.

   b. Facilitate a medical exam with a family care provider to determine if an antihypertensive agent is needed.

3. a. Educate the client about the relationship between caffeine and insomnia.

   b. Teach the client relaxation techniques to utilize at bedtime.

   c. Encourage the client to set alarm clock for 8:00 a.m. daily and to get up.

   d. Advise the client to not take naps.

   e. Suggest that the client use half-caffeinated and half-decaffeinated coffee.

   f. Teach the client that cigarettes will keep him awake (not to smoke after 10:00 p.m.).

4. a. Assist client is setting up a weekly medication box.

   b. Educate the client about using techniques to distract himself from the hallucinations (such as listening to music).

5. a. Assist the client in setting up a schedule to eliminate nicotine use.

   b. Refer client to the Clubhouse Smoking Cessation Program at the clinic.

   c. Educate client in smoking alternatives (nicotine patches, inhalers, gum) or medications that help in smoking cessation (Zyban®, Chantix®), when authorized by his prescriber.

6. a. Teach client stretching techniques to help reduce stiffness and prevent injury while exercising.

7. a. Ensure that client has transportation to the Clubhouse program.

   b. Facilitate a vocational rehabilitation referral.

ADVANCED PRACTICE NURSING: THE CATIE STUDY

With the availability of prescriptive privileges to the APRN, greater emphasis has been placed on good decision-making in the choice of antipsychotic medications and the management of side effects. The CATIE (Clinical Antipsychotic Trials of Intervention Effectiveness) Study funded by the National Institute of Mental Health and completed in 2004, looked at the cost-effectiveness and treatment efficacy of five antipsychotic medications: one traditional and four new generation drugs. Medications included were perphenazine (Trilafon®), olanzapine (Zyprexa®), quetiapine (Seroquel®), risperidone (Risperdal®), and ziprasidone (Geodon®). This double-blind study, done over 3 years, looked at approximately 1500 clients, from 57 community or public health sites or academic settings, to evaluate their time to treatment discontinuation. Only clients with schizophrenia and between 18 and 65 years of age were included. Clients were allowed to discontinue treatment for any reason; most did so for a perceived lack of efficacy or for side effects. Results indicated that 74% of clients overall discontinued their medications prior to 18 months, with the lowest discontinuation rates in the olanzapine group and the highest in the quetiapine group. Clients taking olanzapine had the lowest number of hospitalizations but the greatest discontinuation due to weight gain. Anticholinergic effects, including weight gain, were also high with quetiapine. Weight gain was lowest with ziprasidone and perphenazine. Ziprasidone clients had an improvement in lipid levels, blood glucose, and body weight. Risperidone had the lowest discontinuation rate due to overall side effects. Clients discontinued the traditional antipsychotic perphenazine because of extrapyramidal side effects. There were no differences between the drugs in terms of cardiac QTc intervals, cataract development, suicide ideation, or suicide attempts.

Overall, the CATIE trials demonstrated that, of the five drugs studied, all were equally effective in treating clients with schizophrenia; however, compliance with taking the medications was related to the development of side effects. Older, more traditional antipsychotic medications appeared to offer more in terms of metabolic syndrome management (note: only one drug, Trilafon®, was studied) but are worse in the neurological complications of extrapyramidal syndrome and tardive dyskinesia. The new generation medications are, as a group, better tolerated; however, they are much more expensive and are implicated with increased body weight and increased risk for metabolic syndrome. Ziprasidone (Geodon®) did not increase weight and seemed to reduce lipid levels in some clients. Aripiprazole (Abilify®) and paliperidone (Invega®), both new-generation medications, were not studied in the CATIE trials.

SUMMARY

Schizophrenia is a serious and disabling condition occurring in about 1% of the population. Individuals with schizophrenia typically experience an onset of the disease in their late teens to early 20s, though onset may be later. Women are approximately equal to men in the development of the disorder. Schizophrenia symptoms are divided into positive symptoms, or those that are most responsive to medication treatment (hallucinations, delusions, disorganized thought processes), and negative symptoms, which typically do not respond well to medications (impaired social skills, avolition, decreased use of speech, decreased range of emotional expression). Early antipsychotic medications are highly effective in treating the positive symptoms; however, they are fraught with side effects and are not effective against negative symptoms. New generation antipsychotics have been developed that have beneficial treatment effects on both groups of symptoms and are lower in intolerable side effects. Recently, attention has been paid to weight gain, hyperglycemia, and elevated lipid levels in clients taking antipsychotic medications. When combined with high blood pressure and a sedentary lifestyle, individuals with metabolic syndrome are more susceptible to the development of diabetes and cardiovascular disease. These concerns have led to changes in laboratory monitoring recommendations by the FDA. A new and relatively rare adverse medication event called post-injection delirium/sedation syndrome, or PDSS, was identified in 2009 in association with the long-acting injectable olanzapine medication, Zyprexa Relprevv. Because of PDSS, the FDA requires that all prescribers, pharmacies, healthcare facilities, and patients using this product be registered. Other safety measures include dispensing the product to the facility and not to the client, monitoring clients for 3 hours after each dose, sending the client home with a family member or friend, and recording each injection and each PDSS occurrence in the national database. The nurse's role in patient education, health and wellness management, and monitoring for safety is more important than ever in clients with schizophrenia.

EXAM QUESTIONS

CHAPTER 5
Questions 26-32

Note: Choose the one option that BEST answers each question.

26. An example of what is meant by positive symptoms is

    a. good interpersonal skills and a bright, cheerful affect.

    b. hallucinations and delusions.

    c. poor eye contact and decreased thought content.

    d. rapid response to antipsychotic medication intervention.

27. Negative symptoms include

    a. grandiosity, ideas of reference, and hallucinations.

    b. depressed mood, anhedonia, and suicidality.

    c. somatic delusions and thought disorganization.

    d. emotional flattening, reduced speech, and avolition.

28. A man who believes that the government is spying on him and recording his phone conversations may be experiencing

    a. paranoid delusions.

    b. somatic delusions.

    c. auditory hallucinations.

    d. visual hallucinations.

29. A somatic delusion is a belief that

    a. your spouse is having multiple affairs.

    b. aliens are returning to earth to take you home.

    c. the IRS is plotting a conspiracy against you.

    d. something is gravely wrong with a part of your body.

30. *Terri presents in the emergency department with agitation and pressured speech. She looks to be about 30 years old, and she is very thin and emaciated. She is pacing rapidly and talks illogically of insects that are crawling in her mouth and ears and taking over her brain. Her urine drug screen comes back as positive for cocaine and cannabinoids.*

    The most likely diagnosis for this client is

    a. schizophrenia, disorganized type.

    b. schizoaffective disorder.

    c. brief psychotic disorder.

    d. substance-induced psychotic disorder.

31. The neurotransmitter that is associated with treatment efficacy of traditional antipsychotics as well as with extrapyramidal syndrome effects is

    a. acetylcholine.

    b. dopamine.

    c. serotonin.

    d. gamma-aminobutyric acid.

continued on next page

32. Clozapine, olanzepine, and quetiapine can cause

    a. delusions.

    b. insomnia.

    c. hallucinatons.

    d. sleepiness.

CHAPTER 6

DEMENTIA AND DELIRIUM

CHAPTER OBJECTIVE

At the end of this chapter, the reader will be able to identify the symptoms of dementia and delirium and appropriate nursing measures for promoting safety and maximizing functioning.

LEARNING OBJECTIVES

At the end of this chapter, the reader will be able to

1. identify symptoms of a dementia disorder.

2. differentiate symptoms of dementia from delirium.

3. describe nursing interventions for the client with either a dementia disorder or delirium.

INTRODUCTION

Dementia is a brain-based and progressive disorder that affects all aspects of a person's life. Sometimes described as a "loss of the person," individuals that develop dementia disorders become increasingly distant from their loved ones and in end stages may fail to recognize spouses, children, or others close to them. This can have a devastating effeet on the families, which is compounded by the frequent need to utilize extended care facilities to maintain the safety of the client. Every year it seems that the news media has another report of an older person who has wandered off from home or a care facility and succumbs to hypothermia or is injured in some other type of an accident. Dementia is usually medically managed by a neurologist (rather than a psychiatrist); however, there are many subtypes of dementia that have co-morbid psychiatric symptoms, and it is included in the *DSM-IV-TR* as a psychiatric disorder as well. Medications used in dementia are intended to slow the progression of the disease because no cure currently exists.

Delirium is different from dementia in that it is related to a specific disease, injury, substance, or toxin; it is short-lived (with proper medical treatment); and individuals with delirium also demonstrate signs of psychosis, including hallucinations or delusions. Medical and nursing care for the delirious client focuses first on safety, then on identifying the causative factor and developing treatment related to it.

This chapter will examine the various types of dementia, with an emphasis on Alzheimer's disease, the most common form. Treatment, including medications, will be discussed. Signs and symptoms of delirium are presented with differential criteria. A case study and sample nursing care plan is provided.

ETIOLOGY AND DEVELOPMENT

Dementia refers to the loss of thinking abilities, particularly memory, in combination with disturbances in executive functioning (the ability to think abstractly and to plan and initiate behaviors), aphasia, apraxia, or agnosia. Aphasia is the deterioration in language functioning. Apraxia is defined as "an impaired ability to execute motor activities despite intact motor abilities, sensory function, and comprehension of the required task" (American Psychiatric Association, 2000). A failure to recognize or identify common objects is known as agnosia. Dementia may be progressive, static, or remitting. The most common type of dementia is Alzheimer's disease, which affects approximately 5% of people older than 65 years of age, and nearly half of those older than 85 years of age. As many as 5 million Americans currently have Alzheimer's disease (CDC, 2009).

Alzheimer's disease causes gradual death of brain tissue, which is believed to be related to chemical changes inside individual brain cells. Alzheimer's disease is not the only type of dementia; cerebrovascular accidents (strokes), arteriosclerosis (hardening of the arteries), alcoholism, vitamin deficiencies, serious head injuries, infections such as human immunodeficiency virus (HIV), and other brain assaults, such as seen in an overdose or severe hypoxia may also cause dementia. Pick's disease is a type of dementia that is characterized by a deterioration of the frontal lobe of the brain, with early and fairly profound personality changes and poor response to traditional medications as prominent features.

Neurological disorders, such as Parkinson's disease and Huntington's chorea, may progress to dementia symptoms in late stages. Mad cow disease (Creutzfeldt-Jakob disease) is a dementia related to a parasitic organism, as is end-stage syphilis.

Other changes associated with dementia can include impairment of spatial orientation, poor judgment, and poor insight. Clients may be unaware of the extent of their memory loss or other cognitive abnormalities. Occasionally, disinhibited behavior occurs, resulting in inappropriate language, ignoring societal rules, over-familiarity with strangers, and even dangerous behaviors. Agitation is common as the disease progresses, along with anxiety, mood, and sleep disturbances. Delusions are relatively common and are often paranoid or persecutory in nature. Hallucinations, particularly visual, occur with some frequency as well. Individuals with dementia are highly susceptible to developing delirium with even small changes in medications or physical health status.

CT scans and an MRI may reveal cerebral atrophy, ischemic areas of the brain, focal lesions, or hydrocephalus (fluid in or around the brain), or they may be normal. Most differential diagnosing is focused on ruling-out other diseases before a diagnosis of dementia is made.

The *DSM-IV-TR* categorizes dementia as multiple disorders, with varied etiologies, all of which share common symptomatology. Dementia is broken down into 10 separate disorders, with an 11th, not otherwise specified category, for those symptoms that do not fit easily into any of the 10.

Dementia of the Alzheimer's Type

Dementia of the Alzheimer's type is gradual and involves progressive cognitive decline, not due to another neurological disorder or substance. Brain atrophy may be detected by CT scans or MRIs. Postmortem microscopic examination usually reveals neurofibrillary tangles, plaques, vascular degeneration, neuron loss, and other cellular changes. There is a familial tendency of the disorder that is thought to be associated with chromosome traits. *DSM-IV-TR* diagnostic criteria for dementia of the Alzheimer's type are as follows:

1. The development of multiple cognitive deficits manifested by both

   a. memory impairment; and

   b. one (or more) cognitive disturbances

      i. aphasia

      ii. apraxia

      iii. agnosia

      iv. disturbance in executive functioning

2. The cognitive deficits cause significant impairment in social or occupational functioning, and there is a significant decline from a previous level of functioning

3. Gradual onset and continuing cognitive decline

4. The deficits in criterion 1 are not due to

   a. other central nervous system conditions

   b. systemic conditions (infections, vitamin deficiencies)

   c. substance-induced conditions

5. The deficits do not occur exclusively during a delirium

6. Disturbances not better accounted for by another primary psychiatric disorder (such as major depression or schizophrenia)

Vascular Dementia

Vascular dementia (formerly referred to as "multi-infarct dementia) is less common than dementia of the Alzheimer's type. The onset is typically abrupt, followed by a fluctuating course of deterioration, with sporadic cognitive impairments. To diagnose vascular dementia, there must also be evidence of cerebral or peripheral vascular disease. Longstanding arterial hypertension, as evidenced by elevated blood pressure, an enlarged heart, abnormal heart sounds, or cerebral emboli, may be present. A single cerebrovascular accident (CVA) does not usually result in dementia; rather, the disorder occurs following a series of greater and lesser CVAs, with cognitive deficits more specific to the areas of the brain affected.

CT scans and MRIs typically indicate the extent of damage to the brain in the form of lesions in white and gray matter and focal atrophy. Electroencephalogram (EEG) findings may also support focal lesions. Laboratory tests and electrocardiograms (ECGs) are useful in detecting other, concomitant diseases that may contribute to the dementia (e.g., liver impairment, renal failure). *DSM-IV-TR* criteria for vascular dementia are as follows:

1. Criterion 1 following the same as those of Alzheimer's dementia

2. Criterion 2 following the same as that of Alzheimer's dementia

3. Focal neurological signs and symptoms or laboratory evidence indicative of cerebrovascular disease being present, and related to the disturbance

4. Deficits not occurring exclusively in the course of a delirium

Dementia Due to HIV

Dementia due to HIV occurs as a direct result of HIV infection. Pathological findings postmortem usually reveal multifocal destruction of the white matter of the brain and subcortical structures. There may be an elevation in proteins and WBCs in spinal fluid. Dementia due to HIV often presents with forgetfulness, slowness, poor concentration, and decreased problem-solving abilities. The client may present with apathy and social withdrawal. Delusions, hallucinations, or delirium may be present. Physical examination can indicate tremors, imbalance, ataxia (unsteady gait), hyperreflexia, and other "soft" neurological deficits. Children with HIV infection may also develop dementia, characterized by developmental delays, microcephaly (small brain), flaccidity, and calcifications in the basal ganglia.

Dementia Due to Head Trauma

Dementia can occur as a consequence of a serious head injury. The cognitive impairments seen are directly related to the areas of the brain sustaining the damage. Posttraumatic amnesia is frequently present and is associated with memory impairment. Behavioral symptoms may include aphasia, problems with attention span, anxiety, irritability, depression, or mood swings. Changes in personality are often seen. Dementia due to head trauma is not usually progressive, but repeated injuries (such as those seen in the sport of boxing), may lead to further deterioration (pugilistic dementia). This disorder is most often seen in young men who engage in risk-taking behaviors. Substance abuse or dependence should also be evaluated.

Parkinson's Disease

Parkinson's disease is a slowly progressing neurological condition that is associated with lowered dopamine levels in the brain. It is characterized by tremors, rigidity, bradykinesia, and unsteadiness. Dementia occurs in Parkinson's disease at a rate of 20% to 60%, usually in more advanced cases. Gradually diminishing executive functioning, forgetfulness, and impaired memory occur in conjunction with the motor symptoms of this disease. Parkinson's disease may occur in addition to Alzheimer's disease or vascular or other dementias.

Huntington's Disease

Huntington's disease (also referred to as Huntington's chorea) is an inherited disorder that is transmitted equally to men and women. It occurs as a result of a single autosomal dominant gene on the short arm of chromosome 4. Symptoms usually begin between 30 and 40 years of age; however, both juvenile-onset and late-onset cases have been noted. Early symptoms are elusive and include personality and behavior changes, depression, anxiety, and irritability. Motor symptoms present as fidgeting, then progress to a full lack of motor control. Cognitive changes of impaired memory, decreased judgment, and altered executive functioning occur early in the disorder, with progressive deterioration that includes disorganized speech and psychosis

(hallucinations and delusions). Children of individuals with Huntington's disease have a 50% chance of inheriting the disorder.

Pick's Disease

Pick's disease is a degenerative disease of the brain that specifically affects the frontal and temporal lobes. Personality changes occur early in the course of the illness, with behavioral disinhibition, deteriorated social skills, language abnormalities, and emotional blunting occurring. Other criterion-1 features of dementia occur later. Primitive reflexes (e.g., sucking, grasping) may occur. Apathy or extreme agitation may occur as the disease progresses. Brain imaging may reveal frontal or temporal lobe atrophy. Pick's disease commonly occurs in clients between 50 and 60 years of age.

Creutzfeldt-Jakob Disease

Dementia due to Creutzfeldt-Jakob disease is a direct result of the presence of spongiform encephalopathies, a group of CNS diseases that are caused by agents known as prions, or "slow viruses." These agents are transmitted via infected brain tissue. Cases have been documented related to bovine (cattle) transmission through tainted meat and, recently, deer have tested positive for the prions. There have also been reports of transmission secondary to corneal transplantation and human growth factor injections. Individuals with Creutzfeldt-Jakob disease usually experience fatigue, anxiety, problems with appetite or sleeping, or poor concentration early on, progressing to poor coordination, altered vision, and abnormal gait or other motor movements. The dementia onset is fairly rapid – usually over the course of a few months – and criterion-1 symptoms are present. Up to 25% of clients may have an atypical presentation, and the diagnosis can only be verified at autopsy. The transmissible agent is resistant to ultraviolet radiation, boiling, alcohol, or formalin, but it is susceptible to pressurized autoclaving and chlorine bleach.

Other Dementia Disorders

Other dementia disorders may occur as a result of numerous medical conditions. Table 6-1 presents an overview of some additional dementia disorders.

Substance-induced persisting dementia is a dementia disorder that requires that both criterion 1 and 2 for dementia are met, and that there must be evidence from the history, physical examination, or laboratory tests that the deficits seen are etiologically related to persisting use of a substance or exposure to a toxin. Delirium may be present, but the dementia symptoms must persist even when the delirium has resolved. Blood or urine drug screens may be negative. The age of onset is after 20 years old, and can only occur after prolonged substance exposure. Substance-induced persisting dementia may be related to abused substances such as alcohol, inhalants, sedatives, hypnotics, or anxiolytics; related to medications such as anticonvulsants or methotrexate; or related to toxins, such as lead, mercury, carbon monoxide, organophosphate insecticides, or industrial solvents.

Dementia disorder, not otherwise specified, is the term used for a dementia that does not meet criteria for any of the other disorders. It is commonly used when there is insufficient evidence to determine a more specific type.

THE MINI-MENTAL STATE EXAM

The Mini-Mental State Exam is a structured instrument originally developed in 1975 for the purpose of assessing an individual for the presence or absence of a dementia disorder. It is in widespread use today, many versions of which have been developed into convenient, pocket-sized tools. The Mini-Mental State Exam takes approximately 10 to 15 minutes to administer, and it can be administered by any healthcare provider. Several cognitive domains are assessed, including memory, language, orientation, apraxia, attention, and concentration. Items are scored one point for each correct answer with a total of 30 possible points. A score below 23 usually indicates dementia, although scores from 23

TABLE 6-1: EXAMPLES OF MEDICAL CONDITIONS THAT MAY LEAD TO DEMENTIA DISORDERS

Central Nervous System Disorders	Metabolic Disorders	Cardiopulmonary Disorders	Systemic Illnesses Or Effects	Infections
Multiple Sclerosis	Electrolyte Imbalance	Myocardial Infarction	Pneumonia	Neurosyphilis
Status Epilepticus	Dehydration	Congestive Heart Failure	Septicemia	Herpes
Head Trauma	Severe Anemia	Cardiac Arrhythmia	Urinary Tract Infection	Prions (Creutzfeld-Jacob)
Stroke	Hypoxia	Shock	Sensory Deprivation	Parasitic diseases
Encephalopathy	Hypoglycemia	Respiratory Failure	Temperature Dysregulation	
Pick's Disease	Vitamin B12 Deficiency		Liver or Renal Failure	
Brain Tumor	Hypoalbuminemia			
Brain Lesions				

(American Psychiatric Association, 2000).

to 26 may suggest a well-compensated dementia disorder as well. Clients should be assessed in a quiet environment with the healthcare provider's full attention. (Folstein, Folstein & McHugh, in Schneider et al., 2000) Table 6-2 provides some sample items from the Mini-Mental State Exam.

TABLE 6-2: MINI-MENTAL STATE EXAM SAMPLE ITEMS

Orientation to Time

"What is the date?"

Registration

"Listen carefully. I am going to say three words. You say them back after I stop.

Ready? Here they are...

APPLE (pause), PENNY (pause), TABLE (pause). Now repeat those words back to me."

(Repeat up to 5 times, but score only the first trial)

Naming

"What is this?" (Point to a pencil or pen)

Reading

"Please read this and do what it says." (Show examinee the words on the stimulus form.) CLOSE YOUR EYES

Reproduced by special permission of the publisher, Psychological Assessment Resources, Inc., 16204 North Florida Avenue, Lutz, Florida 33549, from the Mini-Mental State Examination, by Marshal Folstein & Susan Folstein, Copyright 1975, 1998, 2001 by Mini Mental, LLC, Inc. Published 2001 by Psychological Assessment Resources, Inc. Further reproduction is prohibited without permission of PAR, Inc. The MMSE can be purchased from PAR, Inc., by calling (813) 968-3003.

COMMONLY PRESCRIBED MEDICATIONS FOR DEMENTIA

There is no known cure for dementia. The neurotransmitter acetylcholine is involved with memory and cognitive abilities in the brain. The 1970 cholinergic hypothesis of Alzheimer's disease postulated that an acetylcholine deficiency in the brain causes the cognitive impairments. One solution,

then, was to inhibit the enzyme acetylcholinesterase that breaks down acetylcholine, leading to elevated acetylcholine levels in the brain. acetylcholinesterase medications will not cure dementia or reverse the symptoms caused by damaged neurons, but they do have usefulness in slowing the progress of the disease. Acetylcholinesterase medications have also been linked to improved functioning overall and lowering behavioral problems. One non-acetylcholinesterase medication, Namenda,® has been developed to treat moderate to severe Alzheimer's disease. Namenda® works on the N-methyl-D-aspartate (NMDA) receptor as an antagonist. Other NMDA receptor antagonists include the cough syrup Detromethorphan®, the tranquilizer Ketamine®, and Symmetrel® (used to treat Parkinson's disease). An overdose of Namenda® can cause agitation and confusion. Namenda® side effects in clinical trials were low, at approximately 2%, and included dizziness, anxiety or increased agitation, and headache. Medications to treat dementia are listed in Table 6-3.

Side effects of the acetylcholinesterase inhibitors can include nausea or vomiting, decreased appetite, weight loss, and diarrhea. Fatigue or insomnia may develop and headaches are occasionally reported. Starting with a low dosage and titrating slowly can help to reduce many of these problems. Taking once daily Aricept® is more convenient than the twice daily dosing requirements of the other drugs. The acetylcholinesterase inhibitors are only indicated for Alzheimer's-type dementia disorders. Other types of dementia may benefit but clinical studies have not yet supported this. Vascular and other medical-related dementias should be treated as appropriate for those disorders.

Occasionally, clients with dementia develop secondary psychoses and are treated with antipsychotic medications. In 2005, the FDA determined that new generation antipsychotic medications used in clients with dementia and psychosis led to an increased risk

TABLE 6-3: MEDICATIONS USED TO TREAT DEMENTIA				
Brand Name	**Generic Name**	**Dosage**	**Precautions**	**Primary Activity**
Aricept®	donepezil	15 mg daily at bedtime	none	Inhibits enzyme AChE to increase acetylcholine
Reminyl®	galantamine	12 mg twice a day	none	Inhibits AChE Also binds to nicotinic receptors
Exelon®	rivastigmine	6 mg twice a day	none	Inhibits enzyme AChE to increase acetylcholine
Cognex®	tacrine	40 mg four times a day	Elevated liver enzymes in 40% of patients	Inhibits enzyme AChE to increase acetylcholine
NMDA Antagonist				
Namenda®	memantine	20 mg daily Can be taken with AChE products	Caution with NMDA drugs	Antagonizes NMDA receptors
AChE: Acetylcholinesterase NMDA: N-methyl-D-aspartate				

of death (1.6 to 1.7 times the risk) than in clients on placebo or traditional medications. As a result, a Black Box Warning was added to all of the new generation antipsychotics with this caution. Currently, the FDA is considering extending this warning to all antipsychotics, whether new or traditional.

NURSING CARE OF THE CLIENT WITH DEMENTIA

Nursing care of the client with a dementia disorder reflects the areas of deficits observed. Assisting in the assessment process, including administering the Mini-Mental State Exam, getting a good nutritional and substance abuse history, obtaining laboratory tests, and preparing clients for CT scans, MRIs, and EEGs will facilitate a rapid and accurate diagnosis. Education of the client and family is very important early in the disease process.

A good working knowledge of community resources for caregivers of individuals with dementia disorders provides invaluable information to the families. Many Internet resources are available, referrals to adult day care programs may help to decrease caregiver burden, and support groups for caregivers may be helpful.

Maintaining a sense of security and safety for the client becomes increasingly important as the disease state progresses. Nursing interventions to promote safety may include keeping lights on brightly during the day, keeping furnishings and surroundings clean and uncomplicated, and educating families to monitor cooking or other high-risk activities in the home. In the late stages of dementia, a client will need assistance with basic care, such as bathing, dressing, and feeding. Mortality from dementia is secondary to other medical conditions, including opportunistic infections. By keeping the client free from pain and feeling comfortable and providing support for families, the nurse can help the grieving process during terminal care.

In talking with a client with moderate to severe dementia, it is important to remember that the client may become easily frustrated and agitated. The client may make statements that are accusatory or hurtful in nature. It is important for nurses and family members alike, to maintain a calm presentation and not allow personal anger or hurt feelings to affect judgment. Dementia is a progressive disorder. Teaching new information may be an unrealistic goal; in fact the client may be unable to remember information presented only a few minutes before, including names. Repetition and patience are of utmost importance. It is fruitless to engage in a debate to convince a client with dementia of certain facts; rather, the nurse should focus on underlying feelings and continuously reassure the client of his safety. Maintaining eye contact, moving slowly, and approaching the client from the front, while repeating his or her name, will help to diminish fear or prevent startling the client. Choices and options should be upbeat, positive, and limited in range or demands. The nurse should speak slowly and clearly, using simple and easy to understand words. If a client is having difficulty in verbal expression (aphasia or dysphasia), it is useful to revert to close-ended questions that can be answered simply with a "yes" or "no" response; gestures, visual cues, and prompts will help as well. Changing the subject is a useful tool when a client is becoming clearly frustrated.

CASE STUDY: CLIENT WITH DEMENTIA

Chip is a 72-year-old man who is living with his adult daughter and her family. His family physician suspected dementia when Chip began having difficulty in finding his way home from the grocery store. A neurology consult and MRI provided further evidence to support the disorder, and the neurologist prescribed Aricept® 10 mg daily. Most of the time, Chip is oriented to his surroundings and pleasant and cooperative with his family. He has been having increasing problems with confusion in the evening and recently became quite agitated and left the house at 11:00 p.m. "to go to work." Chip is a retired telephone lineman. After one of these episodes, his family physician prescribed 100 mg of amitriptyline (Elavil®) at bedtime, in an attempt to help him

sleep better. Three nights after taking this medication, Chip became extremely agitated and was yelling out, "Get them out of here! Get those men away from those lines before they blow!" His family had to call an ambulance to have him transported to the emergency department, where he was sedated and then admitted to the medical-psychiatric unit. His admitting diagnoses were substance-induced delirium and dementia of the Alzheimer's type. The Elavil® was discontinued and in 2 days he was able to return home to his family with Ativan® 0.5 mg at bedtime for sleep.

Questions

1. What is the name for the bedtime phenomenon that Chip is experiencing?

2. Side effects to monitor with Aricept® are what?

3. What is the rationale for using a benzodiazepine (Ativan®) at bedtime for sleep?

Discussion

Clients with dementia disorders occasionally become increasingly confused as the evening progresses. The mechanism for why this occurs is unknown. This phenomenon is called "sundowning." Families should be educated that this may occur and develop a safety plan for the client. Aricept® works by inhibiting the enzyme that breaks down acetylcholine in the brain. Common side effects to Aricept® include stomach upset, decreased appetite, weight loss, nausea, headache, and insomnia. Chip's delirium was most likely caused by the potent anticholinergic properties of Elavil®. Benzodiazepines do not have anticholinergic properties, and Ativan® is a short-acting benzodiazepine that will reduce bedtime anxiety, aide in sleep onset, and will wear off in 4 to 6 hours. Low doses of medications are safer in elderly individuals because of their reduced liver metabolism and renal clearance.

DIFFERENTIATING DELIRIUM FROM DEMENTIA

The essential feature of a delirium is a change in cognition that cannot be better explained by a pre-existing dementia disorder, accompanied by an alteration in level and state of consciousness (American Psychiatric Association, 2000). There must be evidence from the history, physical examination, or laboratory tests that the symptoms exhibited are a result of a medical condition, substance use (or withdrawal), toxin exposure, or a combination of these factors. In delirium, there is a reduced awareness of others and the environment. Focus and attention are impaired, memory and perceptual experiences may be impaired, and disorientation (especially to time) is present. Language disturbances may be evident as well. The client may present as incoherent and agitated. Hallucinations are not uncommon, along with illusions (misinterpreting items or people in the vicinity) and misperceptions (misunderstanding sights, sounds).

Delirium is often associated with alterations in the sleep-wake cycle. Increased motor activity in the form of restlessness, groping, picking at bedclothes, and sudden movements may occur. Sluggishness, lethargy, and near-stupor may also be seen. Emotional lability can range from fear to irrational anger to inappropriate giggling. Mood shifts can be rapid and unpredictable. Paranoia can lead to aggression or self-injury (falling out of bed, pulling out IV lines). Screaming, crying, calling out, cursing, moaning, and other vocalizations may be heard. Signs of autonomic hyperactivity, such as elevated heart rate, elevated blood pressure, diaphoresis, flushed face, and dilated pupils, are often present. In hepatic encephalopathy (related to liver disease) and other encephalopathies, a flapping movement of the hands known as "asterixis" may occur.

EEG readings are often abnormal, showing either fast activity or a generalized slowing. The symptoms of a delirium can develop over a few hours to a few days. Recovery is closely related to the underlying etiology.

The *DSM-IV-TR* differentiates five types of delirium: delirium due to a general medical condition; delirium due to substance intoxication; delirium due to substance withdrawal; delirium due to multiple etiologies; and delirium, not otherwise specified.

Delirium due to a general medical condition must have demonstrated evidence of the medical condition, and the delirium must be etiologically related to that disorder. Diagnostic criteria include:

1. Disturbance of consciousness with a reduced ability to focus, sustain, or shift attention

2. Change in cognition (such as memory deficit, disorientation, language disturbance) or developing perceptual disturbance, which is not better accounted for by dementia

3. Disturbance developing over a short period of time (hours to days) and tending to fluctuate during the course of the day

4. Evidence from the history, physical examination, or laboratory findings showing disturbance resulting from the direct physiological consequences of a general medical condition

To diagnose a substance-induced delirium, there must be evidence of substance intoxication, toxin exposure, or medication side effects (including drug interactions), in addition to criteria 1 through 3 noted previously. Substance-induced delirium often arises within minutes to hours of exposure to rapid-acting agents, such as cocaine or hallucinogens. Onset can be delayed for longer-acting agents, which may only become toxic when elevated serum levels are reached (e.g., benzodiazepines, such as diazepam, or poisons). Usually the delirium resolves when the offending agent is metabolized and excreted by the body (or dialyzed if necessary). Poor renal or hepatic function will slow resolution of the delirium. Certain medications that are commonly used in psychiatric care have narrow therapeutic ranges versus toxic dosing ranges, and clients may become delirious when overmedicated. These medications include lithium carbonate or lithium citrate, all of the tricyclic antidepressants (e.g., imipramine, desipramine, amitriptyline, nortriptyline), and valproic acid (Depakote®). Delirium is also frequently seen in the postoperative patient, secondary to a combination of anesthesia effects and pain medications, or in individuals abusing high levels of opiate-based pain medications, benzodiazepines, illicit drugs, or alcohol.

Withdrawal associated delirium occurs when substances are cleared by the body. It's usually associated with longer half-life agents or with agents that cause habituation through inducing liver enzymes (e.g., alcohol, diazepam, opiates). The onset and duration of the delirium is associated with the half-life of the agent. Alcohol withdrawal delirium may begin within 24 hours of the last drink, whereas diazepam (Valium®) withdrawal delirium may not start for 3 to 5 days.

Delirium due to multiple etiologies is seen when a client presents with a delirium and there are numerous causative factors. An example of this would be a client with hepatic encephalopathy who is also dependent on alcohol. *DSM-IV-TR* criteria 1 through 3 remain the same; criterion 4 requires that there is evidence that the delirium has more than one etiology.

The term "delirium, not otherwise specified" (delirium, NOS) is used when there is not enough evidence to support the diagnosis of an associated medical condition, substance intoxication, or substance withdrawal. It also includes deliriums associated with unusual causes such as sensory deprivation.

THE TREATMENT OF AGITATED AND AGGRESSIVE CLIENTS

Care must be taken when treating a client who is agitated or aggressive. This behavior is commonly seen with delirium and is often associated with dementia, when the client is undergoing a stressor, such as anxiety, fear, fatigue, insomnia, or a medical illness. The phenomenon of "sundowning" may occur with dementia as well. This involves an increasing confusion and agitation that starts in the late afternoon and becomes more severe as the night progresses. Dangerous behaviors such as wandering into the streets can occur. Nursing care should be focused on maintaining safety and providing reassurance and support. Medications need to be used cautiously, so as not to increase the agitation or induce a worsened delirium.

Medications that have potent anticholinergic properties may increase disorientation and confusion. These include antipsychotics, tricyclic antidepressants, and antihistamines. Benzodiazepines (in low doses) are usually preferable for the acute treatment of a delirious patient. Other medications, such as buspirone (Buspar®) and trazodone (Desyrel®), are also useful. Administering an agent similar to the detoxifying substance, in smaller titrated doses, can help in substance withdrawal delirium. Agitation associated with hallucinogen use can be managed with antipsychotics (while monitoring for emergent extrapyramidal syndrome side effects). New-generation antipsychotics are preferable because the risk of extrapyramidal syndrome is much lower than that of traditional antipsychotics. Several of the new generation antipsychotics are now available in intramuscular formulations (Geodon®, Zyprexa®, and Abilify®). Besides having mild sedative properties, they may also provide earlier antipsychotic treatment.

Occasionally, physical restraints become necessary in the disoriented and agitated client.

Healthcare personnel should be trained in the proper application of the restraints to avoid harm to the client. Soft wrist restraints and vest restraints are preferable to leather restraints. The client should be monitored frequently while in restraints, and there needs to be documented evidence of nursing checks for skin injuries or bruising, opportunities for fluid and nutrition, and opportunities for bowel or bladder elimination. Restraints should be removed as soon as the agitation is reduced to a level that is determined to no longer present a risk to the safety of the client or others.

NURSING CARE PLAN: CLIENT WITH DELIRIUM

Problem Listing

- Potential for injury
- Fear
- Family support needed

Nursing Diagnoses

1. Risk for injury related to drug toxicity, as evidenced by acute delirium and agitation.

2. Fear, secondary to a belief in threat or harm, as evidenced by delusional statements.

3. Caregiver role strain related to increasing illness of client, as evidenced by progressive dementia and attempts to leave the house.

Long-term Goal

Both client and family will receive the level of support needed to ensure ongoing positive relationships while maintaining a high standard of safety.

Short-term Objectives

1. Client will not sustain injury during period of delirium.

2. Client will demonstrate reduced fear by displaying a calmer demeanor and following simple directions.

3. Family will report an increased level of satisfaction with community resource awareness and availability by the time client is ready for discharge.

Nursing Interventions

1. Staff will monitor client closely and administer medications as needed.

2. Staff will assess for the need of temporary, soft wrist restraints during the acute phase of the agitation and delirium.

3. Staff will administer fluids and maintain a patent IV line if needed, while client is hospitalized in the medical-psychiatric inpatient unit.

4. Staff will use a soft, comforting voice tone and inform client of his safety during all procedures.

5. Staff will allow family members to remain at bedside as desired during hospitalization period.

6. Staff will provide social service resources and information on local caregiver support programs to family, prior to client's anticipated discharge date.

ADVANCED PRACTICE NURSING: THE CLIENT WITH DEMENTIA

Treating the client with dementia often triggers ethical issues around the principles of "to do no harm" (see Chapter 2). The prescribing APRN must make decisions about the type and appropriateness of medications, to use to treat the dementia (acetylcholinesterase and NMDA antagonists) as well as to treat other conditions that occur, without potentially causing more harm to the client.

Clients with dementia plus insomnia are challenging in that many of the medications with sedative-hypnotic properties may trigger worsening confusion and pose a safety risk. Antihistamines such as diphenhydramine (Benadryl®) and hydroxyzine HCL (Vistaril®) are commonly utilized for mild insomnia in other clients, but may cause disorientation in the elderly or demented person. Typically, sleeping pills, such as zolpidem (Ambien®) or temazepam (Restoril®), may be too strong and contribute to nocturnal falls and injuries. The sedative triazolam (Halcion®) has been associated with psychosis. Tricyclic antidepressants are occasionally prescribed to aide in sleep (e.g., Elavil®); however, such medications are risky to administer because of increasing confusion caused by anticholinergic side effects as well as increased risks for delayed QTc intervals, leading to cardiac arrhythmias. Other options for sleep-inducing may include short-acting benzodiazepines, low dose buspirone (Buspar®), or trazodone (Desyrel®).

In treating the client with dementia plus psychotic symptoms, care and consideration must be made in regards to the Black Box Warnings for new generation antipsychotics (1.6 to 1.7 times increased risk for death). This has to be weighed against the potential neurological complications (extrapyramidal syndrome and tardive dyskinesia) associated with the more traditional antipsychotics. No matter which medication chosen, doses should be adjusted to approximately 50% that of a typical adult.

Agitation and aggression may be the most common reasons that clients with dementia are admitted to inpatient psychiatric settings. Geropsychiatric units have sprung up throughout the country to provide for just this type of short-term intensive care. Length of stay is usually 2 weeks or less (extended care facilities must hold bed space for 14 days) and the focus is on stabilization and reducing aggression. Medications such as valproic acid (Depakote ER®) have been found useful in reducing aggressive outbursts, as are the new generation antipsychotic medications. Sometimes, aggression is a result of a medical problem, such as a urinary tract infection or pain. This should always be considered when working with a client who has dementia. Additionally, anxiety may translate into a fight-or-flight response

and the clinician should consider whether the client may be anxious. Selective Serotonin Reuptake Inhibitor (SSRI) antidepressants in low doses are effective in treating anxiety. These include escitalopram (Lexapro®), citalopram (Celexa®), sertraline (Zoloft®), fluoxetine (Prozac®), and others.

Finally, an APRN working in geropsychiatric care must have a good knowledge base of medical disorders and medical drug treatment. Drug-to-drug interactions account for a number of emergency room visits and hospitalizations and are a major cause of delirium in the elderly client. This is complicated by the large number of individual medications that older persons are prescribed. Understanding these issues and actively looking for potential drug interactions is a sign of high quality nursing care that keeps the client's health needs foremost.

SUMMARY

Providing care to the client with a dementia disorder is challenging. Differentiating dementia from delirium is an essential nursing skill. This chapter examined Alzheimer's disease and other dementia disorders and provided both a case study and a sample nursing care plan for the client with dementia. Medications for dementia primarily work on increasing the available acetylcholine by inhibiting the enzyme that starts its metabolism. The extra acetylcholine slows down the progression of dementia, but is not a cure. One medication, memantine HCL (Namenda®), works differently by antagonizing the transmitter NMDA and can be used in addition to acetylcholinesterase products for a dual-activity approach. Many medications are also used to treat comorbid conditions found in dementia disorder, but care must be taken to minimize the risk for drug-to-drug interactions. Delirium may initially present as confusion and disorientation, but it is clearly different from dementia in its causation, intensity, duration, and treatment. In both dementia and delirium, safety issues are common nursing care problems.

EXAM QUESTIONS

CHAPTER 6
Questions 33-38

Note: Choose the one option that BEST answers each question.

33. Dementia of the Alzheimer's type has a

    a. rapid onset and rapid decline in functioning.

    b. gradual onset and progressive decline in functioning.

    c. gradual onset with no decline in functioning.

    d. rapid onset with no decline in functioning.

34. A required criterion for the diagnosis of both Alzheimer's dementia and vascular dementia is

    a. protein and white cells in cerebrospinal fluid.

    b. a fluctuating course of disorientation.

    c. history of cerebrovascular disease.

    d. an impairment in memory.

35. The nurse working with a client who has a moderate degree of dementia should

    a. be prepared to repeat instructions patiently.

    b. educate the client thoroughly about his medications.

    c. expect clients to remember healthcare facility routines.

    d. encourage the family to institutionalize the client for safety.

36. *Charlie is a 52-year-old man who is arrested with a breathalyzer test of .26 for public intoxication. He is incarcerated until his family can be found to bail him out. 48 hours after his arrest, he tells the jail matron that his skin is crawling and he keeps seeing spiders crawling across the ceiling. Within 4 hours, the staff finds him screaming incoherently and cowering in the corner. He looks "twitchy," sweaty, and flushed.*

    The most likely cause of these symptoms is

    a. untreated paranoid schizophrenia.

    b. hallucinogen overdose (acquired from his cell mate).

    c. delirium associated with alcohol withdrawal.

    d. a manipulative attempt to get out of jail and into a hospital.

37. A medication group that may precipitate a delirium at therapeutic or recommended doses in a susceptible client is

    a. antibiotics.

    b. tricyclic antidepressants.

    c. non-steroidal anti-inflammatory drugs (NSAIDS).

    d. multivitamins.

38. A priority for nursing care of the client with a dementia disorder or a delirium is

    a. promoting self-esteem.

    b. reorienting to reality.

    c. maintaining safety.

    d. educating about the illness.

CHAPTER 7

ALCOHOL AND SEDATIVE ABUSE
AND DEPENDENCE

CHAPTER OBJECTIVE

At the end of this chapter, the reader will be able to discuss alcoholism and sedative, hypnotic, and anxiolytic dependence in American society, including the recognition and treatment of withdrawal syndromes.

LEARNING OBJECTIVES

At the completion of this chapter, the reader will be able to

1. describe signs of alcohol, sedative, hypnotic, and anxiolytic intoxication and withdrawal.

2. discuss medical and nursing care for withdrawal from alcohol, sedatives, hypnotics, and anxiolytics.

3. recognize medical disorders that are associated with alcohol dependence.

4. discuss therapy and family issues that occur in the alcohol-addicted client.

INTRODUCTION

Alcohol abuse and dependence will be discussed in this chapter as well as typical withdrawal symptoms, commonly referred to as "D.T.'s" (delirium tremens). Sedatives, hypnotics, and anxiolytics (medications used to treat anxiety) create responses in persons very similar to alcohol, both in intoxication and withdrawal. Withdrawal from dependency on sedative, hypnotics, and anxiolytics mimics withdrawal from alcohol, but can be more complicated due to extended half-lives of the drugs. Nursing care of the individual intoxicated with alcohol or sedatives, and during withdrawal from those substances, will be discussed and the reader will be provided with a sample nursing care plan and case study of treating a client with alcoholism.

ALCOHOL DEPENDENCE

We, of Alcoholics Anonymous, are more than one hundred men and women who have recovered from a seemingly hopeless state of mind and body...the only requirement for membership is an honest desire to stop drinking. We are not allied with any particular faith, sect or denomination, nor do we oppose anyone (Alcoholics Anonymous, 1976).

This quote is from the first edition of the 1939 printing of Alcohol's Anonymous' The Big Book. By 1955, membership in Alcoholics Anonymous had grown to over 150,000 individuals in nearly 6,000 groups and was no longer located solely in the United States. By 1976, there were over 28,000 groups made up of over 1 million members.

In 2007, 51% of Americans reported being current alcohol users with 23% of these persons reporting regular binge drinking, defined by the consumption of 5 or more drinks in one day, within the past month. Heavy drinking, defined as binge drinking on at least 5 days within the past month, was reported in 6.9% of the population (approximately 17 million people). In young adults between ages 18 and 25 years of age, binge drinking was reported in 41.8% of the population, and heavy drinking rates were 14.7%. Rates of alcohol use in children between 12 and 17 years of age were 15.9%, with binge and heavy drinking rates at 9.7% and 2.3% respectively. Problems related to the excessive consumption of alcohol costs society an estimated $185 billion dollars annually (SAMHSA, 2008).

Alcohol dependence has both genetic and environmental components. The National Longitudinal Alcohol Epidemiologic Study found that adolescents who begin drinking by 15 years of age have a four-fold incidence of developing alcohol dependence in their lifetime, as compared to those who do not begin drinking until 21 years of age, despite parental alcohol patterns. Contributing environmental factors may include cultural attitudes toward drinking, the availability (and legality) of alcohol, the effects of alcohol on mood and behavior, and perceived levels of stress (National Institute on Alcohol Abuse and Alcoholism, 2008).

Alcohol dependency in the United States is 5.4% in men and 2.3% in women, regardless of ethnicity. Rates are almost doubled for Native Americans (8.4% in men; 4.4% in women) and are lowest in Asian Americans (3.6% in men; 1.3% in women). Black men have a slightly higher incidence of dependency on alcohol than do Hispanic/Latino men (5.0% compared to 5.9%) and Hispanic/Latino women are significantly less likely to be dependent on alcohol (1.9%) (SAMHSA, 2008).

ALCOHOL INTOXICATION

Alcohol intoxication is characterized by behavioral or psychological changes, such as mood lability, mild euphoria, reduced inhibitions, impaired judgment, or aggression, that develops shortly after ingestion of alcohol. Other symptoms may include slurred speech, poor coordination, unsteady gait, impaired memory, decreased attention span, nystagmus of the eyes and, possibly stupor or coma. The amount of alcohol required to produce these changes varies in an individual, based on such factors as gender, age, body mass, and genetic vulnerabilities, but most healthy adults can metabolize approximately one drink (one beer, glass of wine, or shot of hard liquor) an hour. Impaired judgment begins at a blood alcohol level of 0.08% to 0.1%. Blackouts, or episodes where the intoxicated individual is awake and functioning but has no memory of the time spent, usually occur at a high blood level in the occasional drinker, but may occur at a very low blood level in the alcohol dependent person.

Metabolism of alcohol occurs in the liver where it is broken down first into acetaldehyde and hydrogen and then into acetic acid, which later ends up as carbon dioxide and water. Acetaldehyde is toxic to the liver, where it impairs normal cellular functioning, interferes with the absorption of vitamins, and increases fat storage. Tolerance to alcohol is probably associated with elevated liver enzyme levels and cellular adaptation.

ASSESSMENT OF ALCOHOL DEPENDENCE

Assessment tools are useful to guide the healthcare provider in determining the severity of use, making an appropriate formal diagnosis, planning treatment, and in monitoring ongoing progress. Most assessment tools are simple, standardized questionnaires that can be self-administered or administered by a healthcare provider; more than 100 such tools are available, many of which are free of charge.

The 10-item revised Clinical Institute Withdrawal Assessment for Alcohol (CIWAA-Ar) can be completed and scored in ten minutes or less (Bayard, McIntyre, Hill, & Woodside, 2004). It is available in the article on the American Academy of Family Physicians Website (http://www.aafp.org/afp/20040315/1443.pdf).

Paolo DePetrillo and Mark McDonough developed the Alcohol Withdrawal Syndrome Type Indicator in 1999 to provide a simple assessment tool for alcohol withdrawal syndrome (AWS) symptoms. The AWS Type Indicator uses a simple "yes" or "no" rating scale and it divides withdrawal symptoms into three subtypes: A, B, and C. Subtype A (4 items) addresses CNS excitation symptoms, such as anxiety, restlessness, or hypersensitivity to light and sound. Subtype B (7 items) evaluates adrenergic nervous system activity, including nausea or vomiting, tremors, sweating, blood pressure and heart rate readings, and apical pulse irregularities. Subtype C (9 items) assesses signs of delirium, including confusion, disorientation to person-place-time, and psychosis. The AWS Type Indicator takes about 3 minutes to administer. It is available free of charge for noncommercial use from the Focused Treatment Systems at www.sagetalk.com or by calling 1-800-728-6799 (DePetrillo & McDonough, 1999).

The 22-item Michigan Alcoholism Screening Test (MAST) is a self-scoring test that consists of all "yes" or "no" questions. 3 to 5 points indicate early or moderate drinking issues, whereas 6 or more indicate problem drinking. It is free and available at http://counsellingresource.com/quizzes/alcohol-mast/index.html as well as through many other online resources.

The CAGE Questionnaire is quickly administered and consists of the following four questions:

1. Have you ever felt you should **C**ut down on your drinking?

2. Have people **A**nnoyed you by criticizing your drinking?

3. Have you ever felt bad or **G**uilty about your drinking?

4. Have you ever had an **E**ye-opener in the morning to steady your nerves or get rid of a hangover?

The CAGE Questionnaire is available at http://counsellingresource.com/quizzes/alcohol-cage/index.html

ALCOHOL WITHDRAWAL

Alcohol withdrawal symptoms begin as soon as the body begins to metabolize the alcohol into acetaldehyde. Often, these early symptoms are masked as the individual continues to imbibe. After a night of sleeping a hangover may be experienced, which is characterized by irritability, headache, nausea, vomiting, and dizziness. Repeated intoxication leads to alcohol tolerance and then to dependence. Withdrawal effects for the dependent person begin when the serum alcohol level begins to drop. In chronic alcohol abusers, withdrawal effects may occur at levels much higher than zero; therefore, the nurse should rely on clinical signs and symptoms and not just on laboratory or breathalyzer values. The detoxification process may continue for 3 to 5 days. Table 7-1 presents an overview of initial, intermediate, and severe signs of alcohol withdrawal.

Alcohol withdrawal management usually consists of liberal use of benzodiazepine agents as soon as symptoms are seen. An elevated blood pressure and pulse reading are the best indicators; however, consideration should be made for the client with primary hypertension, in which case an elevated pulse rate alone is a more sensitive measure. Benzodiazepines work to alleviate the associated anxiety and restlessness, through a tranquilizing

TABLE 7-1: ALCOHOL WITHDRAWAL SYMPTOMS (UNTREATED)

Initial

- Elevated heart rate
- Elevated blood pressure
- Headaches
- Mild nausea
- Subjective sensations of anxiety or restlessness
- Cravings
- Sleep disturbances

Intermediate

- Severe cravings
- Hand or whole body tremors
- Hot, flushed skin
- Diaphoresis
- Significantly elevated blood pressure and pulse
- Nausea, vomiting, diarrhea, stomach cramps
- Dizziness or light-headedness
- Dehydration (low grade temperature & thirst)
- Irritability, hostility

Severe

- Illusions or hallucinations
- Delusions
- Delirium
- Panic level anxiety
- Agitation or assaultiveness
- Seizures (grand mal)

(Bayard et al., 2004).

effect, and to reduce the risk of seizure development and delirium tremens, a psychotic state characterized by hallucinations (usually visual) and paranoid delusions. The more physiologically dependent a client is on alcohol, the more difficult and uncomfortable the detoxification period will be. Medications commonly used include lorazepam (Ativan®), chlordiazepoxide (Librium®), and diazepam (Valium®). Diazepam is particularly useful in the emergency department because it can be administered IV. A primary safety issue in the detoxifying client is the risk of seizures, which may compromise breathing or contribute to aspiration and respiratory distress. Prolonged grand mal

seizures can lead to brain damage that is caused by a lack of oxygen to the brain. Nursing care for the person experiencing withdrawal from alcohol is discussed more fully later in this chapter.

Cross-tolerance is a phenomenon where a client develops tolerance for agents similar to the drug-of-choice. It is not unusual to find a cross-tolerance effect between alcohol and benzodiazepines. The nurse may need to administer relatively high doses of benzodiazepines (as ordered) early in the detoxification process to manage this problem. Other comfort medications may be given, such as promethazine (Phenergan®) for nausea and trazodone (Desyrel®) to aid in sleep. Acetaminophen should be avoided because of its extensive metabolism in the liver. Similarly, aspirin is contraindicated because of the risk of increased bleeding times associated with liver disease as well as esophageal and gastric ulcerations. Ibuprofen is a better choice for minor aches and pains. Vitamin administration is usually an automatic part of alcohol detoxification. In particular, the water soluble B vitamins should be administered, including thiamine, niacin, and folic acid, because of the metabolic problems with vitamin absorption in a fatty liver.

MEDICATIONS FOR ALCOHOL DEPENDENCE

No medications are indicated primarily to treat alcohol dependence; however, several agents are useful in reducing cravings or preventing relapses (see Table 7-2). Naltrexone (Revia®) is an opioid receptor site antagonist that reduces alcohol cravings. It is believed to block some of the pleasure responses induced by alcohol in the brain by occupying the endorphin receptors in the neurons. Naltrexone induces immediate narcotic withdrawal in an individual who has been using opioids; therefore, the healthcare provider needs to assess the client carefully for other substance dependencies. Naltrexone has long been

TABLE 7-2: MEDICATIONS USED TO TREAT ALCOHOL DEPENDENCY

Brand Name	Generic Drug	Dosing	Indication	Comments
Revia®	Naltrexone	50 mg orally once daily	Reduce alcohol use; reduce opioid effects	Will cause opioid withdrawal when taken
Vivitrol®	Naltrexone XR	380 mg IM monthly	Reduce alcohol relapse rates	Will cause opioid withdrawal when taken
Campral®	Acamprosate calcium	333 mg orally 3 times a day	Reduce alcohol relapse rates	Expensive but well-tolerated
Antabuse®	Disulfiram	250 mg orally once daily	Severe alcohol dependence (converts alcohol to acetaldehyde)	Cannot be used with any alcohol products, including topical preparations

used in emergency care under the name Narcan® as a treatment for opioid (e.g., heroin, morphine) overdose. A formulation of naltrexone extended-release, Vivitrol®, given in a monthly injection, was demonstrated to reduce alcohol relapses by 32% in combination with psychosocial therapy, as compared to 11% in clients receiving therapy alone (www.vivitrol.com).

Disulfiram (Antabuse®) is a drug that inhibits the breakdown of acetaldehyde in the brain. When alcohol is consumed in the presence of disulfiram, the individual experiences an immediate reaction, which may include such symptoms as flushing, sweating, nausea, vomiting, tachycardia, hypotension, headache, heart palpitations, tremors, and weakness. Disulfiram alone can be stressful on the liver, and monitoring of liver enzymes is recommended. Disulfiram and alcohol together can induce cardiac arrhythmias, seizures, myocardial infarction, and cardiac failure. The purpose of disulfiram is to act as a behavioral deterrent for the client. Presumably, when taking disulfiram, the client will be less likely to succumb to the desire to drink because of a fear of becoming ill.

Acamprosate calcium (Campral®) helps clients who are alcohol dependent to maintain abstinence from alcohol. Its mechanism of action is unclear, but it is thought to work in the glutamate/GABA system to regulate neuronal excitability and inhibition. Campral® does not affect withdrawal from alcohol. It is taken orally three times a day and is contraindicated in individuals with severe renal disease. Nausea and diarrhea are the most common side effects reported in rates greater than a placebo.

Another clinical approach has been to utilize selective serotonin reuptake inhibitors (SSRIs) in the treatment of clients who are alcohol dependent. Drugs such as fluoxetine (Prozac®), sertraline (Zoloft®), paroxetine (Paxil®), and escitalopram (Lexapro®) have shown some usefulness in helping to alleviate depressive and anxiety symptoms in these clients. Although SSRI's are not considered sedating, it would be prudent to wait to begin their use until the client has nearly completed detoxification. It is unclear whether the substance abuse is a contributing factor to the mood symptoms or whether the mood problems are a result of the substances themselves; however, most clients report improved moods and decreased relapse-inducing cravings when they are taking SSRIs. Additionally, SSRIs are nonaddictive, easy to dose, and relatively low in side effects. The nurse should keep in mind, however, that SSRI's are not a treatment for alcohol dependence; rather, they are used to help in maintaining sobriety when relapses may be associated with depression or anxiety disorders.

MEDICAL COMPLICATIONS OF ALCOHOL DEPENDENCE

Alcohol is a CNS depressant. Every year, young men and women die of alcohol poisoning, from ingesting amounts of alcohol that are too much for the liver to metabolize before respiratory suppression and cardiac problems result. Alcohol is also a vasodilator, which predisposes individuals to frostbite and death from hypothermia. The combination of alcohol and other substances can be particularly lethal.

Alcoholic hallucinosis is a condition that may be experienced by the client who is alcohol dependent. In alcoholic hallucinosis, the client develops psychotic symptoms (hallucinations and delusions) while intoxicated. Psychosis can also occur during alcohol withdrawal, commonly known as delirium tremens.

Wernicke-Korsakoff syndrome is an alcohol-induced, persistent dementia disorder that is characterized by memory deficits, a foggy or clouded consciousness, peripheral neuropathies and, often, confabulation (making up events or answers to fill in memory gaps). Wernicke-Korsakoff syndrome is closely related to thiamine and niacin deficiencies in the brain, along with chronic toxicity secondary to acetaldehyde.

Administration of B-complex vitamins and thiamine injections at the time of detoxification may help to reverse some of the cognitive problems, but the dementia experienced is usually irreversible.

Liver disease (fatty liver, cirrhosis) leads to obstructed blood flow through the liver. This causes portal hypertension, ascites (fluid in the abdominal cavity), and esophageal varices (swelling of the arteries supplying blood to the esophagus, secondary to portal hypertension). Ascites puts pressure on the diaphragm and makes breathing more difficult. Esophageal varices may rupture and cause death by exsanguination (bleeding) or asphyxiation.

Decreased liver functioning contributes to prolonged blood clotting time, elevated ammonia levels in the serum, elevated bilirubin levels, and low albumin (protein) levels and predisposes the individual to confusion, jaundice, malnutrition, and edema.

Alcohol is an irritant to tissues and mucous membranes. As an irritant, the stomach responds by increasing production of hydrochloric acid, which then results in gastric and duodenal ulcers. Hemorrhage from ulcers can be dangerous, if not life threatening.

A variety of other medical complications can develop that are associated with alcohol dependence. Thiamine deficiencies contribute to peripheral nervous system problems that are experienced as chronic pain and a tingling sensation in the extremities. Pancreatitis and diabetes mellitus are seen at higher rates in the client who is alcohol dependent. Skeletal and cardiac muscle damage can occur, leading to myopathies and enlargement of the heart. Night vision and peripheral vision may be reduced by damage to the eyes. Prolonged alcohol abuse in men decreases testosterone levels and may result in impotence.

Alcohol use during pregnancy, especially in the first trimester, can result in fetal alcohol syndrome. Infants born with this disorder often have varying degrees of mental retardation. Physical defects may also be present. Two key characteristics of fetal alcohol syndrome are poor social skills and a high level of impulsivity in behaviors. The ability to distinguish between right and wrong (moral development) is also often impaired.

THE AA MODEL

A physician named William Silkworth first conceived the idea of Alcoholics Anonymous (AA) in 1935, after the treatment of a stockbroker from New York. The stockbroker described a spiritual epiphany as instrumental in his recovery. The stockbroker shared his recovery story during a business trip with a physician in Akron, Ohio, who was also an alcoholic. He stopped drinking as well, and the concept that one alcoholic could help another was born. The basic tenets of moral inventory, confession of personality defects, restitution to those harmed, helpfulness to others, and the belief in and dependence upon a higher power still make up the AA model today. AA meetings are supportive in nature. There is not an identified leader (although members may choose to help organize meetings). Sharing is on a first-name only basis. Testifying, or telling one's story, is encouraged. Members are encouraged to deal with life one day at a time, and tokens are given out for number of days of sobriety. Members who are further along in their recovery process are encouraged to become sponsors for new members. A sponsor's role is to be available for support and to give advice during times of vulnerability or temptation. The AA model is structured around 12 steps to recovery; in fact, various support groups are now often referred to as 12-step programs, in deference to the success of the AA model. These 12 steps are illustrated in Table 7-3.

MOTIVATIONAL INTERVIEWING

Motivational interviewing is an evidence-based technique for enhancing motivation to change in clients who are ambivalent about making changes. First developed in 1983 by William Miller, PhD, motivational interviewing is a client-centered approach to overcome ambivalence and promote change. It is particularly helpful in clients with addictive disorders. With motivational interviewing, clients are asked to examine how their behaviors interfere with their life goals. The clinician is non-confrontational and uses open-ended and reflective questions and statements while talking with the client. Approaches include expressing empathy (e.g., "I know how difficult it must be for you to be expected to come to daily groups when you have no driver's license."), pointing out discrepancies between current behavior and future goals (e.g., "It's hard for me to understand how you plan to go back to work full-time when you are drinking every night."), and promoting self-efficacy (e.g., "You can make your own decisions – all we can do is to offer you choices"). Motivational interviewing has been

---

TABLE 7-3: 12 STEPS OF ALCOHOLICS ANONYMOUS

1. To admit that we are powerless over alcohol and our life has become unmanageable

2. To believe that a Power greater than ourselves can restore us to sanity

3. To make a decision to turn our will and our lives over to the care of this higher Power

4. To make a searching and fearless moral inventory of ourselves

5. To admit to our higher Power, ourselves, and to another human being the exact nature of our wrongs

6. To be ready to have our higher Power remove all these defects of character

7. To humbly ask Him to remove our shortcomings

8. To make a list of all persons we harmed, and become willing to make amends to them all

9. To make direct amends wherever possible, except when to do so would injure the other person(s)

10. To continue to take personal inventory and admit when we are wrong

11. To seek through prayer and meditation to improve our conscious contact with our higher Power and for knowledge and strength to carry out His will

12. To carry the message to other alcoholics, and to practice these principles in all of our affairs

(Alcoholics Anonymous, 1976)

extensively researched and discussed since 1983 with numerous published articles reviewing its effectiveness and implementation (http://www. motivationalinterview.org).

STAGES OF CHANGE MODEL

In 1983, psychologists James O. Prochaska and Carlo DiClemente developed the Stages of Change Model (a.k.a., the Transtheoretical Model) to try and explain why individuals had so much difficulty in giving up cigarette smoking. Six distinct phases were identified. Today, these stages are well-recognized and taught in other forms of substance dependence, including alcoholism and tobacco cessation.

The following is a discussion of the Stages of Change Model, with suggested nursing interventions for each step:

Precontemplation

In this stage, individuals are not even thinking about changing their addictive behaviors. They may not believe they have a problem, or they may feel that others are unnecessarily concerned. Precontemplation is associated with four broad rationales: reluctance, rebellion, resignation, and rationalization. Reluctant individuals do not want to consider change; rebellious precontemplators do not like to be told how to act, and they want to make their own decisions; resigned persons feel overwhelmed by the problem and have given up hope; and rationalizing precontemplators have many reasons why the substance isn't really a problem in their lives.

Nursing Interventions:

1. *Reluctance* – educating the client may help him or her to overcome initial reluctance. Help the client to explore factors influencing his or her hesitation to make the necessary changes. Identify barriers to change, such as finances or stigmatization.

2. *Rebellion* – provide the rebellious client with some sense of control over his or her own decision-making. Offer choices and encourage him to consider his options and possible consequences. Use open-ended questions and reflective statements. Motivational-interviewing approaches are very useful in this stage.

3. *Resignation* – encourage the client to be hopeful and forward thinking. Assist the client in setting some goals for himself or herself and to focus on the long-term positive outcomes of making a change.

4. *Rationalization* – use gentle confrontation to help the client see how his or her behavior has impacted others or caused problems in his life. Ask the client to make lists of positives and negatives to a) continuing the current behavior and b) changing the targeted behavior.

Contemplation

In this stage, the individual is ready to consider the possibility that a change may be necessary. There is often a high level of ambivalence, and change is not yet assured. The healthcare provider can assist the person in weighing the pros and cons of making a change.

Nursing Interventions: Engage the client in group learning activities with others who have similar problems. Provide literature and information for the client. Involve family members and other support persons. Implement interventions to overcome rationalization (as noted above), including lists of pros and cons to making the change.

Preparation/Determination

The preparation stage signals the beginning of a commitment to change. Individuals begin to research options and gather information, such as calling treatment providers or reading Internet resources.

Nursing Interventions: Provide structured activities such as smoking cessation or coping skills groups. Assist the client and his or her support systems in obtaining information and finding out about community resources. Discuss financial needs such as the costs of nicotine-withdrawal patches, and help client to apply for financial assistance programs. Communicate with other healthcare providers to let them know of the client's imminent plans to change, as appropriate (in case changes involve starting or stopping new prescriptions or affect the health status of the client).

Action

Individuals in this stage are able to implement plans to make changes. Success is not guaranteed, but they have moved closer to their goals by making some definitive decisions and acting on those choices.

Nursing Interventions: Provide consistent and regular support and encouragement. Be available between sessions for consultation and advice.

Maintenance (Relapse and Recycling)

During the maintenance stage, individuals may go through a series of relapses. Building new patterns of behavior is difficult and can be emotionally charged; change can take up to 6 months to complete. Family dynamics and relationships with friends are all affected. Relapsing in and of itself is a learning experience – individuals can be helped by learning triggers to relapse and how to substitute other activities in the future.

Nursing Interventions: Help the client to develop a relapse prevention plan. Remain nonjudgmental and recognize that relapsing is a part of any significant, self-directed behavioral change.

Termination

The final stage of change is referred to as termination. In this stage, the addict no longer finds that the substance is a temptation and no longer desires its use.

Nursing Interventions: Provide the client and his support system with community resource information (Prochaska & DiClemente, 1983).

TREATMENT INTERVENTIONS AND FAMILY ISSUES

Therapeutic Interventions

Treatment for alcoholism (and other drug dependencies) begins even before the acute detoxification period. An intervention may be the first step to recovery. In an intervention, selected family, friends, and significant others come together in a supportive setting (usually the client's home) and confront the client about the alcohol or drug usage and how it has negatively impacted each of the people in the room. Interventions are highly emotionally-charged events and are best when facilitated by a trained specialist. After the people in the room express themselves, the target client is given an opportunity to respond. An intervention is not completed until a plan is in place for the next step, which is usually some type of detoxification program. At the end of the intervention, the client should feel supported by family, friends, and significant others and not abandoned or rejected.

Treatment Programs

Following detoxification, clients experience a wide range of emotions and treatment options. Intensive programs (24-hour facilities, 12-hour day programs) are geared to immersing in the recovery process by allowing the client to essentially suspend normal daily activities, such as employment or school, and to focus on education, self-awareness, and recovery. Intensive outpatient programs usually run 2 to 3 hours, three times a week and they may follow the residential or day programs. Intensive outpatient programs allow the client to gradually reintegrate into normal activities, while still maintaining a pronounced emphasis on recovery. Weekly groups and individual therapy sessions may follow intensive outpatient programs. Cognitive behavior (or rational-emotive) therapists work to help clients to understand the events, behaviors, and thoughts that led to drinking (or drug-using) occurrences, and then to "unlearn" these self-destructive patterns and replace them with more adaptive strategies.

Family Issues

Children of alcoholics sometimes grow up to become alcoholics or drug abusers or to marry individuals with addictions. Many theories exist as to why this occurs – certainly, human beings are drawn to others with whom they feel familiar, but there may be deeper psychological drives in place (e.g., a need to repair childhood traumas through rehearsal and repetition). Family studies suggest pronounced genetic and familial inheritance factors with alcoholism as well. Breaking the pattern of addictions within a family requires a tremendous amount of awareness and patience. Children of addicted parents are more likely to be abused or neglected or to end up in foster care or residential placements (due to their own behaviors or to the incarceration or residential treatment of their parents). Clients who use alcohol or other substances to excess have little time left over for partnership or parenting responsibilities. Family life is almost always disrupted and chaotic. Numerous supports programs exist, including Children of Alcoholics (COA), Adult Children of Alcoholics (ACOA), Al-ANON, and Codependents Anonymous (CA), and families should be encouraged to attend the program appropriate for them. Codependency is a recognized phenomenon in which the non-using partner or spouse of an addict behaves in ways that subtly allow the addiction to continue, such as lying to the client's employer about not showing up to work, making excuses for negative behaviors to others (e.g., "Mommy's sick" when the addicted person has a hangover or "You didn't mean to hit me, it was the alcohol talking!"), or even purchasing alcohol or drugs for the client with illogical rationales such as "He'll get it somewhere, it might as well be at home." Codependent partners need to be helped to realize the part they play in encouraging the addictive

behavior to continue. Family therapy may be essential in rebuilding trust and positive relationships within the family.

SEDATIVE, HYPNOTIC, AND ANXIOLYTIC ABUSE AND DEPENDENCE

Benzodiazepines, benzodiazepine-like substances, barbiturates, and barbiturate-like substances make up the class of sedatives, hypnotics, and anxiolytics. This class includes all prescription sleeping pills and all prescription antianxiety agents with a benzodiazepine-like action (buspirone is not included). Drugs with important other uses, such as antiepileptics, may also be included, depending their abuse and dependence potential. Similar to alcohol, these categories of substances are CNS depressants. They may be prescription or "street" acquired. All can cause tolerance, dependency, and withdrawal syndromes. CNS depressants are extremely dangerous if taken in an overdose, especially if combined with other medications, street drugs, or alcohol. Table 7-4 presents an overview of sedative, hypnotic, and anxiolytic drugs commonly seen. One particular benzodiazepine, flunitrazepam (Rohypnol®), has been labeled the "date rape" drug because of its potent sedative and amnesic actions. It is not legally available in the United States.

Benzodiazepines and barbiturates work by enhancing the effects of the neurotransmitter gamma-aminobutyric acid (GABA). The action of GABA is to open chloride channels at the cellular level, which make a neuron less responsive to other neurotransmitters, such as serotonin, norepinephrine, and dopamine. The overall effect is a slowing down of neuron firing. Benzodiazepines and barbiturates contribute to this brain-inhibition effect and slow down excitability, agitation, nervousness and, often, alertness, attention span, concentration, and

TABLE 7-4: SELECTED SEDATIVES, HYPNOTICS, AND ANXIOLYTICS

Classification	Generic Name	Trade Name	Common Usage	Comments
Benzodiazepines	alprazolam	Xanax®	Anxiolytic	Duration 2-4 hrs.
	oxazepam	Serax®	Anxiolytic	Duration 1-2 hrs.
	lorazepam	Ativan®	Anxiolytic	Duration 4-6 hrs.
	diazepam	Valium®	Anxiolytic, status epilepticus	Duration 10-12 hrs.
	clonazepam	Klonopin®	Anxiolytic, antiepileptic, bipolar disorder	Duration 10-12 hrs.
	chlordiazepoxide	Librium®	Anxiolytic, alcohol detoxification	Very long half-life
	clorazepate	Tranxene®	Anxiolytic	Seldom used
	estazolam	Prosom®	Sedative, hypnotic	Newer on market
	temazepam	Restoril®	Sedative, hypnotic	Duration 8-12 hrs.
	flurazepam	Dalmane®	Sedative, hypnotic	Long duration
	triazolam	Halcion®	Sedative, hypnotic	Associated with psychosis
	flunitrazepam	Rohypnol®	Sedative, hypnotic, amnesic	Illegal in U.S.
Non-benzodiazepine	zolpidem	Ambien®	Sedative, hypnotic	Less dependency
	zaleplon	Sonata®	Sedative, hypnotic	Less dependency
Chloral derivation	chloral hydrate	Noctec®	Sedative, hypnotic	Short-term use only
Barbiturate	secobarbital	Seconal®	Sedative, antiepileptic	
	pentobarbital	Nembutal®	Sedative, antiepileptic	Dental anesthetic
	amobarbital	Amytal®	Sedative, amnesic, anesthetic	"Truth serum"
	butabarbital	Butisol®	Sedative, antiepileptic	
	phenobarbital	Luminal®	Antiepileptic, sedative	
	thiopental	Pentothal®	Anesthetic, sedative	Used frequently in surgery
	methohexital	Brevital®	Anesthetic, sedative	
Miscellaneous	meprobamate	Equanil® Miltown®	Anxiolytic, sedative	High abuse potential
	methaqualone	Quaalude®	Sedative, hypnotic	High abuse potential

decision-making abilities. GABA receptors are located on approximately 40% of all neurons. GABA receptors are required for benzodiazepines to have an inhibitory effect. Barbiturates enhance and imitate GABA, so receptor availability is not as important. Of the two groups, barbiturates are far more lethal than benzodiazepines (Keltner et al., 2007).

The *DSM-IV-TR* identifies four key criteria for identifying intoxication secondary to a sedative, hypnotic, or anxiolytic.

1. Recent use of the sedative, hypnotic, or anxiolytic.

2. Significant maladaptive behavioral or psychological changes that develop during or after use.

3. One or more of the following signs:
   a. Slurred speech
   b. Incoordination
   c. Unsteady gait
   d. Nystagmus of the eyes
   e. Impaired memory or attention
   f. Stupor or coma

4. The symptoms are not due to a general medical condition or another mental disorder.

Intoxication signs and symptoms of a sedative, hypnotic, or anxiolytic are almost identical to those of alcohol and differentiation should be made using a Breathalyzer® or blood alcohol test. In the presence of a sedative, hypnotic, or anxiolytic, a urine drug screen will test positive for benzodiazepines or barbiturates.

SEDATIVE, HYPNOTIC, AND ANXIOLYTIC WITHDRAWAL

The timing and severity of withdrawal syndromes are positively correlated with the pharmacokinetics and pharmacodynamics of the substance used. Withdrawal from short-acting agents (e.g., alprazolam) can begin within hours.

Withdrawal from longer-acting agents (e.g., clonazepam) may not begin for 1 to 2 days, or even longer. Withdrawal symptoms may include the following: increased heart rate; increased blood pressure; sweating; hand tremor; insomnia; nausea or vomiting; visual, tactile, or auditory hallucinations; agitation; anxiety, including panic attacks; and grand mal seizures. Withdrawal from benzodiazepines and barbiturates often requires medical intervention and supervision. Administering gradually decreasing doses of the offending agent, or a similar substitution, is accepted practice. Detoxification may occur in either an inpatient or an outpatient setting; however, in an outpatient setting the client must exercise a great deal of self-control and discipline to maintain the weaning schedule. The more rapid the weaning schedule is, the more uncomfortable and potentially dangerous it is for the client. A weaning schedule of up to 2 weeks (sometimes longer) is recommended.

NURSING CARE OF THE CLIENT DETOXIFYING FROM ALCOHOL, SEDATIVES, HYPNOTICS, OR ANXIOLYTICS

Recognition of the signs of withdrawal and appropriate treatment is foremost when caring for a client withdrawing from alcohol, sedatives, hypnotics, or anxiolytics. Often, protocols are in place that allow the nurse to medicate the clients based on set criteria, such as blood pressure and pulse. Ignoring the client's objective symptoms or subjective complaints will result in a worsening of withdrawal symptoms and an increased potential for a seizure. In the first 1 to 2 days of detoxification, fairly liberal use of withdrawal agents is recommended. Seizure precautions are an important nursing safety concern because of the risk of neuron excitability. Assessing the client for other medications that may lower his or her seizure threshold is important (e.g., buproprion, traditional antipsychotics, clozapine). Other safety concerns include monitoring for the emergence of psychotic symptoms, agitation, aggression, or suicidal thoughts and treating as necessary. Clients who present with significant withdrawal complications may require physical restraints for protection of themselves and the healthcare providers. Supporting fluid and electrolyte status through oral and intravenous routes may be necessary. Administering a bland diet and antiemetics helps in controlling nausea and vomiting. Encouraging the client to maintain bed rest as much as possible for the first 24 hours also aids in the recovery process. It may be necessary to limit visitors in an inpatient setting to facilitate a quiet and nonstressful environment. Assessing for, and assisting in the treatment of, concomitant medical problems should be ongoing.

Client Education

When the acute phase of physical detoxification is completed, the nurse can begin to focus on other appropriate interventions. Assessing the client's readiness to change (Stage of Change) and developing a plan of care based on this assessment is important. Educating the client about the importance of self-help programs and providing information about local resources can help the client to develop a sober support network in the community. Incorporating family members and significant others in the recovery process is important because clients as well as their significant others need to understand the dynamics of addictions and addictive behaviors. A nonjudgmental approach, with practical and supportive information, is most useful. Discharge planning from inpatient care should include referrals to outpatient treatment providers as well as to AA or NA (Narcotics Anonymous). Many outpatient programs exist, ranging from once-weekly therapy, to group therapy three times a week (an intensive outpatient program), to residential care with 12 hours of programming daily.

CASE STUDY: CLIENT WITH ALCOHOL DEPENDENCE

Maggie is a 38-year-old woman who has been employed as a real estate agent for the past 10 years. She graduated high school and completed 4 years of a business degree before landing this lucrative position for a large company. In high school, Maggie drank some with her friends. She had her first blackout at her senior prom; later she found out that she was dancing on the tables and making a fool of herself. In college, she attended various fraternity parties and had another blackout episode. This time she awoke to find herself naked and in bed with two men. She had no memory of the preceding events. Maggie continued to drink socially on weekends, and then she started taking prospective customers out during the week. Soon, she found herself having wine with lunch, a cocktail or two after work, then several more in the evening at home. After Maggie's mother suddenly died of an aneurysm, her drinking escalated further to the point that she started to call in sick to work or go home early. She got her first DUI arrest while driving back to the office after showing a house. Her second DUI arrest (while at work) 2 months later cost her both her job and her driver's license. Unemployed, her drinking started to spiral out of control and she was always either intoxicated or sick. One night, Maggie started to vomit blood in copious amounts. Frightened, she called 911 and was rushed to the emergency department where she had surgery to repair ruptured esophageal varices. She was detoxified after 5 days and started attending AA meetings while in the hospital. Maggie learned that she was an alcoholic and would always be an alcoholic. She agreed to see a therapist and continue to attend AA meetings once discharged. Maggie relapsed three more times before she was able to reach 2 years of sobriety and become a sponsor for another woman.

Questions

1. Is Maggie demonstrating alcohol abuse or alcohol dependence?

2. What is an alcoholic blackout?

3. What are some signs of alcohol withdrawal?

Discussion

Maggie initially abused alcohol, but when she continued to use, despite clear, negative consequences, she became alcohol dependent. A blackout is experienced when an individual appears to be awake and oriented, but has no memory of the events that occurred. Signs of alcohol withdrawal include an elevated blood pressure and heart rate, tremors, anxiety, sweating (diaphoresis), nausea and vomiting, hallucinations, and a high risk for seizures.

NURSING CARE PLAN: ALCOHOL DEPENDENCE

Problem Listing

- GI Bleeding
- Tremors
- Ineffective coping
- Poor nutrition
- Dizziness
- Insomnia
- Anxiety
- Diaphoresis
- Elevated blood pressure and heart rates

Priority Nursing Diagnosis

Potential for harm due to alcohol withdrawal, as evidenced by tremors, elevated vital signs, anxiety, diaphoresis, and dizziness.

Long-term Goal

Client will be safely detoxified in a medically supervised setting.

Short-term Objectives

1. Client will have a consistent blood pressure reading of less than 130/90 within 5 days of admission.

2. Client will have a heart rate of less than 100 beats per minute.

3. Client will report less anxiety and fewer tremors.

4. Client will not develop hallucinations or other signs of psychosis.

Nursing Interventions

1. Assess blood pressure, heart rate, and respirations every 2 hours and as needed.

2. Administer ordered benzodiazepines liberally every 2 hours and as needed.

3. Administer antiemetics as needed.

4. Encourage sipping of electrolyte replenishing fluids continuously.

5. Monitor intake and output.

6. Assess for blood in emesis and in stools.

7. Provide a bland, light diet for the first 48 to 72 hours of detoxification (unless on nothing by mouth status).

8. Keep environment quiet and nonstressful by turning down lights, keeping temperature at a comfortable level, and keeping noise to a minimum.

9. Restrict visitors if necessary.

10. Meet with the client daily to provide emotional support.

11. Educate the client about processes of alcohol addiction (tolerance, dependence, withdrawal) daily until discharged.

12. Make referrals to continuing care treatment providers and resources, including AA meetings.

ADVANCED PRACTICE NURSING: MANAGING A DETOXIFICATION PROTOCOL

Advanced practice nurses are involved in alcohol and substance dependency treatment from the beginning detoxification stages, to the ongoing therapy and treatment, to educational and aftercare programs. For the purposes of this section, specific information is provided on detoxification from alcohol and sedatives, hypnotics, and anxiolytics. Detoxifying programs are usually carried out in hospital or residential settings because of the safety risks inherent in treating alcohol, sedative, and anxiolytic dependence as well as the strict discipline required of the client not to re-use. Clients with a history of withdrawal seizures, serious dehydration, or existing delirium tremens should be detoxified in a hospital, where emergency care is readily available. Having specific protocols is helpful when planning a residential or outpatient detoxification.

Alcohol withdrawal takes from 3 to 5 days in general (longer when impaired liver function is present). Clients should have their blood pressure and heart rates checked at least every 2 hours and should be given a long-acting benzodiazepine such as chlordiazepoxide (Librium®) at the first sign of elevation. Doses of 25 to 50 mg may be given every few hours if necessary, as long as the client is awake, alert, oriented, and feeling distressed. Lorazepam (Ativan®) can also be used; however, it has a shorter half-life. For clients with existing hypertension, for which they take medications, blood pressure and heart rate may not be reliable indicators. In these situations, it is prudent to medicate for anxiety symptoms for the first 24 hours. Ancillary treatment measures are also helpful. These include anti-nausea medications such as promethazine (Phenergan®), usually administered in injection form or suppositories; ibuprofen for headaches; and antihistamines to sleep. Anything that elevates seizure risk is best avoided, including chlorpromazine (Compazine®), a common anti-nausea medication. Some clinicians prefer to give high-risk clients antiepileptic medications such as phenytoin (Dilantin®) to help prevent seizures (liver disease should be considered when using antiepileptics).

Benzodiazepine withdrawal mimics alcohol withdrawal in its blood pressure and heart rate elevations, anxiety, tremors, nausea and other symptoms; however, the duration of the withdrawal varies based on the agent used. The simplest way to manage an outpatient detoxification is to give the client controlled but weaning doses of the medication over a period of time. For example, a client who is taking alprazolam (Xanax®) 2 mg three times per day should have the dosage reduced by 0.25 to 0.5 mg daily until off of the medication. This will take approximately 2 to 3 weeks to finish, but anxiety will be minimized as well as the risk of seizures. The prescribing APRN can give the client limited (1 week) prescriptions or daily prescriptions, if needed, and check his or her vital signs each time he or she comes in to pick up the prescription. Supportive measures to help with nausea or sleep will improve compliance.

SUMMARY

Clients intoxicated or addicted to alcohol, sedatives, hypnotics, or anxiolytics present particular challenges to the healthcare professional. Frequently uncooperative, such clients may be in denial, angry, agitated, delirious, confused, anxious, or combative. Recognizing the offending agent and planning appropriate treatment interventions is essential in the acute phases of care. Numerous useful assessment tools are available at no charge to the nurse. After assessment and identification of the problem, rapid medicating and providing a safe, non-stimulating environment are essential. Medical complications may be present in alcohol dependence, including chronic conditions that may result from long-term use (liver disease, esophageal varices, and Vitamin B 12 deficiencies) as well as acute problems, such as dehydration, hypertensive crises, and seizures. When detoxification is complete, clients and their families should be encouraged to participate in therapy and self-help programs, such as AA or Al-Anon. Therapeutic models that are helpful in alcohol and substance recovery include Motivational Interviewing and Stages of Change. Self-help programs provide clients and families with community resources and support that aide in maintaining sobriety and reducing relapse rates.

EXAM QUESTIONS

CHAPTER 7
Questions 39-44

Note: Choose the one option that BEST answers each question.

39. Symptoms indicative of sedative or alcohol intoxication include

    a. restlessness, pacing, rapid speech.

    b. perceptual alterations, euphoria.

    c. slurred speech, impaired memory, unsteady gait.

    d. a sense of peacefulness, relaxation, increased appetite.

40. Alcohol detoxification can last

    a. 6 to 12 hours.

    b. 1 to 2 days.

    c. 2 to 3 days.

    d. 3 to 5 days.

41. Medications commonly used to treat withdrawal symptoms, such as tremors, anxiety, and an increased seizure risk, are

    a. benzodiazepines.

    b. antidepressants.

    c. anticholinergics.

    d. opiate receptor antagonists.

42. A medical complication caused by portal vein hypertension is

    a. esophageal varices.

    b. gastric ulcers.

    c. pancreatitis.

    d. peripheral neuropathies.

43. Family members of the client with an alcohol addiction

    a. are generally mentally healthy and well-adjusted.

    b. can develop alcohol or drug addictions as well.

    c. should separate from the client as soon as possible.

    d. have no impact on the recovery process.

44. A nursing safety concern that is paramount in alcohol and sedative, hypnotic, and anxiolytic detoxification is

    a. preventing the development of seizures.

    b. educating families and clients.

    c. providing thorough discharge referrals.

    d. administering antiemetics and a bland diet.

CHAPTER 8

SUBSTANCE ABUSE AND DETOXIFICATION

CHAPTER OBJECTIVE

At the end of this chapter, the reader will be able to discuss drug dependency in American society, including the recognition and treatment of withdrawal syndromes.

LEARNING OBJECTIVES

At the completion of this chapter, the reader will be able to

1. recognize signs of substance abuse and dependence.

2. differentiate symptoms of intoxication and withdrawal from opioids, amphetamines, cocaine, inhalants, hallucinogens, and nicotine.

3. discuss medical and nursing treatment for substance dependence and withdrawal.

INTRODUCTION

In 2008, an estimated 20.1 million Americans 12 years of age and older were current illicit drug users, using one or more abusive substances. This estimate represents 8% of the U.S. population who are older than 12 years of age. Of these individuals, 15.2 million had used marijuana within the past month, 6.2 million had used prescription medications in an abusive manner, 1.9 million had used cocaine, 1.1 million had used hallucinogens (other than marijuana), 600,000 had abused inhalants, 200,000 had used heroin, and approximately 100,000 had used methamphetamines (SAMHSA, 2008).

Opioid use and abuse continue to be at peak prevalence rates (Johnston, O'Malley, Bachman, & Schulenberg, 2009). Complications related to opioid dependence accounted for 18% of all substance abuse hospital admissions in 2001. Over an 8-year period (1994-2002), hospital admissions involving oxycodone dependence or abuse jumped 450% and admissions involving hydrocodone dependence or abuse went up 170% (SAMHSA, 2006).

SUBSTANCE USE AND DEPENDENCE

The *DSM-IV-TR* differentiates substance abuse from substance dependence and substance-related disorders (which may include heavy metals, pesticides, poisons, or over-the-counter agents). The essential feature of substance abuse is a maladaptive pattern of substance use that is associated with recurrent and significant negative consequences related to the use of the substance. There must be repeated use during a 12-month period, which results in a failure to fulfill major role obligations at work, school, or home; or use in situations in which it is dangerous or hazardous (e.g., operating a motor vehicle); or substance-related legal problems such as arrests; or persistent social or interpersonal problems caused by the substance use. Substance dependence incorporates the criteria for substance abuse, but also requires that at least three of the following criteria are met.

1. Tolerance

    a. A need for increasing amounts of the substance to achieve intoxication; or,

    b. Markedly diminished effect with continued use of the same amount of the substance.

2. Withdrawal

    a. A withdrawal syndrome characteristic to the substance used; or,

    b. The substance, or a closely related substance, is taken to relieve or avoid withdrawal symptoms.

3. The substance is often taken in larger amounts or over a longer period than was intended.

4. There is a persistent desire or unsuccessful efforts to reduce or control substance use.

5. A great deal of time is spent in activities necessary to obtain the substance, use the substance, or recover from its effects.

6. Important social, work, or recreational activities are given up or reduced because of substance use.

7. The use is continued despite knowledge of having a physical or psychological problem that was likely caused or exacerbated by the substance.

Substance withdrawal syndromes are currently recognized for alcohol, amphetamines and related substances, cocaine, nicotine, opioids, and sedatives, hypnotics, and anxiolytics. Withdrawal develops when the amount of the substance being used is reduced or discontinued. The use of multiple substances complicates the clinical picture significantly because detoxification protocols may be necessary for each individual substance, and physical signs and symptoms may be complex.

OPIOID ABUSE AND DEPENDENCE

Opioids include commonly prescribed pain medications (both oral and intramuscular), intravenous drugs used on the streets, and certain anesthetics. Examples of opioid substances include opium, heroin, methadone (Dolophin®), morphine, codeine, hydromorphone (Dilaudid®), meperidine (Demerol®), hydrocodone (Lortab®), and oxycodone (OxyContin®, Percodan®, Percocet®, Tylox®). An opioid partial agonist used to treat opioid addiction is buprenorphine HCL/naltrexone HCL (Suboxone®). Opioids work by stimulating naturally occurring endorphin receptor sites in the brain and producing an overall sense of euphoria, accompanied by an increased tolerance to pain and reduced anxiety. Side effects of opioids include drowsiness, respiratory depression, constipation, decreased gastric secretions, urinary retention, hypotension, and pinpoint pupils. An excess amount of opioids (overdose) produces CNS depression, seizures, respiratory depression, stupor, coma, and possibly death. Naltrexone (Narcan®, Revia®, Vivitrol®), an opioid antagonist, is used to treat opioid overdose. Vivitrol® is an intramuscular injection used to prevent alcohol relapses. Taking opioids with other CNS depressants, such as alcohol, benzodiazepines, or barbiturates, is especially lethal and can cause death due to respiratory suppression. Urine drug screens test positive for opioids and assist in determining other drugs that may also be present.

It is estimated that 55% to 94% of infants born to women who are addicted to opioids experience withdrawal symptoms at birth, which may include respiratory depression, CNS irritability, jitteriness, tremor, diarrhea, vomiting that may lead to electrolyte imbalances, and seizures. (American Academy of Pediatrics: Committee on Drugs, 1998).

Nursing Care of the Client with Opioid Withdrawal

The *DSM-IV-TR* definition of opioid withdrawal includes the following:

a. cessation or reduction of opioid use that has been heavy and prolonged; or,

b. administration of an opioid antagonist after a period of opioid use (i.e., naltrexone)

Three or more of the following, developing within minutes to several days after use is stopped or after an opioid antagonist is administered:

a. dysphoric mood

b. nausea or vomiting

c. muscle aches

d. lacrimation (tears) or rhinorrhea (runny nose)

e. pupillary dilation, piloerection (goosebumps), or sweating

f. diarrhea

g. yawning

h. fever

i. insomnia

The symptoms cause significant distress or impairment but they do not occur due to a general medical condition or another mental disorder.

Nursing care should be focused on supporting the client and providing reassurance. Opioid intoxication and overdosage are life threatening, but withdrawal is rarely dangerous unless other medical conditions are present. It is, however, uncomfortable for the client. Administering nonsteroidal analgesics such as ibuprofen can help relieve the muscle aching and leg cramps reported by the client. Nonaddictive sleep aides such as trazodone (Desyrel®) are also useful. Monitoring and maintaining fluid and electrolyte statuses, as well as urinary output and bowel functioning helps to avoid complications.

The desire to use (cravings) can be overwhelming, and clients may make elaborate arrangements to obtain drugs to alleviate their symptoms. Monitoring visitors may be required with clients who are detoxifying from opioids. Some clinicians may prescribe clonidine (Catapres®, Catapres-TTS®) in oral or topical form to treat the discomfort associated with withdrawal from opioids. Clonidine is an alpha-adrenergic agonist that reduces impulses in the sympathetic nervous system, resulting in a decrease in blood pressure, heart rate, and cardiac output and the prevention of pain signal transmission, anxiety, and hyperactivity. Another medication that may help to prevent relapse, but is not FDA-approved for this use, is buproprion (Wellbutrin SR®, Wellbutrin XL®, and Zyban®). Buproprion increases the amount of dopamine, serotonin, and norepinephrine in the brain, which appears to reduce the cravings associated with substances, such as opioids, cocaine, and nicotine.

COCAINE AND AMPHETAMINE USE

Cocaine is found naturally in the leaves of the coca plants. It was introduced to the West as an anesthetic in the mid-1800s. Cocaine was once used in soft drinks (Coca-Cola®), but its use was eliminated in 1906. Cocaine is a powerful stimulant with significant euphoria that is associated with its actions to block the reuptake of the neurotransmitter dopamine in the brain. Cocaine also depletes the neuronal stores of norepinephrine, causing an adrenalin-like rush. Cocaine rapidly crosses the blood-brain barrier and is rapidly metabolized by the healthy liver, resulting in a short length of action (2 to 4 hours). Effects of cocaine use include an increase in alertness, strength, endurance, sexual stimulation, motor activity, heart rate, and blood pressure. There is a decreased need for sleep, and appetite is reduced. Inhibitions are also reduced. Because of its extensive abuse, medical use of cocaine has ceased to be practiced. A relatively new form of less expensive cocaine is available on the streets. Mixing cocaine with baking soda and water, then heating it and allowing it to harden produces "crack" cocaine. It can then be smoked for an immediate high, which is followed by a significant crash. The depression experienced may lead to suicide attempts.

Amphetamines have been available since the late 1800s and have a variety of legitimate medical uses, including the treatment of attention deficit hyperactivity disorder and narcolepsy. Some drugs that are used to treat obesity are chemically similar to amphetamines (sibutramine). Therapeutic amphetamines are administered orally or via a transdermal skin patch; however, illicit uses may include sniffing or intravenous use. Amphetamines include such drugs as phentermine (Adapex®), dextroamphetamine (Dexedrine®), mixed amphetamine salts (Adderall®, Adderall XR®), lisdexamfetamine (Vyvanse®), and methamphetamine (Desoxyn®) and related substances methylphenidate (Ritalin®) and Ecstasy. Amphetamines may also be "cooked up," or produced in a homemade lab, making products such as "crank," "crystal meth," or "CAT" (methcathinone). Amphetamines are sometimes combined with heroin and injected in a "speed ball" – a particularly lethal combination. Amphetamines work by causing the release of norepinephrine and dopamine from nerve endings and blocking their reuptake, resulting in higher norepinephrine and dopamine brain levels. Side effects of amphetamines include alertness, improved concentration, increased energy, restlessness, insomnia, decreased appetite, and mood changes.

Too much amphetamine or cocaine at one time, or chronic usage, can result in severe agitation, tachycardia, cardiac arrhythmias, hypertension, increased respirations, and psychosis. Paranoid delusions and visual hallucinations may occur. Death is usually due to sudden cardiac arrest (seen primarily after intravenous use). Long-term use may result in malnutrition, gastrointestinal prob-

lems, chronic insomnia, and anxiety disorders. Sniffing or snorting the drugs can cause nasal septum perforations and chronic nosebleeds. Intravenous use may result in phlebitis, cellulitis, and infections that can ultimately lead to gangrene and tissue necrosis.

Cocaine and Amphetamine Withdrawal

One of the main concerns with cocaine and amphetamine withdrawal is a "crash" in mood symptoms, probably related to the exhaustion of norepinephrine and dopamine transmitters. Depression and suicide ideation can occur and may last for several weeks. Safety of the client is a primary nursing concern. Other withdrawal symptoms include irritability, fatigue, insomnia or hypersomnia, nightmares, increased appetite, and psychomotor retardation or agitation.

Khat

A relatively new focus of the U.S. Drug Enforcement Administration (DEA) has been on the prevention of the importation and selling of Khat (pronounced "cot"). Khat is a shrub native to East Africa and the Arabian Peninsula that is chewed like tobacco. It produces an amphetamine-like response with increased energy, loss of appetite, insomnia, hypertension, and tachycardia. It can also lead to exhaustion, violence, mania, hallucinations, or suicidal depression. In 2006, the DEA indicted a 44-member international Khat smuggling ring that was responsible for bringing in more than 25 tons ($10 million dollars) of Khat to the United States (U.S. Drug Enforcement Administration, 2006).

Methamphetamine

Methamphetamine (Figure 8-1), or "meth" as it is commonly called, is an increasing public health problem in the United States. Methamphetamine addicts can develop a number of health problems, and children raised in homes where methamphetamine is manufactured or abused may suffer from physical problems, neglect, and safety risks.

FIGURE 8-1: METHAMPHETAMINE

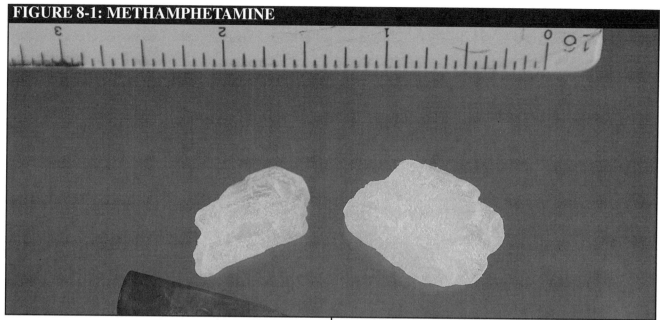

Homemade methamphetamine, or "meth labs" as they are commonly called, use a number of common household chemicals plus ephedrine or pseudoephedrine to produce methamphetamine. Chemicals that may be used in addition to pseudoephedrine and ephedrine include isopropyl (rubbing) alcohol, toluene (brake cleaner), ether (engine starter), red phosphorus (matches or road flares), sodium chloride (table or rock salt), iodine, lithium (batteries), trichloroethane (gun cleaner), sodium metal, methanol (gasoline additives), muriatic acid, anhydrous ammonia (fertilizer), sodium hydroxide (lye), acetone, and cat litter. Many of these chemicals are highly volatile and explosive; 15% of meth labs are discovered after they explode. Severe burns or death are not uncommon.

Meth labs may be built in a home, a camper, a storage unit, or even in the trunk of a car. Remote, rural areas are popular. In 2008, 6,783 meth labs were discovered by the DEA (Figure 8-2) with the highest number found in the Midwestern states of Missouri (1,471), Indiana (724), Tennessee (553), and Kentucky (416).

Signs of a methamphetamine lab may include an inordinate amount of laboratory equipment (beakers, flasks, tubing, etc.) on the property, a strong chemical odor in the area, windows covered with stained blankets or sheets, excessive trash, increased nocturnal activity, and prepayment of rent in cash.

Children exposed to methamphetamine manufacturing are at risk for chemical contamination, secondary methamphetamine smoke inhalation, injuries caused by spills or burns, death due to explosions, neglect, abuse, and exposure to other hazardous living situations, such as exposed wires, lack of hot water or electricity, and aggressive guard dogs. Additionally, little is known about the incidence of brain damage or learning disabilities for children who are exposed to meth labs. In many U.S. states, children found during a meth lab drug "bust" are automatically put into foster care until they can be evaluated medically and a safe and suitable living situation is found (U.S. Department of Justice, 2007).

Nursing Care of the Client Using Amphetamines

Clients who use amphetamines or cocaine may present for treatment for malnutrition, vitamin deficiencies, electrolyte imbalances, cardiac arrhythmias, poor dental care with related oral infections, skin lesions, agitation, hostility, hallucinations, or paranoia. Initial care of the amphetamine intoxicated person is focused on maintaining safety,

FIGURE 8-2: TOTAL OF ALL METH CLANDESTINE LABORATORY INCIDENTS INCLUDING LABS, DUMPSITES, CHEM/GLASS/EQUIPMENT, CALENDAR YEAR 2008

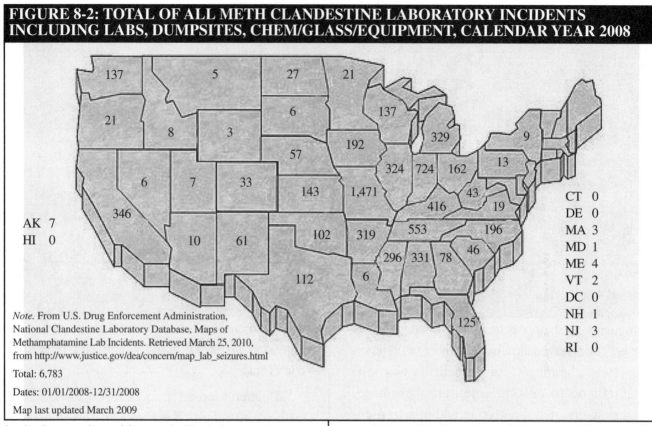

Note. From U.S. Drug Enforcement Administration, National Clandestine Laboratory Database, Maps of Methamphatamine Lab Incidents. Retrieved March 25, 2010, from http://www.justice.gov/dea/concern/map_lab_seizures.html

Total: 6,783

Dates: 01/01/2008-12/31/2008

Map last updated March 2009

hydration, and nutrition and alleviating anxiety or psychosis. Medications may be ordered that are sedative in nature for short-term use. IV fluids and gradual reintroduction to nutritious foods may be necessary. ECG's are recommended for complaints of chest pain or tachycardia or abnormal heart sounds. A dental consult is recommended for any long-term amphetamine user. After the initial detoxification period, the nurse can be instrumental in educating the client and family in the effects of amphetamines on the body and in setting up referrals to treatment providers and support programs (see the discussion of nursing care of the addicted client in Chapter 7).

HALLUCINOGENIC AGENTS

Hallucinogens are agents that induce hallucinations. Natural hallucinogens include psilocybin (hallucinogenic mushrooms), mescaline or peyote (derived from cactus), and marijuana (from the cannabis sativa plant). Synthetic substances include lysergic acid diethylamide (LSD), phen-cyclidine (PCP) or "angel dust," and Ecstasy (3, 4-methylenedioxymethamphetamine or MDMA). Hallucinogens result in a heightened awareness of reality, followed by distorted perceptions, and then visual, auditory, or tactile hallucinations. Colors, tastes, and musical sounds may seem more intense or vivid. Time may seem to be slowed down or speeded up. Emotional sensations range from euphoria and a sense of peacefulness and wonder to fear, panic, confusion, and paranoid reactions. Hallucinogens do not produce any physiological dependence, although a hallucinogen persisting perception disorder ("flashbacks") may occur. This is defined by the *DSM-IV-TR* as a recurrence of disturbances in perception similar to those experienced while under the influence of the drug. The symptoms must cause clinically significant distress and cannot be due to a general medical condition or other mental disorder such as schizophrenia. Episodes may occur repeatedly and they usually abate after several months.

Mescaline and psilocybin have traditionally been used in Native American religious practices. Hallucinogenic effects last up to 12 hours for mescaline and 8 hours for psilocybin. In addition to hallucinogenic effects, they dilate the pupils and increase heart rate, blood pressure, and body temperature. Occasionally psilocybin will cause a skin tingling sensation and involuntary movements.

LSD was initially developed as a potential treatment for schizophrenia. It has potent serotonin binding effects and can cause dramatic hallucinations that last up to 12 hours. Side effects of LSD ingestion include tachycardia, increased blood pressure, trembling, dilated pupils, sense of unreality, perceptual alterations, confusion, impaired judgment, and synesthesia. Synesthesia is the hallucinatory experience that causes an individual to feel as though he can "smell" colors or "taste" music. Severe emotional reactions may occur, including panic and paranoia. LSD intoxication has been attributed to a number of suicides.

PCP has been used traditionally in veterinary medicine as a tranquilizer and anesthetic. PCP can be taken orally, intravenously, nasally, or smoked. Effects last up to 8 hours after use. PCP causes an initial euphoria with perceptual distortions. Side effects include increased blood pressure and heart rate, staggering, vomiting, increased salivation, bizarre behaviors, muscular rigidity, and violent outbursts. The aggression and strength of PCP users is legendary in emergency department settings. Another anesthetic, Ketamine® ("Special K") has also been used for its dissociative effects. Ketamine® has been implicated in date rapes due to its amnesic properties.

Ecstasy (MDMA) has been around since the 1900s when it was synthesized primarily as an adjunct to psychotherapy. Its common use is in nightclubs and "Raves." At low doses, it increases affection and a sense of closeness to others. Higher doses result in an amphetamine-like response with euphoria, increased sexuality, and disinhibition.

Mild hallucinogenic effects may also occur. Side effects are amphetamine-like with teeth grinding, tachycardia, dry mouth, and decreased appetite. Memory impairment may also occur. Deaths have been reported secondary to hyperthermia, dehydration, rhabdomyolysis, and renal failure.

Nursing Care of the Client Using Hallucinogens

An overdose of hallucinogens is not usually fatal; however, deaths may occur secondary to dangerous or risk-taking behaviors. Suicides and homicides are most likely to be associated with LSD and PCP respectively. Nursing care should focus on maintaining a calm, quiet environment. Antipsychotics may be indicated for persistent hallucinations. Chemical and physical restraints may be necessary. Benzodiazepines are useful for reducing panic and anxiety as well as educating and modeling relaxation techniques with the client.

MARIJUANA

Marijuana cultivation has taken place for over 5,000 years. It varies in potency, depending on the soil and growth conditions and varieties harvested. The active ingredient in marijuana, tetrahydrocannabinol (THC) is stored in fatty tissues in the body for up to 6 weeks after use. Marijuana is typically smoked; although it can be ingested as well. Effects from smoking last 2 to 4 hours, whereas effects from ingestion may last up to 12 hours. Marijuana produces a sense of well-being and relaxation. It increases hunger and also has antiemetic properties, which is why it may be useful for individuals undergoing chemotherapy for cancer or HIV-related diseases. Marijuana has also been indicated in reducing intraocular pressure associated with glaucoma. Side effects of use include impaired short-term memory and concentration, dry mouth, sore throat, increased heart rate, bloodshot eyes, and dilated pupils. Smoking marijuana can lead to bronchitis. There is some evidence to support reduced testosterone levels and sperm counts. Emotional reactions, other than a mild euphoria, may include anxiety, panic, and paranoia.

Marijuana users may experience extreme irritability, insomnia, restlessness, and increased activity during withdrawal.

INHALANT ABUSE AND DEPENDENCE

Inhalants such as gasoline, glue, paint thinners, and hydrocarbons found in cleaning solutions, correction fluid, and spray-can propellants (as well as a variety of other substances) are inexpensive and readily accessible. This leads to their abuse in children as young as elementary school. CNS effects include dizziness, euphoria, slurred speech, lethargy, depressed reflexes, psychomotor retardation, tremor, muscle weakness, blurred or double vision, nystagmus, incoordination, stupor, and coma. Other effects may include respiratory problems, coughing, sinus discharge, mouth ulcers, nosebleeds, headaches, gastrointestinal problems, confusion, and a loss of appetite. Inhalants can cause both central and peripheral nervous system damage. Memory problems, decreased problem-solving abilities, generalized weakness, and peripheral neuropathies are prominent. Recurrent use may lead to hepatitis, cirrhosis, or renal failure. Sudden death can occur from respiratory or cardiovascular depression, acute arrhythmias, hypoxia, asphyxiation, or electrolyte abnormalities. The odor of paint or solvents may be detected on the individuals clothing or breath or a rash may be present around the nose and mouth.

CAFFEINE INTOXICATION AND WITHDRAWAL

Caffeine is an insidious and ubiquitous drug. It is legal and widely available in coffee, tea, chocolate, soft drinks, and new energy drinks. Caffeine is added to many over-the-counter drug products, including some aspirins (Excedrin®), cold remedies, and diet aids. Caffeine tablets (No-Doz®) are easy to obtain. Table 8-1 provides an overview of some sources of caffeine along with average milligram dosages. People of all ages, even young children or infants, consume caffeine.

TABLE 8-1: SOURCES OF CAFFEINE	
Source	**Dosage in Milligrams**
Coffee, brewed	100-140 mg per cup
Coffee, instant	65-100 mg per cup
Tea, black	40-100 mg per cup
Tea, green	30-50 mg per cup
Soda/Soft drink	45 mg per 12 oz. can
Energy drinks	200-250 mg per can
Chocolate bar	5 mg per bar
OTC Analgesics	25-50 mg per tablet
OTC Cold remedies	25-50 mg per tablet
Diet aids	75-200 mg per tablet
OTC: Over the counter	

Caffeine intoxication is characterized by at least five (or more) of the following symptoms that develop following the consumption of caffeine:

- restlessness
- nervousness
- excitement
- insomnia
- flushed face
- diuresis
- gastrointestinal disturbance
- muscle twitching

- rambling flow of thought and speech

- psychomotor agitation

- tachycardia or cardiac arrhythmia

- periods of inexhaustibility

(American Psychiatric Association, 2000).

Most Americans consume some caffeine daily. Intoxication symptoms of rambling thoughts, psychomotor agitation, tachycardia, and arrhythmias usually occur at 1,000 mg or above, although symptoms may not be present if tolerance through repeated use has developed. Higher doses have produced ringing in the ears, flashing lights, severe headaches, and anxiety. Doses of 10,000 mg or more have resulted in grand mal seizures and respiratory failure, leading to death (usually seen in overdoses).

The *DSM-IV-TR* describes caffeine withdrawal as evidenced by the occurrence of marked fatigue or drowsiness, marked anxiety or depression, or nausea and/or vomiting following the abrupt cessation (or reduction) in caffeine intake. Symptoms may persist for 1 to 2 days after discontinuation.

Caffeine-induced sleep disorder typically produces insomnia at a dose-dependent effect (e.g., the higher the dose of caffeine, the worse the sleep problems). A client may experience insomnia secondary to caffeine, even when other symptoms of caffeine use (alertness, increased energy) are not present.

NICOTINE DEPENDENCE AND WITHDRAWAL

Increased interest has been shown in the past few years to the issue of nicotine use and dependence. Nicotine dependence can develop with all forms of tobacco and with prescription nicotine-withdrawal preparations (skin patch, gum). Nicotine dependence is associated with cardiovascular risk. Smoked nicotine (in the form of tobacco) is associated with diminished pulmonary function tests, cough, chronic obstructive pulmonary disease, lung and oral cancers, ulcers, and excessive skin wrinkling.

The *DSM-IV-TR* recognizes nicotine dependence and withdrawal as a major health problem. Criteria for nicotine withdrawal include:

1. Daily use of nicotine for at least several weeks.

2. Abrupt cessation or reduction, followed (within 24 hours) by at least four of the following symptoms:

    a. dysphoria or depressed mood

    b. insomnia

    c. irritability, frustration, or anger

    d. anxiety

    e. difficulty concentrating

    f. restlessness

    g. decreased heart rate

    h. increased appetite or weight gain.

3. The symptoms cause significant distress or impairment.

4. The symptoms do not occur due to a medical or other mental disorder.

Nursing Care of the Client with Nicotine Withdrawal

Withdrawal from nicotine, though uncomfortable, does not necessitate hospitalization. The reader is encouraged to review the six stages of change that an individual may experience discussed in Chapter 7 – a brief review of these stages follows. Precontemplation (stage 1) occurs when the client is not yet ready to change nor does he or she want to change. Reluctance, rebellion, resistance or rationalization may be present. During contemplation (stage 2), the individual is thinking about stopping smoking, but has not yet made a commitment to stop. The preparation and determination stage (stage 3) begins the process of research into support and treatment programs for the client. Once ready, a plan of action is put into place (stage 4). Clients should be educated as to the detrimental effects of nicotine use and then counseled on an ongoing basis to support efforts to stop. The use of nicotine transdermal skin patches, nicotine inhalers, and nicotine gums may assist in helping the client to overcome the smoking (or chewing) habit; the dosage of nicotine is gradually reduced at a later time. Another alternative is to set up a smoking schedule during which the client agrees to limit smoking to one cigarette an hour for several days, then one every 2 hours, and so forth, until discontinuing smoking entirely. Cognitive behavioral therapy is very beneficial; it helps the individual to recognize certain events or situations that trigger a desire to smoke, then to change those behaviors into actions that are less harmful. Maintenance of recovery (stage 5) can be extremely difficult and cigarette smokers may relapse repeatedly. Finally, termination occurs when the client no longer desires or even wants to be around cigarette smoking or any form of nicotine use (stage 6).

Two non-nicotine medications are now approved to assist in nicotine cessation. Zyban® (buproprion SR) is an antidepressant medication that acts by boosting the brain's natural dopamine and serotonin levels. This action reduces cravings for nicotine and helps to prevent relapse. Zyban® is the same product as Wellbutrin SR® and has the same precautions, which include a risk for increased agitation or suicidal thoughts (especially in adolescents) and a lowered seizure threshold. It is contraindicated in individuals with a history of epileptic or withdrawal seizures or with anorexia nervosa. Chantix® (varenicline) is a synthetic nicotine agonist that binds with nicotine receptors in the brain; thus, not allowing nicotine from tobacco products to be taken up by neurons. In effect, the person's brain is tricked into believing that he or she has already used tobacco. Over a period of several weeks, cravings are reduced and smoking cessation is facilitated. In individuals taking Chantix® in its research trials, 44% were able to stop smoking within 12 weeks, as opposed to 18% taking a placebo. However, Chantix® has demonstrated some significant post-trial psychiatric side effects

to be monitored, including agitation, mania, depression, increased psychosis or suicidality, which has led to a Black Box Warning in its package insert about the possibility of these symptoms. More common side effects to Chantix® include nausea, vomiting, vivid or strange dreaming, sleep problems, constipation, and bloating. Neither Zyban® nor Chantix® contain nicotine, so are not contraindicated in clients who are continuing to smoke intermittently; they also can be used in combination with nicotine patches, gum, or inhalers.

CASE STUDY: SUBSTANCE ABUSE AND WITHDRAWAL

Simon is a 40-year-old man with a long history of back problems. He worked as a bricklayer for 20 years and injured his back through repeated heavy lifting. The resultant back spasms caused him to be bedridden for days at a time. Simon's family physician placed him on the muscle relaxant cyclobenzaprine (Flexeril®) 10 mg four times per day and hydrocodone 5mg/acetaminophen 500 mg (Lortab® 5/500) tablets to take daily as needed. Simon had some initial pain relief, but soon found that the Lortab® stopped working. He increased his dose to every 4 hours, and then he started to take 2 tablets at a time. He quickly ran out and his physician refused to prescribe more, but offered him a referral to a pain management clinic. Feeling anxious, Simon called his dentist to report chronic pain secondary to an infected tooth. The dentist called in a prescription for oxycodone (Percocet®) until Simon could be seen. After getting the prescription, Simon cancelled the dental appointment. Soon he was taking up to 30 tablets of painkiller a day – some were his wife's old prescriptions and some were purchased from friends. Simon also made appointments with four different physicians to have his back pain evaluated. All of them gave him pain pills – some with 2 or 3 refills. When Simon was running out, he would go to the local emergency department and be given a meperidine (Demerol®) injection and oral prescriptions. This pattern of behavior continued despite family concerns, until Simon began vomiting and turned sallow in color. He was again taken to the emergency department, but this time his diagnosis was acute hepatitis secondary to acetaminophen overdosage. In the emergency department, Simon was given naltrexone (Narcan®) and had a nasogastric-tube placed for a stomach lavage. He was then hospitalized and placed on oral acetylcysteine (Mucomyst®) every 4 hours around the clock for 3 days twice daily with acetaminophen levels and daily liver enzymes. Simon reported feeling "like I've been hit by a Mack truck." He was tremulous and diaphoretic and alternated between chills and flushing. He experienced nausea, vomiting, diarrhea, muscle cramps, and back spasms so intense that he was in tears much of the first 2 days. After he became more medically stable, the physician prescribed pregabalin (Lyrica®) for his chronic pain and gave him some ibuprofen for generalized discomfort and trazodone (Desyrel®) to aid in sleep. On discharge, a referral was made to a pain clinic, where Simon received physical therapy, combined with steroid injections, topical analgesics (lidocaine patches), heat, massage, and education regarding the importance of activity and weight loss to reduce his pain.

Questions

1. What was the substance to which this client became addicted and how was this demonstrated?

2. What was the purpose for the drug naltrexone (Narcan®) given in the emergency room?

3. What were the withdrawal symptoms experienced by this client?

Discussion

Simon became physically dependent on opioids. He developed tolerance and required increased dosages to achieve the same desired effect,

he engaged in irrational drug-seeking behaviors that included lying and manipulation, and he experienced acute withdrawal symptoms when the opioids were withdrawn. Naltrexone (Narcan®) is a potent opioid antagonist that effectively displaces the opioid from the receptor neuron. Signs of opioid withdrawal include chills, shaking, diaphoresis (sweating), nausea, tremors, gastrointestinal distress, body aches, muscle cramps and insomnia similar to a flu (but with no, or only a low grade, fever).

NURSING CARE PLAN: OPIOID DEPENDENT CLIENT

Problem Listing

- Chronic pain
- Inadequate coping responses to deal with pain
- Opioid withdrawal symptoms
- Insomnia
- Potential for injury
- Drug-seeking behaviors

Priority Nursing Diagnosis

Ineffective coping with chronic pain as evidenced by drug-seeking behaviors and opioid addiction.

Long-term Goal

Client will successfully utilize more adaptive means of dealing with chronic pain, without the use of addictive substances.

Short-term Objectives

1. Client will verbalize an understanding of the dangers of overuse of prescribed medications.

2. Client will report a decrease in pain to a level that does not interfere with the enjoyment of life and daily activities.

3. Client will attend narcotics anonymous support groups at least once a week.

Nursing Interventions

1. Educate the client and family as to the processes of addiction (tolerance, dependency, withdrawal).

2. Assess clients level of readiness to change, based on the Stage of Change model.

3. Utilize motivational interviewing to address client's level of readiness to change.

4. Help the client to develop a list of pros and cons to using opioids to treat his pain.

5. Discuss with the client alternative pain management techniques that may be useful, including heat, massage, gentle exercise, and stretching.

6. Assist the client in scoring or rating pain on a scale of 1 to 10, so that the client can better communicate how it feels to healthcare providers (and himself).

7. Assist the client in identifying and listing diversional activities to use at home.

8. Teach the client various relaxation techniques to be utilized when the pain level is increasing, prior to seeking out medication relief.

9. Provide resources for the client's use in eliminating opioid dependence.

10. Monitor and support the client's avoidance of opioids.

ADVANCED PRACTICE NURSING: DEALING WITH A DRUG-SEEKING CLIENT

Advanced practice nurses are in a unique position to be able to manage a client's detoxification and recovery, utilizing such therapeutic principles as Motivational Interviewing and Stages of Change Models. Prescribing APRNs working with clients who have addictive behaviors must be vigilant about the possibility of drug diversion or misuse of prescriptions. Clients may not be completely aware that their behaviors are inappro-

priate when they are so entrenched in an addictive lifestyle. An example is the relatively common practice of sharing medications, such as giving pills to friends that are in pain or nervous, without consideration that this could be potentially dangerous or could trigger drug interactions in the other person. Some medications have a wide therapeutic index, whereas other medications can be very dangerous if taken in excess (such as tricyclic antidepressants). Prescription drug combinations of anxiolytics, opioid pain medications, and hypnotics for sleep are a potentially lethal combination. APRNs who prescribe controlled substances (laws vary on this state to state) may want to consider utilizing prescription contracts with clients. Most clinicians are very strict about authorizing early refills or dealing with reported lost prescriptions. Police reports may be required for claims of stolen medications. Some states have internet-based controlled substance registries. For example, Indiana has a program called INSPECT that records all controlled substance use (data is provided by pharmacies) that includes prescriber, pharmacy, and the, medication dispensed including the amount given and date. This program is accessible to the prescriber and the pharmacist for checking on clients for whom substance abuse is suspected.

SUMMARY

Substance abuse and dependence is present in over 8% of American society. Marijuana is the most popularly used substance overall. Other drugs used include cocaine, methamphetamine, and khat; hallucinogens such as LSD and psilocybin; ecstasy; heroin; inhalants; and prescription drugs. Opioid abuse has increased dramatically since 2002 and now accounts for a significant portion of hospital drug abuse admissions. Nicotine and caffeine are legal, but are also habituating; individuals develop tolerance, increasing use, and withdrawal symptoms. Each product of abuse has its own signs of intoxication and withdrawal, some more painful and difficult than others. Substance abuse and intoxication are costly; for example, in terms of lost wages and increased health care costs. Other costs are not as obvious and may include family conflicts, family violence, poor parenting (neglect, abuse, failure to protect children from harm), poor living circumstances, and a lack of productive participation in society. Nursing care plans for clients with substance dependence disorders often focus on maintaining safety for the client and others; evaluating for comorbid health conditions such as cardiac arrhythmias (amphetamines or cocaine); assessing for psychiatric complications, such as depression, panic levels of anxiety, suicidal thoughts, paranoia or other forms of psychosis; administering medications to treat symptoms of withdrawal; educating the client and family on the process of addictions and on specific drugs; teaching relaxation techniques; and working with the client in a non-judgmental manner to promote and enable more positive behaviors and coping skills.

EXAM QUESTIONS

CHAPTER 8
Questions 45-51

Note: Choose the one option that BEST answers each question.

45. Which of the following is an oral opioid that is prone to abuse and addiction?

    a. Buproprion (Wellbutrin)

    b. Clonidine (Catapres)

    c. Naltrexone (Narcan)

    d. Oxycodone (Oxycontin)

46. One indication of substance dependence (as opposed to abuse) is that the client

    a. becomes intoxicated every weekend.

    b. demonstrates a need for increasing amounts of the substance to achieve intoxication.

    c. maintains a full-time job while using marijuana every evening.

    d. uses an amphetamine to stay awake and study for an exam.

47. An excess of amphetamines may cause

    a. stupor and coma.

    b. paranoid delusions and hallucinations.

    c. orthostatic hypotension.

    d. bradycardia and respiratory depression.

48. A safety concern during cocaine or amphetamine withdrawal is

    a. patient education.

    b. excessive sleepiness.

    c. malnutrition.

    d. suicide risk due to rebound depression.

49. Hallucinogens cause the following CNS responses:

    a. dilated pupils, perceptual distortions, and sense of unreality.

    b. euphoria, increased energy, and hyperactivity.

    c. sluggishness, slowed hand-eye coordination, and ataxia.

    d. improved concentration, increased alertness, and insomnia.

50. *Tommy, a 12-year-old boy, comes to the healthcare facility for complaints of headaches, dizziness, and nosebleeds. He is noted to be staring off into space and he frequently answers questions with, "Huh?" or "What?" Tommy's mother is afraid he may have a brain tumor because he has had problems recently with forgetfulness and poor grades at school. While checking his blood pressure, you notice a faint chemical odor.*

    Your nursing assessment should consider that Tommy

    a. may have a brain tumor and an MRI is needed.

    b. may have diabetes and the odor is from ketoacidosis.

    c. may be abusing inhalants and a substance abuse evaluation is necessary.

    d. has poor hygiene and his mother is being overly dramatic and attention seeking.

continued on next page

51. Characteristics of nicotine withdrawal are

   a. sluggishness and respiratory depression.

   b. decreased appetite, nausea, and vomiting.

   c. muscle aches, lacrimation, and tremors.

   d. irritability, frustration, and anger.

CHAPTER 9

MAJOR DEPRESSION AND RELATED DISORDERS

CHAPTER OBJECTIVE

At the end of this chapter the reader will be able to describe symptoms of depressive disorders and relevant treatment modalities, including therapy and medications.

LEARNING OBJECTIVES

At the end of this chapter, the reader will be able to

1. describe the symptoms of depression.

2. differentiate major depression from other types of depressive disorders.

3. discuss antidepressant medications and their side effects.

INTRODUCTION

The Centers for Disease Control and Prevention (CDC), a branch of the Department of Health and Human Services, reported in 2008 that 1 in 20 persons 12 years of age and older have depression, with rates highest between 40 and 59 years of age (7.3%), in women (6.7%), and in African-Americans (8.0%). In individuals living at or below the poverty level, rates of depression in those between 40 and 59 years old go up to 22.4%. Depression is second only to hypertension as the most common chronic condition encountered in healthcare settings. Depression can lead to signifi-

cant impairments in functionality, with 35% of men and 22% of women reporting difficulties with getting things done at work, getting things done at home, or getting along with other people. Despite the problems experienced with depression, only 29% of individuals with mild to moderate symptoms reported seeking services from a qualified mental health provider. This number went up to 39% for severe depression symptoms (Pratt & Brody, 2008). Despite its relatively high prevalence rate (up to 10% in the United States), depression continues to be stigmatized in our culture, unless a person is perceived as having a good reason to be depressed (such as the loss of a job or death of a family member). Current psychiatric theories on the causes of depression certainly take into consideration environmental stressors; however, neurobiological changes in the brain (particularly involving the transmitters serotonin and norepinephrine) have a significant impact on the severity and treatment responses of the disorder. A family history of depression is a major risk factor in the development of the disorder.

Mortality associated with depression is significant. In 2004, suicide was the 11th leading cause of death in the United States (National Institute of Mental Health, 2009). Rates in males are nearly four times the rates in females. Suicide is highest in persons with a diagnosis of depression and depression accompanied by substance abuse. Suicide risk is highest in men who are older than 65 years of age, particularly if they are single, divorced, separated, or widowed. Suicide tends to be higher in white males, with severe physical illness a contributing factor. Rates are second highest in American Indian and Alaskan Native populations, followed in descending order by Hispanics, Asian Americans and Pacific Islanders, and African Americans (despite higher rates of depression overall). Women are more likely to take poison or a drug overdose to commit suicide, and men are more likely to use firearms. Intentional death by suffocation is approximately equal between genders. Panic attacks and severe anxiety symptoms are also associated with increased suicides.

Five commonly recognized forms of depression will be discussed in this chapter: major depression disorder, dysthymic disorder, seasonal affective disorder, premenstrual dysphoric disorder, and postpartum depression. Antidepressant medications will be reviewed, and a case study with nursing care plan is provided.

MAJOR DEPRESSION DISORDER

Major depression is characterized by either a loss of interest or pleasure in nearly all activities or a significantly depressed or irritable mood that lasts for at least 2 weeks. Children and adolescents tend to experience grouchiness and irritability much more frequently than overt sadness. Table 9-1 provides *DSM-IV-TR* criteria for major depression.

The symptoms must cause clinically significant distress for the client and interfere with functioning in social or family, academic, or occupational areas. Major depression cannot be diagnosed during an expected course of bereavement, unless the symptoms persist for longer than 2 months or are accompanied by marked impairments, morbid pre-

occupations, suicidal thoughts, psychosis, or severe psychomotor retardation.

The moods associated with major depression are often described as hopeless or feeling as if "in a black hole." Occasionally, individuals report feeling numb or without emotion. Children may say that they never really feel happy or that they think the family would be better off if they had never been born. Clients appear to stop caring about hobbies or social interactions, including with loved ones. Mild to moderate depression may stimulate the appetite in some clients and cause weight gain. Severe depression almost always results in a loss of appetite or complaints that food tastes funny or is without taste. Typical sleep disturbances with depression consist of normal to slightly delayed onset of sleep, followed by middle of the night wakening. Some experience an increase in need and duration of sleep (hypersomnia). Sleep is described as not restful and children may report nightmares or be found wandering about the house. Fatigue and poor energy is pronounced. Thought changes include ruminations, obsessions, poor concentration, impaired decision-making abilities, worry, guilt and, occasionally, psychosis. A phenomenon known as *pseudodementia* may occur during the course of a depression, particularly in older clients. Pseudodementia is the rapid onset of memory and concentration problems accompanying depression that may cause others to think that the client is developing a dementia disorder.

Psychotic symptoms including hallucinations, delusional beliefs, or gross disorganization can also occur in major depression. Clients who have psychotic symptoms during an episode of depression have a poorer prognosis than those who do not, and the symptoms may be indicative of the development of a bipolar disorder (especially when the symptoms are present in young children). The reader is referred to Chapter 10 for a more in-depth discussion of bipolar disorder. Clients with psychotic depression must be treated aggressively with

TABLE 9-1: CRITERIA FOR MAJOR DEPRESSION		
The client must endorse a depressed mood (in adults) or an irritable mood (in children/adolescents); or a loss of interest and pleasure in most activities.		
The client must also endorse 4 or more of the following symptoms during a 2-week period:	YES	NO
Weight loss (without dieting); Weight gain (more than 5%); or a significant change in appetite		
Insomnia or Hypersomnia		
Restlessness/agitation or slowing/retardation observable by others		
Fatigue or loss of energy		
Feelings of worthlessness or excessive guilt		
Difficulty concentrating or thinking clearly or indecisiveness		
Recurrent thoughts of death, suicidal ideation, or a suicide attempt		
(American Psychiatric Association, 2000)		

antidepressants and antipsychotics because of the increased risk of harm to self or others.

Certain medications and medical conditions may aggravate or trigger an episode of depression. Endocrine diseases, such as hypothyroidism or diabetes mellitus, can have a dramatic effect on moods and precipitate major depression, as can brain disorder, such as dementia, epilepsy, multiple sclerosis, cerebrovascular accidents, or tumors; infectious or inflammatory diseases; electrolyte disturbances; severe nutritional deficiencies; toxins, such as lead or other heavy metals, alcoholism and drug abuse. Many medications list depression as a possible side effect. Well-known problem medications include corticosteroids such as prednisone, birth control pills, opioid pain pills, and some antihypertensives. An acne medication, Accutane®, has been implicated in suicides of adolescents; however, clinical data has not yet been sufficient to have the FDA remove it from the market. Antimalarial agents such as chloroquine can sometimes precipitate depression or psychosis in susceptible individuals, with reports of suicide attempts and violence.

PSYCHOTHERAPY

Several psychotherapeutic models have been used in the treatment of depression. Until the advent of antidepressant medications in the 1950s, therapy was the sole treatment option. Clients could be depressed for periods of months to years. Today, therapy plus medication is the optimum management strategy. 80% to 90% of individuals with major depression can eventually achieve remission and return to their former levels of functioning (National Alliance on Mental Illness, 2006). Medication alone results in remission of symptoms in about 40% of cases, with another 20% to 30% achieving a 50% reduction in symptoms (Markley, 2008, p. 315). See Chapter 4 for a more complete discussion of counseling and therapy options, including complementary treatments.

MEDICATION INTERVENTIONS

Four broad categories of medications are utilized in the treatment of major depression: tricyclic antidepressants, monoamine oxidase inhibitors (MAOIs), selective serotonin reuptake inhibitors (SSRIs), and miscellaneous or combination agents. Three of the newer generation antipsychotics/mood stabilizers have now been approved for the adjunct treatment of depression or for depression associated with bipolar disorder. One "medical food" has been approved as an adjunct treatment for depression as well. Drug combinations may also be used to treat depression – most commonly, two antidepressants or an antidepressant plus a mood stabilizer. Tables 9-2 through 9-6 provide an overview of the most commonly prescribed antidepressants in these groups along with significant side effects or precautions. A general discussion of these medications follows.

Tricyclic Antidepressants

Tricyclic antidepressants (TCAs) were the first medications developed to treat depression. Imipramine (Tofranil®) was synthesized shortly after the antipsychotic chlorpromazine (Thorazine®) and it is similar in molecular structure and side effects. TCAs work by blocking the reuptake of the neurotransmitter monoamines norepinephrine and serotonin, thus prolonging their activity in the brain. TCAs have a number of side effects. Sedation can be pronounced in some clients. In low doses, TCAs are useful for their sedative actions but clients may report worsened daytime fatigue and lethargy. TCAs also stimulate appetite and can cause weight gain. CNS side effects include tremors, potentiation of other sedatives, and cognitive clouding. Confusion and disorientation may occur, particularly in older clients. Clients can also exhibit pseudoparkinsonism symptoms such as those seen with traditional antipsychotic medications.

TABLE 9-2: TRICYCLIC ANTIDEPRESSANTS

Generic Name	Trade Name(s)	Sedation	Weight Gain	Blood Pressure Changes	GI Upset	Dry Mouth Constipation Urinary Retention	Comments	Precautions for all Tricyclic Antidepressants
Amitriptyline	Elavil® Endep®	+++	+++	+++	–	+++	Useful in chronic pain	May cause Q-Tc cardiac conduction delays
Nortripyline	Pamelor® Aventyl®	++	++	++	–	+++		
Imipramine	Tofranil®	++	++	++	–	+++	Useful for enuresis	
Desipramine	Norpramin	++	++	++	–	+++	Derivative of nortriptyline	
Clomipramine	Anafranil®	++	++	++	–	+++	Useful for obsessive-compulsive disorder	
Doxepan	Sinequan®	+++	++	+++	–	+++	Sedating	

+++ High   ++ Moderate   + Low   – Negligible

TABLE 9-3: MONOAMINE OXIDASE INHIBITORS

Generic Name	Trade Name(s)	Sedation	Weight Gain	Blood Pressure Changes	GI Upset	Dry Mouth Constipation Urinary Retention	Comments	Precautions for all Monoamine Oxidase Inhibitors
Phenelzine	Nardil®	+	++	+++	–	+++		Dangerous drug-drug interactions
Tranylcypromine	Parnate®	+	++	+++	–	+++		
Isocarboxazid	Marplan®	+	++	+++	–	+++		Dangerous drug-food interactions
Moclobemide	Manerix®	+	++	++	–	+++	Less interaction with tyramine	
Selegeline	Emsam®	+	++	+++	–	+++	Transdermal skin patch	Risk for hypertensive crisis

+++ High   ++ Moderate   + Low   – Negligible

TABLE 9-4: SELECTIVE SEROTONIN INHIBITORS

Generic Name	Trade Name(s)	Sedation	Weight Changes	Blood Pressure Changes	GI Upset	Dry Mouth Constipation Urinary Retention	Comments	Precautions for all Selective Serotonin Inhibitorss
Fluoxetine	Prozac® Sarafem®	–	+	–	+	–	Approved for major depressive disorder in children & adolescents ages 8-18; Approved for obesessive-compulsive disorder in children & adolescents ages 7-17. Sarafem® & Prozac® Weekly are approved for adult use only.	Risk of increased suicidal thoughts and behaviors in children & adolescents.
Paroxetine	Paxil®	+	++	–	+	–		
Sertraline	Zoloft®	+	+	–	++	–	Approved for obsessive-compulsive disorder in children & adolescents ages 6-17.	
Citalopram	Celexa®	++	+	–	+	–		
Escitalopram	Lexapro®	–	–	–	+	–		

+++ High   ++ Moderate   + Low   – Negligible

TABLE 9-5: MISCELLANEOUS ANTIDEPRESSANTS

Primary Neurotransmitters	Generic Name	Trade Name(s)	Sedation	Weight Gain	Blood Pressure Changes	GI Upset	Dry Mouth Constipation Urinary Retention	Comments
Serotonin & Dopamine	Buproprion Buproprion SR	Wellbutrin® Wellbutrin SR® Wellbutrin XL® Zyban®	–	–	–	+	–	Contraindicated in seizure disorder, alcoholism, and anorexia nervosa Zyban® is for smoking cessation
Serotonin & Norepinephrine	Venlafaxine Venlafaxine XR	Effexor® Effexor XR®	–	+	++	+	–	More serotonin in low doses; more norepinephrine in higher doses
	Duloxetine	Cymbalta®	–	+	–	++	–	Also approved for pain in fibromyalgia and diabetic peripheral neuropathies
	Desvenlafaxine	Pristiq®	–	–	–	+	–	Not metabolized extensively in the liver
Miscellaneous	Mirtazapine	Remeron® Remeron SolTab®	+++	++	–	–	–	Moderately sedating SolTab is dissolvable
	Trazodone	Desyrel®	+++	++	–	–	–	Extremely sedating Often used off-label for sleep induction
"Medical Food"	L-methylfolate	Deplin®	–	–	–	+	–	Approved as an adjunct to antidepressants Equivalent to 52 mg folic acid

+++ High   ++ Moderate   + Low   – Negligible

TABLE 9-6: MOOD STABILIZERS APPROVED FOR ADJUNCT TREATMENT OF DEPRESSION

Generic Name	Trade Name(s)	Sedation	Weight Changes	Blood Pressure Changes	GI Upset	Dry Mouth Constipation Urinary Retention	Comments	Precautions for & Risks of all Medications
Aripiprazole	Abilify®	++	++	–	–	++	Approved in low doses as an adjunct treatment to antidepressants	Risk of hyperglycemia Risk of hyperlipidemia Risk of extrapyramidal syndrome or tardive dyskinesia Increased death when used in elderly clients with dementia
Quetiapine	Seroquel	+++	+++	++	–	++	Approved for depression in bipolar disorder at 300 mg, bipolar mania at 600 mg	
Olanzapine/ Fluoxetine	Sybyax®	+++	+++	–	+	++	Combination of Zyprexa® and Prozac® in each dose	

+++ High   ++ Moderate   + Low   – Negligible

Anticholinergic effects consist of dry mouth and eyes, urinary hesitancy, blurred vision, and slowing of the gastrointestinal (GI) tract leading to constipation. Cardiac and peripheral vascular effects can be pronounced with TCAs. Vasodilation can lead to orthostatic hypotension that is exhibited by dizziness, reflex tachycardia, and fainting. Delayed cardiac electrical conduction can lead to cardiac arrhythmias, including premature ventricular contractions and ventricular tachycardia. Several deaths in children taking TCAs have been reported because of arrhythmias. TCAs have a narrow therapeutic versus toxic range; monitoring serum levels is indicated. Other medications that are extensively metabolized in the same manner as TCAs (cytochrome P450, 2D6, 1A2 and 3A4 pathways) may have an additive effect and elevate blood levels of TCAs into a toxic range. Some of these medications include cimetidine (Tagamet®), fluoxetine (Prozac®), traditional antipsychotics, quinidine and other cardiac antiarrhythmics, levadopa, and some blood pressure medications. Using TCAs with monoamine oxidase inhibitors (MAOIs) is particularly dangerous.

TCAs should be used cautiously in clients who have a history of suicide attempts or who are currently suicidal because they are highly toxic in an overdose.

Monoamine Oxidase Inhibitors

MAOIs have been available almost as long as TCAs. Originally a derivative of the tuberculosis drug isoniazid, MAOIs work by inhibiting the enzyme that breaks down monoamines (serotonin and norepinephrine), thus making them more available in the brain. MAOIs are rarely used today because of extensive drug-to-drug and drug-to-food interactions. When MAOIs are taken in the presence of the amino acid tyramine (a product of tyrosine, which is a precursor to dopamine, norepinephrine, and epinephrine), the client may experience a hypertensive crisis with blood pressure readings upward of 210/120. Cerebrovascular accidents, from hemorrhaging, and death can occur. Foods that are high in tyramine levels are listed in Table 9-7. Drug interactions can be pronounced and the client should avoid all medications that have a

TABLE 9-7: FOODS HIGH IN TYRAMINE

Aged Cheeses and Milk
- Cheddar, blue, brie, mozzarella
- Sour cream
- Yogurt

Aged or Pickled Meats
- Bologna
- Liver
- Pickled herring
- Sardines
- Salami (luncheon meats)
- Most dried fish

Alcoholic Beverages
- Beer, alcohol-free beer
- Sherry wine
- Chianti wine

Fruits and Vegetables
- Bananas
- Figs
- Avocados
- Fava beans
- Sauerkraut

Miscellaneous
- Soy sauce
- Aged sauces
- Yeast
- Chocolate
- Licorice
- Caffeinated beverages

stimulant activity (including over-the-counter cold remedies), SSRIs, TCAs, and numerous antihypertensives. CNS depressants may be intensified in the presence of MAOIs. Less dangerous side effects of MAOIs are related to increased activation in the brain. Clients complain of jitteriness, hyperactivity, anxiety, agitation, restlessness, insomnia, and euphoria. A drop in blood pressure normally occurs with MAOIs; for some clients this can be significant. Other side effects include dry mouth, blurred vision, constipation, and urinary hesitancy.

Selective Serotonin Reuptake Inhibitors

SSRIs have been the medications of choice for treating depression since fluoxetine (Prozac®) was first introduced in 1986. SSRIs are effective and generally well tolerated by clients. They work by blocking the reuptake of serotonin (and other neurotransmitters to a lesser degree) in the brain's neurons. Most of them only require once a day dosing, and

serum levels are not necessary because of their relative safety in an overdose. SSRIs are mildly activating for most clients. Side effects include stimulation, insomnia, jitteriness, and stomach upset. Headaches and dizziness may occur. Some clients have sexual performance issues or decreased libido. Stimulants can potentiate the activating effects of SSRIs (including caffeine). A few of the SSRIs have mild antihistamine-like activity that causes them to be sedating, rather than stimulating, and to increase appetite (citalopram [Celexa®], paroxetine [Paxil®]). SSRIs are generally weight neutral – although some clients report a mild weight loss with fluoxetine (Prozac®) and weight gain with paroxetine (Paxil®) and sertraline (Zoloft®). SSRIs can have drug interactions with many other drugs – in general, they potentiate the activity of medications that are highly protein-bound (e.g., TCAs) or that are extensively metabolized by cytochrome P450 such as, benzodiazepines, antipsychotics, and some antihypertensives. A new SSRI, desvenlafaxine (Pristiq®), bypasses liver metabolism and is not affected by (nor does it affect) P450 enzyme metabolized drugs. Pristiq® is also helpful in clients with liver disease; however, it must be used in caution with clients who have renal disease.

Two serotonin-related syndromes have been identified: serotonin syndrome and serotonin withdrawal. Serotonin syndrome occurs when there is too much serotonin in the brain, which may be seen with certain drug interactions (MAOIs, St. John's Wort) or in an overdose situation. Symptoms include restlessness or agitation, muscle twitching or jerking, sweating, shivering, tremors, abdominal cramps, diarrhea, nausea, headaches, ataxia, and hypomania or confusion and agitation. Hospitalization may be necessary because deaths have been contributed to this syndrome. Treatment consists of stopping the medications and supporting the client with IV fluids. Symptoms usually resolve in 24 to 72 hours. Serotonin syndrome has occurred in clients taking medications with potent serotonergic activity in

TABLE 9-8: MEDICATIONS WITH SEROTONERGIC PROPERTIES AND THEIR INDICATIONS

Selective serotonin reuptake inhibitors, such as fluoxetine, paroxetine, and sertraline – antidepressants

Selective norepinephrine reuptake inhibitors, such as duloxetine, and venlafaxine – antidepressants

5-HT1 receptor agonists (Triptans), such as, sumatriptan (Imitrex®), and rizatriptan (Maxalt®) – migraines

Monoamine oxidase inhibitors, such as, phenelzine, tranylcypromine, and selegiline – antidepressants

Tricyclic antidepressants, such as, amitriptyline, doxepan, and imipramine – antidepressants

Dextromethorphan – "DM" or "Tuss" – cough medications

Amantadine (Symmetrel®) – anticholinergic for Parkinson's disease

Bromocriptine (Parlodel®) – antilactation

Buspirone (Buspar®) – anxiolytic

Meperidine (Demerol®) – acute pain management

Nefazodone (Serzone®) – antidepressant

Mirtazapine (Remeron®) - antidepressant

Tramadol (Ultram®) – chronic pain management

Sibutramine (Meridia®) – appetite suppressant

Phentermine (Adipex®) – appetite suppressant

Linezolid (Zyvox®) – antibiotic

Tryptophan – amino acid (nutritional)

Lithium (Eskalith®, Lithobid®) – antimanic

Amphetamines (various types) – central nervous system stimulant

Cocaine/LSD/MDMA (Ecstasy) – illegal drugs

St. John's Wort – herbal treatment for depression

(Indiana Medicaid Drug Utilization Review Board Newsletter, 2008)

combination with one another or with antidepressants. Table 9-8 provides a list of medications with serotonergic properties that should be used with caution in clients who are taking them in combination.

Serotonin withdrawal can occur when brain levels of serotonin are allowed to drop precipitously. Symptoms are described as flu-like, with dizziness, aching joints and muscles, a feeling of detachment, fatigue, and dizziness. Serotonin withdrawal occurs more predominantly with high-potency medications such as paroxetine and less with longer half-life products such as fluoxetine. Symptoms can be avoided by weaning off the medication over several days. Children rarely exhibit these problems. Serotonin withdrawal is uncomfortable, but not dangerous.

Miscellaneous Agents

Miscellaneous antidepressant agents are medications that have varied activity on neurotransmitters. Buproprion (Wellbutrin®, Wellbutrin SR®, Zyban®) is a selective dopamine reuptake inhibitor. It is low in side effects with stimulation or activation being the chief complaint of clients. Mild increases in heart rate may occur. The primary concern with buproprion is that it lowers the seizure threshold and may precipitate seizures in susceptible individuals. Buproprion should not be given to a client with epilepsy, an eating disorder, or during alcohol detoxification. Two interesting other actions of buproprion are that it reduces cravings (it's been approved for use in smoking cessation in the form of Zyban®) and it tends to increase libido (whereas SSRIs have a tendency to cause sexual dysfunction). Buproprion may be beneficial in treating attention-deficit problems as well.

Venlafaxine (Effexor®, Effexor XR®) is an antidepressant that acts like an SSRI in lower doses, but inhibits the reuptake of norepinephrine at higher doses. It is effective for chronic depression with an anxiety component. Side effects are low and primarily include GI upset. There have been some problems with venlafaxine elevating blood pressure in some clients, thus caution should be used in clients with primary hypertension. Desvenlafaxine (Pristiq®) was developed in 2008 to eliminate some of the variable dosing issues of venlafaxine. Pristiq® is given once a day in two dosage options and it is not metabolized extensively by the liver. This gives it the added benefits of being a safer option in clients with liver disease or alcoholism and lowers the risk of drug interactions with other medications metabolized in the liver.

Duloxetine (Cymbalta®) is an SSRI and SNRI with approximately equal effects on both of these neurotransmitter systems. It is approved for the treatment of major depression, generalized anxiety disorder, peripheral neuropathy associated with diabetes mellitus, and fibromyalgia. Duloxetine is one of the only antidepressants approved for these pain disorders in the absence of a mood or anxiety disorder. Primary side effects to duloxetine include dizziness, nausea and headache.

Nefazodone (Serzone®) and trazodone (Desyrel®) are serotonin reuptake inhibitors plus receptor blockers. They are both good for depression that is associated with anxiety and insomnia. Trazodone is extremely sedating at therapeutic doses, so its usefulness is often limited to an adjunct treatment for depression-related insomnia. Trazodone can also cause the unusual side effect of priapism, which is a painful and persistent penile erection. Surgical intervention has been needed in some men. Nefazodone is well tolerated but has a number of drug-to-drug interactions, along with a Black Box Warning of the risk of hepatic failure. A small percentage of clients cannot metabolize nefazodone well, and they experience a serotonin-like syndrome at low doses or even with the initial dose. Nefazodone is rarely used because of these problems.

Mirtazapine (Remeron®, Remeron SolTab®) works by blocking the feedback mechanisms for regulating serotonin and norepinephrine, thereby increasing their levels. It also has potent antihistamine activity. It is effective for insomnia and weight loss related to depression. Side effects other than sedation are quite low. Remeron SolTab® is a rapidly dissolving formulation that disintegrates on the tongue in less than 30 seconds. It is extremely useful in the extended-care facility setting.

Adjunctive Medication Treatment

Adjunctive antidepressant medication treatment may be needed when a single agent is insufficient. Clinicians may prescribe two antidepressants from different categories to target the brain chemistry in as many ways as possible. Several new-generation antipsychotics/mood stabilizers have been approved for the treatment of depression as an adjunct to antidepressants (aripiprazole [Abilify®]) or for depression in bipolar disorder (quetiapine [Seroquel®], Symbyax®). An antipsychotic such as ziprasidone (Geodon®) can be helpful for severely treatment-resistant clients due to its potent serotonin activity. Mood stabilizers (covered in Chapter 10) may be used adjunctively, which include lithium carbonate, lamotrigine (Lamictal®), and valproic acid (Depakote®). CNS depressants such as benzodiazepines may provide short-term anxiety relief, but excess use will result in cognitive dulling and potentially worsened depression. Sedative-hypnotic medications are commonly prescribed for insomnia in depressed clients. There has been some research into the adjunctive use of modafinil (Provigil®), a CNS stimulant indicated for narcolepsy, fatigue associated with obstructive sleep apnea, or shift-work sleep disorder. It may have some usefulness for clients with depression who have responded to antidepressant medications but still complain of daytime fatigue and lethargy. One "medical food" exists that is approved by the FDA for the adjunctive treatment of depression. L-methylfolate (Deplin®) acts as a regulator of a co-factor for trimonoamine neurotransmitter synthesis. This co-factor boosts the antidepressant actions of known medications. Deplin® is a highly concentrated form of folic acid.

Most folic acid supplements are 1 mg. Pregnant women are recommended to take 4 to 5 mg daily. Deplin® is approximately equivalent to 52 mg of folic acid.

DYSTHYMIC DISORDER

A dysthymic disorder is characterized as a chronically depressed mood nearly every day for over 2 years. Children may be irritable rather than sad, and the duration requirement is only 1 year. While depressed, at least two of the following other symptoms are present: poor appetite or overeating, increased sleep or insomnia, low energy or fatigue, low self-esteem, poor concentration or difficulty in making decisions, and feelings of hopelessness. Clients with dysthymic disorder are often self-critical and may see themselves as uninteresting. Dysthymic disorder is differentiated from major depression in that the intensity is less severe; the client may still be able to function in social, occupational, or academic areas; and there are no suicidal thoughts or urges. Dysthymic disorder is not diagnosed if there is a history of mania or if the symptoms are associated with a psychotic disorder, substance abuse, a general medical condition, or a side effect of a medication.

Treatment for dysthymic disorder consists primarily of counseling (cognitive behavioral techniques in particular) and antidepressant medications. SSRIs and miscellaneous agents are preferable because of their lower occurrence of side effects.

SEASONAL AFFECTIVE DISORDER

Seasonal affective disorder (SAD) is a depression that occurs primarily through the winter months. It tends to be more like a dysthymic disorder in severity; however, it may reach the level of major depression, especially if there is a history of depressive disorders in clients or their families.

SAD appears to be related to the hormone melatonin, which is produced by the body in response to sunlight. When melatonin levels are low, depression can result. The disorder is more prominent in the northern countries, and it occurs more frequently in women.

Treatment for SAD may include antidepressant medications, but clients may also choose to utilize full-spectrum light exposure through the use of special light bulbs designed for this purpose.

PREMENSTRUAL DYSPHORIC DISORDER

The criteria for a premenstrual dysphoric disorder (PMDD) are marked depressive moods, anxiety, and irritability, with a decreased interest in activities, that regularly occurs during the week prior to the onset of menses and is relieved when menses begins. The symptoms must be significant enough to interfere with functioning (work, school, and other activities) and must be completely remitted for at least a week after the menstrual cycle. PMDD seems to be associated with the sex hormones, in particular the rising progesterone phase of the menstrual cycle.

Initial treatment for PMDD may be the utilization of birth control pills or hormone replacement therapy to try and balance the estrogen and progesterone levels. If hormones are ineffective, poorly tolerated, or the client does not want to take them, then SSRI antidepressants are helpful. Fluoxetine, in particular, has been shown to be effective in treating PMDD, and it is marketed under the name Sarafem® specifically for this purpose.

POSTPARTUM DEPRESSION

Depression with a postpartum onset usually occurs in the client within 4 weeks of the birth of the child but it can be delayed if depression becomes more serious. Postpartum "blues" are relatively common; however, postpartum depression is significantly more serious and may have an impact on the safety of the mother and infant. Postpartum depression occurs in about 10% of newly delivered mothers. Infanticide can occur as a result of postpartum depression with psychosis; afterward, mothers have reported that they believed their children to be possessed by demons, or that the children were doomed from the beginning. Postpartum depression with psychosis occurs in 1 in every 500 to 1,000 deliveries, usually within 2-weeks of delivery (Mayo Clinic Staff, 2008). Women with a history of major depression or previous postpartum depression are at the highest risk (30% to 50%) (American Psychiatric Association, 2000). Other behaviors toward the infant that are seen during episodes of postpartum depression may include disinterest, fearfulness of being left alone with the baby, anxiety, panic attacks, or overly-intrusive behaviors (such as waking the baby frequently). Prolonged depression in a new mother may be associated with problems in bonding with the child.

Treatment for postpartum depression starts with prenatal education. Expectant mothers and their families need to know that this is a real medical condition, and they need to be informed as to the symptoms that may be experienced (see criteria for major depression). If depression occurs, the mothers should be encouraged to seek treatment immediately, which may consist of a combination of therapy and antidepressant medications. Antipsychotics should be utilized for any psychotic symptoms. If the mother refuses to take medications, serious consideration should be made as to the safety of leaving the child in the home.

Clients with a history of major depression or postpartum depression should probably initiate antidepressant treatment during the third trimester of pregnancy. A study of 86 children (Nulman et al., 2002) looked at child development following prenatal exposure to both TCAs and fluoxetine and found that there were no significant deficits in cognition, language development, or the temperament of the children of mothers who took these medications. In fact, untreated depression in mothers was associated with less cognitive and language achievement in the children. Recommendations were that antidepressants be provided when needed during pregnancy.

NURSING INTERVENTIONS FOR CLIENTS EXPERIENCING DEPRESSIVE DISORDERS

Symptoms of depression affect nearly every body system, social relationship, and even an individual's personal sense or spirituality. Nursing care must be planned to take into consideration the whole client. Physical care may include treatment interventions to help alleviate insomnia or a loss of appetite. Diet education and nutritional supplements may be recommended. Clients who are depressed may not care for other medical conditions; therefore, a thorough evaluation of these is necessary. Activities of daily living as basic as bathing and brushing one's teeth may be ignored by the severely depressed client. It is important to assist in structuring the client's day to try to maintain some contact with others and some degree of cognitive stimulation. Safety should be assessed because suicide risk and the incidence of other self-harm behaviors can be extremely high. It may be necessary to initiate an emergency detention and hospitalize a client who refuses treatment and is expressing suicidal ideation because hopelessness may cause the client to feel that there is nothing that can be done to help. Supporting and educating families is equally important. Depression can be very stressful on a family, and suicide is devastating. Significant others should be educated that depression is a medical disorder and that there is effective treatment available. Family counseling may be necessary. Clients with depression who are employed may have medical leave benefits which help ease some of the financial pressures experienced by the family. Spiritual support, in the form of encouraging usual religious practices, can be helpful. Every effort should be made to allow hospitalized clients access to clergy, if they so desire.

CASE STUDY: MAJOR DEPRESSION

Debra is a 54-year-old woman with no significant mental health history. She recently saw her family physician for vague complaints of fatigue, restlessness, and insomnia, which she felt were attributed to "going through the change." Her physician recommended light exercise and a hormone replacement medication. One week later, Debra's husband noted that she no longer had any desire to go places with him and she seemed listless and apathetic. Her sleep problems worsened and she found herself waking at 2:00 or 3:00 a.m. and unable to return to sleep. Her appetite started to decrease and she frequently "forgot" to make the family's evening meal while complaining of exhaustion. Debra started experiencing intense headaches nearly every day, causing her to always keep the curtains drawn and the lights low. Her symptoms exacerbated rapidly following the death of her favorite cat from old age. She began crying uncontrollably and refused to go out in public. Her husband noticed that she was in the house either pacing in an agitated, purposeless manner or she was staring off into space; even television could no longer distract her. Over the course of a month, she lost 15 lb. She started to talk to her husband about "the hereafter" and what to do with her possessions "once I am gone." He insisted she see a therapist who immediately referred Debra for an evaluation with a psychiatric APRN. The APRN obtained a thorough history to rule out any concomitant illnesses or drug or alcohol abuse, and ordered some baseline laboratory tests, including a thyroid panel. The tests showed only a mild dehydration, but were otherwise normal. She then prescribed escitalopram (Lexapro®) 10 mg once daily for depression and as needed temazepam (Restoril®) 15 mg at night for insomnia. The therapist continued to work with Debra to teach her some cognitive strategies to deal with day-to-day stressors. Debra reported an improved mood and sleep within a week. By the fourth week, her husband stated she was "nearly back to herself." At the end of 6 weeks, Debra felt "normal" again and was able to terminate therapy, but agreed to continue taking the antidepressant. She no longer needed the sleeping medication.

Questions

1. What were the symptoms of depression demonstrated by this client?

2. Why did the APRN order a thyroid panel?

3. What type of medication is escitalopram (Lexapro®)?

Discussion

Depression has numerous characteristic symptoms that can help to make the diagnosis. Early symptoms may include fatigue, restlessness, and insomnia. Appetite changes are common. Some clients experience physical aches and pains. Clients have difficulty with concentration or focus and may be agitated. In more severe phases, recurrent thoughts of death or dying can occur. Hypothyroidism may mimic depression, with both disorders having low energy, fatigue, and sluggishness as symptoms. Thyroid levels should be checked in any client with suspected major depression. Escitalopram (Lexapro®) is a SSRI that is indicated for the treatment of major depression and generalized anxiety disorder.

NURSING CARE PLAN: CLIENT WITH MAJOR DEPRESSION

Problem Listing

- Fatigue
- Dysmenorrhea
- Insomnia
- Weight loss
- Crying episodes
- Impaired decision-making
- Changes in activities of daily living
- Hopelessness
- Suicidal thoughts
- Altered family relationships
- Poor concentration
- Socially isolating self

Priority Nursing Diagnosis

Self-care deficit related to persistent depressed mood, as evidenced by fatigue, hopelessness, poor hygiene, and social isolation.

Long-term Goal

Client will return to her previous functioning level.

Short-term Objectives

1. Client will not remain in bed all day.
2. Client will resume previous activities with husband (e.g., flea markets) within 2 weeks.
3. Client will resume household responsibilities (e.g., cooking meals) within 2 weeks.

Nursing Interventions

1. Assist the client in making a daily living schedule and post this in a prominent place in the home.
2. Help the client and her husband to identify places to go for diversional recreation no less than twice a week.
3. Provide medication education to the client and her husband.
4. Assist the client in evaluating sleep patterns and develop a sleep hygiene plan (e.g., reduced caffeine, getting up at the same time every day, hour of sleep sedatives) to facilitate improved sleeping patterns.
5. Instruct the client to engage in 20 to 30 minutes of brisk walking daily (preferably outdoors if the weather is permitting).
6. Instruct the client in a healthy diet with plenty of fruits and vegetables. Daily multivitamins can be recommended.
7. Encourage the client to continue her regular church attendance.

ADVANCED PRACTICE NURSING: MEDICATION MANAGEMENT OF TREATMENT-RESISTANT DEPRESSION (THE TEXAS MEDICATION ALGORITHM PROJECT)

Approximately 60% of people respond positively to the first antidepressant they are given; the remaining 40% have intolerable side effects or don't find the medication to be effective. Beginning in 1995, the state of Texas, in collaboration with a number of pharmaceutical companies and the University of Texas, implemented the Texas Medication Algorithm Project (TMAP), which looked at treatment recommendations and medication decision trees for a number of psychiatric illnesses, including depression. Published In 2008, the *TMAP procedural manual: Major depressive disorder algorithms* became available through their Web site (http://www.dshs.state.tx.us/mh programs/pdf.TIMA_MDD_Manual_0806 08.pdf). Some general clinical management strategies include treating the client with medications that are best tolerated (as opposed to most cost-effective) to increase adherence and compliance to the medication, providing medication at adequate dosages over sufficient periods of time, and treating for a minimum of 6 to 9 months to achieve remission (Suehs et al., 2008).

TMAP medication treatment indicates that the client should initially be given any one of the SSRIs, SNRIs, or the miscellaneous drugs buproprion or mirtazapine, presented earlier in this chapter, for a period of 4 to 6 weeks. Partial responders should have augmentation with another one of the drugs within that group but not in the same family (i.e., fluoxetine and buproprion; escitalopram and mirtazapine) or with buspirone (Buspar®) or thyroid supplementation. Non-responders should be cross-titrated over to a different drug within that group and given another month to respond. If the client is still significantly depressed, then such strategies as changing to an MAOI, using combination SSRI/SNRI or miscellaneous drugs, adding a tricyclic antidepressant, or adding lithium, buspirone, or a dopamine agonist (Abilify®) to the initial antidepressant should be considered. Clients who are still not responding may be given antipsychotic medications first and then referred for ECT or a VNS implant. VNS implants typically augment medication therapy for clients who are severely treatment resistant. Psychotherapy is indicated for all clients (Suehs et al., 2008).

SUMMARY

Major depression is a serious illness that can be disabling to the individual, devastating for a family, and lead to death by suicide if left untreated. Societal costs, for example, because of lost wages and decreased productivity, are extremely high. Depression may be related to circadian rhythms (seasonal affective disorder), pregnancy and delivery (post-partum depression), menstrual cycles (premenstrual dysphoric disorder), or it may occur at a lower, more chronic level (dysthymic disorder). Depression is familial and may have some genetic origins as yet to be determined. Environmental events or trauma may activate or trigger an episode of depression, or there may be no discernible cause. If possible, the treatment of depression always includes some component of therapy, especially in cases of first onset, childhood or post-partum depression, or severe impairment. Complementary treatments may be recommended, including the use of full-spectrum sun lights, herbal remedies (St. John's Wort), exercise, and diet. Medications are almost always effective in reducing depression symptoms within 6 weeks. The primary neurotransmitters involved in depression alleviation appear to be serotonin and norepinephrine, with lesser effects from dopamine promoting agents. Concomitant treatment may also be indicated, including anxiolytics or sleep aides. Nursing care of clients who are depressed should focus on safety (preventing suicide), sleep and nutrition support, promoting regular activities of daily living, and psychosocial assistance.

EXAM QUESTIONS

CHAPTER 9
Questions 52-57

Note: Choose the one option that BEST answers each question.

52. Significant symptoms of depression include

    a. mood changes, fatigue, and sleep and appetite disturbances.

    b. euphoria, restlessness, and irrational spending sprees.

    c. agitation, confusion, and bizarre or unusual behaviors.

    d. paranoid delusions and reports of persistent hallucinations.

53. Tricyclic antidepressants

    a. are the current medications of choice in the treatment of depression.

    b. have few side effects.

    c. are not sedating.

    d. can cause serious cardiac arrhythmias.

54. Selective serotonin reuptake inhibitors and selective norepinephrine reuptake inhibitors

    a. have numerous dangerous side effects.

    b. are the current pharmacological treatment of choice.

    c. can cause significant cardiac arrhythmias.

    d. have a high risk for drug-food interactions.

55. Dysthymia in adult clients is a depressive disorder characterized by

    a. chronic symptoms of depression lasting over 2 years.

    b. short-term depressive episodes lasting a few months.

    c. symptoms of suicidal ideation or self-injury.

    d. cyclic mood changes corresponding with the weather.

56. Depression that occurs in the winter but remits in the summer is called

    a. seasonal affective disorder.

    b. major depression.

    c. dysthymic disorder.

    d. bipolar depression.

57. Postpartum depression usually occurs

    a. immediately after delivery.

    b. 1 week after delivery.

    c. in the first 4 weeks after delivery.

    d. several months after delivery.

CHAPTER 10

BIPOLAR SPECTRUM DISORDERS

CHAPTER OBJECTIVE

At the end of this chapter the reader will be able to discuss symptoms of bipolar spectrum disorders and appropriate nursing care and medication treatment.

LEARNING OBJECTIVES

At the end of this chapter, the reader will be able to

1. describe symptoms of bipolar disorder.

2. discuss mood stabilizing medications and their side effects.

3. describe nursing interventions for the client with mania.

INTRODUCTION

Bipolar disorders have been recognized since Emile Kraepelin first developed his classification and labeling system in the late 1800s. Descriptions of elevated and expansive moods, alternating with periods of sluggishness or lethargy were described, along with stationary or fundamental non-impairing baseline states. Kraepelin called these disorders "manic-depressive," a term that persisted until the *DSM-IV* revision in 1994, when the name was changed to bipolar disorder. The prevalence of bipolar spectrum disorders is between 1% and 5% in the general population. Bipolar II disorder has not been well described and there actually may be more cases than previously recognized. Depression is often the presenting symptom in bipolar II disorder, with diagnosing delays of up to 12 years and a history of three to four different psychiatric consultations before the disorder is recognized. Bipolar disorder NOS (not otherwise specified) is often used to describe mood instability and atypical symptoms of bipolar disorder in children and adolescents. Bipolar I disorder is more clearly recognizable by clinicians because the symptom presentation is often overt mania that may not be associated with psychosis. Bipolar spectrum disorders have a familial association: First-degree relatives have rates of bipolar I disorder from 4% to 24%, and of bipolar II disorder from 1% to 5%, suggesting a strong genetic component in these disorders (American Psychiatric Association, 2000). The causes for bipolar spectrum disorders are unclear but they are believed to be related to an imbalance of chemicals in the brain called neurotransmitters.

Substance abuse is common in clients with bipolar disorders, at approximately 68% in those with bipolar I disorder and 48% in those with bipolar II disorder. These substance abuse rates are higher than in clients with schizophrenia (47%), major depression (27%), or anxiety (24%) (Vornik and Brown, 2007).

DIAGNOSIS OF BIPOLAR DISORDER

Mania

To be diagnosed with a bipolar disorder, the client must demonstrate manic, hypomanic, or mixed manic/depressive moods, alternating between periods of depression. Some clients may report that they have never felt depressed, though this is unusual. Symptoms of mania are listed in Table 10-1.

TABLE 10-1: SYMPTOMS OF MANIA IN BIPOLAR DISORDER
1. The individual must have a period of abnormal and elevated, expansive, or irritable mood lasting at least 1 week (or less if hospitalization is required).
2. Three or more of the following symptoms must be present (four if the mood is predominantly depressed): a. inflated self-esteem or grandiosity. b. reduced need for sleep (3 to 4 hours or even none at all for days). c. pressured speech or talkativeness. d. racing thoughts or flight-of-ideas. e. distractibility. f. increased activity (either goal-directed or purposeless). g. high-risk behaviors (e.g., sexual indiscretions, spending sprees, bizarre business investments).
(American Psychiatric Association, 2000)

The manic symptoms must be significant enough to cause impairment in functioning (social relationships, work situations, or school settings). Manic symptoms also may not be associated with, or the result of, substance abuse (e.g., amphetamines or cocaine), a general medical condition (e.g., hyperthyroidism or adrenal gland tumor), or with medications (e.g., corticosteroids or antimalarials).

Hypomania

The symptoms of hypomania are essentially the same as for mania, but to a lesser degree and is commonly seen in clients with bipolar II disorder. The client must have a period of persistently elevated, expansive, or irritable moods that last at least 4 days and that are a distinct change from baseline moods and behavior. Three or more of the criterion-2 symptoms listed in Table 10-1 must be present (four if the mood is predominantly irritable). The changes in moods and behaviors have to be easily recognized by others, but they cannot be severe enough to warrant hospitalization. Psychotic symptoms do not occur with hypomania. If psychosis is seen, then the diagnosis is bipolar I disorder, or substance abuse should be considered.

Mixed

Mixed manic/depressive symptoms have to be present for at least 1 week. Criteria for both mania and major depression are met nearly every day during this period. Individuals may demonstrate rapidly alternating mood shifts (anger, euphoria, sadness), agitation, insomnia, appetite problems, psychotic symptoms, or suicidal thoughts. Suicide attempts are high in this population because the high level of distress felt by the client, as opposed to mania and hypomania in which clients generally feel little distress, although others report significant problems with the erratic behaviors. Mixed presentations are more common in children and adolescents.

BIPOLAR I DISORDER

A bipolar I disorder is diagnosed when a client experiences one or more clearly manic or mixed manic/depressive episodes. Often, the client has a history of depression that has chiefly resolved. Bipolar I disorder is cyclical; manic states will be alternated with periods of normal functioning and episodes of depression. These cycles are not necessarily proportionate, and clients may experience two to three manic episodes for every depressed state or numerous depressive episodes with more rare mania cycles; nor are the cycles always predictable. Some individuals may cycle regularly every 6 months (usually in the fall and the spring), but in others, no clear pattern can be distinguished. Psychotic symptoms may occur that are usually characterized by delusions of grandeur, paranoid delusions, ideas of reference, or auditory hallucinations. Individuals with bipolar I disorder can be significantly disabled by the condition, or they may be highly functional and hold esteemed positions in fields such as law, medicine, or business.

BIPOLAR II DISORDER

Bipolar II disorder is characterized by the occurrence of one or more significant depressive episodes, alternating with at least one occurance of hypomania. Hypomania is most likely to occur immediately following an episode of depression. Clients with bipolar II disorder may have difficulty differentiating hypomania from feeling good; often the sleep disturbance associated with hypomania is the clue. Reports from family members or significant others help to establish the diagnosis. Clients with bipolar II disorder who are treated solely with antidepressants may report difficulties in remaining at baseline, describing such symptoms as "moodiness," "mood swings," or "irritability" when they are not feeling depressed.

CYCLOTHYMIC DISORDER

Clients with cyclothymic disorder present with a history of chronic, fluctuating moods, with numerous periods of hypomanic and depressed symptoms, none of which require hospitalization, reach the point of psychosis, or meet the criteria for major depression. Cyclothymic disorder persists for at least 2 years (1 year in children and adolescents) and the client may be described by others as moody, unpredictable, or temperamental. Cyclothymia is of a lesser degree or intensity than bipolar II disorder and may be more of an underlying personality trait.

BIPOLAR DISORDER IN CHILDHOOD

Children with bipolar disorders almost always have a mixed presentation. Cycling of moods is less clear than in adult clients, and the presentation of mania may be less euphoric and more agitated, with explosive anger outbursts and violent episodes occurring. These outbursts can be triggered with little provocation (e.g., "No. You can't have another cookie."), and both the degree of the outburst and its duration may be extremely frightening for those around the child. Temper tantrums in children are usually self-limiting and respond to firm directives ("Go to your room now!"). Outbursts seen in a child with a bipolar disorder are much more intense and may involve hitting or kicking adults (including schoolteachers or administrators), attempting to bite, throwing things, destroying property, attacking pets or younger children, or using weapons (such as a dinner fork) against others. The duration of these episodes can last from 30 minutes to several hours and they usually don't end until the child exhausts himself. Children with this type of behavior are often diagnosed as bipolar disorder, not otherwise specified, or mood disorder, bipolar type. Bipolar disorders are strongly associated with attention deficit hyperactivity disorder (ADHD) of childhood and share many of the same symptoms. Four key symptoms are present in children with bipolar disorder that are not typically present in children with ADHD. These include a decreased need for sleep, grandiose ideas about the self, affective "storms" (sometimes called rage attacks), and preoccupation with issues of sexuality.

Classic bipolar I disorder is also seen in childhood. The presentation of bipolar I disorder in a child is similar to an adult's, with pronounced sleep problems and an elevated or expansive mood, accompanied by either euphoria or irritability. Children with bipolar I disorder commonly experience some psychotic symptoms, including delusions of grandeur ("I'm Spiderman and I can shoot webs out of my hands!") or hallucinations ("Grandpa came as an angel to my room to talk to me last night.")

TREATMENT INTERVENTIONS

Management of a client with a bipolar spectrum disorder must be responsive to the state experienced by the client at that point in time. During episodes of major depression, the client may need activity of daily living support, cognitive behavior or supportive therapy, and monitoring of nutrition or physical health (review Chapter 9: Major Depression and Related Disorders). During manic or hypomanic phases, staff may have to be firm and set limits on inappropriate behaviors. Clients in the throes of full-blown manic episodes are usually hospitalized for their own protection (to prevent them from carrying out fantastic plans or behaving bizarrely in the community) or for the protection of others (to prevent direct or indirect harm to others because of the client's irrational or delusional beliefs). The ethical issue of liberty versus respect for the client arises when a healthcare provider makes difficult decisions when caring for a client who is overtly manic. Such clients are also unpredictable; assaultive behavior can occur rapidly and without apparent provocation. The family may not understand the illogical thoughts and actions of the client, and they can experience feelings of anger, disbelief, or denial. Clients with hypomania are highly productive in the workplace or at home. Clients with mania are at risk for losing employment because of their symptoms and often need to be encouraged to take a medical leave-of-absence until their symptoms are remitted. During baseline states, education is paramount for the client and family. Understanding mania, hypomania, and mixed symptoms as a psychiatric disorder helps the family to avoid feeling hurt or betrayed when the client cycles again. Helping the client to develop an increased awareness of the specific symptomatology (which is often consistent for each episode of mania/hypomania) helps to manage the disorder more effectively. Clients should also be instructed that insight is frequently lacking during hypomanic/manic cycles and that they may have to trust others, rely on their opinions, and follow their advice when manic symptoms are developing.

MEDICATION INTERVENTIONS

Antidepressants

Antidepressants are utilized during the major depression component of a bipolar I or II disorder. Tricyclic antidepressants SSRIs are powerful mania-inducers, when used in the absence of a mood stabilizer in client with bipolar disorder. Buproprion (Wellbutrin SR®) is sometimes preferred because of its prominent dopamine activity. Bipolar disorder (particularly type II) frequently is not diagnosed until after a client has been exposed to antidepressants and the client rapidly develops hypomanic or full-blown manic symptoms. Client education with antidepressant medications must always include informing the client and family of this possibility. Mood stabilizers are necessary to prevent or reduce the occurrence and intensity of manic symptoms. An overview of mood stabilizing medications is provided in Table 10-2 and a discussion of the medications follows.

TABLE 10-2: MEDICATIONS FOR MOOD STABILIZATION IN BIPOLAR SPECTRUM DISORDERS (1 OF 2)

Category	Generic Name	Trade Name	Sedation	Weight Gain	Hepatic Risk	Renal Risk	Blood Disorder Risk	Serum Monitoring Recommended (annual and as needed)	Comments
Lithium	lithium carbonate lithium citrate	Eskalith CR® Lithobid®	+	++	–	+++	–	Lithium level, blood urea nitrogen, thyroid stimulating hormone	Risk of hypo-thyroidism; dehydration may lead to toxicity
Anti-epileptics	divalproex valproic acid	Depakote® Depakote ER® Depakene®	+++	++	+++	–	+	valproate, serum, glutamic oxaloacetic transaminase, serum glutamic pyruvic transaminase, complete blood count, amylase, as needed	Liver impairment in children; risk of pancreatic problems; associated with polycystic ovarian syndrome; GI Irritation
	carbamezapine	Tegretol® Equetro®	++	+	–	–	+++	CBC, carbamazepine levels	Risk of white blood cell (WBC); risk of Stevens-Johnson syndrome; high in drug interactions
	oxcarbazepine	Trileptal®	++	+	–	–	–	None	Not U.S. Food & Drug Administration (FDA) approved for bipolar disorder
	topiramate	Topamax®	+	May cause weight loss	–	–	–	None	Not FDA approved for bipolar disorder; cognitive complaints
	gabapentin	Neurontin®	++	–	–	–	–	None	Not FDA approved for bipolar disorder; used in chronic pain
	lamotrigine	Lamictal®	+++	+	–	–	–	None	Risk of Stevens-Johnson rash
	tiagabine	Gabitril®	+++	–	–	–	–	None	Not FDA approved for bipolar disorder; benzodiazepine-like effects
Anti-psychotics	olanzapine	Zyprexa® Zydis® Symbyax®	+++	+++	+	–	–	Liver function tests, hemoglobin A1c, fasting blood sugar, lipid panels	Rapid onset of action; weight gain can be major problem
	risperidone	Risperdal®	+++	++	+	–	–	Same as above	Approved for use in children; may elevate prolactin levels
	quetiapine	Seroquel® Seroquel XR®	+++	++	+	–	–	Same as above	Also approved for bipolar depression
	ziprasidone	Geodon®	+	–	+	–	–	Same as above	Induces hypomania in low doses

continued on next page

TABLE 10-2: MEDICATIONS FOR MOOD STABILIZATION IN BIPOLAR SPECTRUM DISORDERS (2 OF 2)

Category	Generic Name	Trade Name	Sedation	Weight Gain	Hepatic Risk	Renal Risk	Blood Disorder Risk	Serum Monitoring Recommended (annual and as needed)	Comments
Anti-psychotics continued	aripiprazole	Abilify®	++	+	+	–	–	Same as above	Approved for use in children & in depression as adjunct treatment
	paliperidone	Invega®	++	+	+	–	–	Same as above	Not FDA approved for bipolar disorder
	clozapine	Clozaril®	+++	+++	+	–	+++	Frequent WBC & absolute neutrophil counts	Some positive data in schizoaffective disorder
	paliperidone	Invega®	++	+	+	–	–		Not FDA approved for bipolar disorder
Benzodiaz-epine	clonazepam	Klonopin®	+++	–	+	–	–	–	Dependency is a problem

+++ High Risk   ++ Moderate Risk   + Low Risk   – Negligible Risk

Lithium

Lithium was discovered in 1817, when it was touted as a cure for gout and epilepsy. In 1949, it was first utilized in the treatment of manic/depressive symptoms in clients in Australia, but it was not available in the United States until 1970, because of the deaths of two cardiac patients who received lithium chloride as a salt substitute. Lithium has traditionally been the treatment of choice for the client with bipolar disorder since the 1970s. It is effective predominantly for mania states and can be helpful as an adjunctive treatment to antidepressants. Lithium is a naturally occurring mineral that displaces sodium at the cell membrane, but how this treats and prevents mania is unknown. It is well absorbed orally and primarily excreted via the kidneys. Lithium has a narrow therapeutic versus toxic range. Serum monitoring of blood urea nitrogen, serum creatinine, and thyroid stimulating hormone is required when initiating this drug and annually thereafter. Lithium competes with antidiuretic hormone in the renal collecting tubules and can precipitate diabetes insipidus. A significant number of clients on lithium maintenance treatment develop hypothyroidism. Long-term lithium usage has been associated with renal insuf-

ficiency. Common side effects of lithium, even at therapeutic levels, include nausea, diarrhea, tremor, weight gain, polyuria, mild drowsiness, and a perception of cognitive dulling. Some clients may also have problems with fluid retention. Lithium toxicity most frequently occurs when the balance of fluids and electrolytes (particularly sodium) become abnormal and dehydration results. Excessive diarrhea or vomiting, sweating, or the use of diuretics such as furosemide can precipitate lithium toxicity. Clients who are lithium toxic will display worsened diarrhea and vomiting, ataxia (staggering gait), restlessness, confusion, and agitation. Emergency care is indicated to avoid renal failure. Clients taking lithium may also experience a polygenic polydipsia (excess and unquenchable thirst) that can cause so much free fluid to be taken in that sodium and potassium levels drop dangerously, resulting in cardiac arrhythmias. Fluid restrictions in a hospital setting are the treatment for this disorder. Lithium is contraindicated in cardiac disease and in pregnancy because of an increased risk of fetal heart defects.

Antiepileptics

Lithium is used less frequently today than are antiepileptics in the treatment for bipolar disorder. In general, the antiepileptic drugs are better tolerated and safer than lithium, with similar treatment efficacy (see Table 10-2). Levetiracetam (Keppra®) and phenytoin (Dilantin®) are antiepileptic drugs that do not have any positive treatment effects for bipolar disorder; in fact they may be associated with worsening irritability and anger problems.

Divalproex/valproic acid (Depakote®, Depakote ER®, Depakene®) has been used since the 1960s to treat epilepsy. During the course of its use, it was noted to have a calming effect in clients. The FDA approved it for use as a primary agent for bipolar disorder in the late 1990s. It is generally well tolerated by the client. Valproic acid (Depakene®) causes more problems with GI upset than does divalproex (Depakote®, Depakote ER®), so it is rarely prescribed. Common side effects include nausea, diarrhea, sedation, weight gain, tremor, and hair loss. Multivitamins with chromium are sometimes recommended when clients notice hair thinning. Elevations in liver enzymes can occur. Pancreatitis and liver failure have been associated with divalproex/valproic acid, especially in young children. Toxicity can occur at serum levels higher than 125 mg/ml, which cause ataxia, confusion, slurred speech, and delirium. Serum monitoring of liver function enzymes is recommended at baseline, when a therapeutic dose is achieved, and annually thereafter. Divalproex dosage also can be determined through serum level checks. Depakote ER® is also approved for migraine headache prevention at low, once-daily doses. Additionally, Depakote® and Depakote ER® have been utilized for agitation and aggression in the dementia population with good results. Divalproex and valproic acid are teratogenic and should not be used during pregnancy because of increased risk of neural tube defects such as spina bifida.

Carbamazepine (Tegretol®, Equetro®) also has been shown to be effective in bipolar I disorder. Although it is generally well tolerated, side effects include nausea, sedation, drowsiness, and occasional loss of appetite. The significant risk of agranulocytosis in clients taking carbamazepine requires that serum monitoring of WBCs and CBCs be done initially, when a therapeutic dose is reached, and annually thereafter. Any signs of cold or infection in a client taking carbamezepine should prompt an immediate CBC. If blood dyscrasias occur, the medication must be stopped. There are a number of drug-to-drug interactions that occur with carbamazepine.

A new medication related to Tegretol® is oxcarbazepine (Trileptal®). Trileptal® can have the same GI and sedation side effects as Tegretol®, but it does not appear to cause decreased WBCs or other blood changes. Serum testing is not recommended for Trileptal®. It may be more effective for bipolar II disorder than bipolar I, but its use is still fairly early in the mental health setting. Drug-to-drug interactions are low with Trileptal®; however, it may interfere with estrogen-based birth control prevention (pills, injections, or through other delivery systems), and clients should be counseled about the increased risk of pregnancy. Additional birth control methods such as condoms are recommended.

Topiramate (Topamax®) is gaining popularity because of its anorectic side effects. Overweight clients have reported significant weight loss when adding Topamax® to their other medications as an adjunctive treatment. Topamax® has not been well studied as a single agent for bipolar disorder. Its side effects are relatively low with some complaints of dizziness and GI distress. Topamax® is mildly activating; some clients may report insomnia, anxiety, or restlessness. The most significant problem with utilizing Topamax® is the necessity for gradual titration because of problems with cognitive clouding or dulling. Serum level monitoring is not recommended for Topamax®.

Gabapentin (Neurontin®) is an antiepileptic that has treatment efficacy for mild bipolar disorder (primarily type II) as well as chronic pain conditions and peripheral neuropathies; however, it is not FDA-approved for any of these uses. Neurontin® has some activity on the anxiety-related neurotransmitter gamma aminobutyric acid (GABA), which also gives it anxiolytic properties. Neurontin is well tolerated with side effects of dizziness and sedation. Titration is usually required to avoid excessive fatigue or staggering gaits. Serum level monitoring is not necessary with this product.

Lamotrigine (Lamictal®) has shown treatment efficacy in rapid cycling and mixed mood states of bipolar disorder. Side effects of Lamictal® include insomnia, jitteriness, headache, and occasional activation or hypomania. Side effects are generally mild. Concerns over a progressive, autoimmune-mediated, excoriating rash, known as Stevens-Johnson syndrome, have led clinicians to use caution with Lamictal®. The caveat is to start low and go slow when titrating this drug.

New Generation Antipsychotics

The newer generation antipsychotics include clozapine (Clozaril®), risperidone (Risperdal®), olanzapine (Zyprexa®), quetiapine (Seroquel®), ziprasidone (Geodon®), aripiprazole Abilify®), and paliperidone (Invega®). These products demonstrate some antimanic properties, and all but clozapine and paliperidone have now received FDA approval for their use as primary agents in bipolar disorder. Serum medication levels are not necessary with these antipsychotic medications because their potential for toxicity is low. Pregnancy studies have not been completed, but there is no clear evidence of fetal toxicity (as seen with lithium and valproic acid). The medications do have class warnings in two areas: There is an increased risk of hyperglycemia with these products (less with Geodon®), thus blood sugar monitoring is advisable, and there is an increased risk of death when used in elderly patients with dementia-related psychosis (see discussion in Chapter 6).

Olanzapine (Zyprexa®, Zydis®) rapidly reduces the agitation and increased motor activity seen in manic clients and it stabilizes moods for ongoing use. Side effects of olanzapine include sedation, occasionally restlessness, and increased appetite. Weight gain associated with olanzapine has been pronounced, with up to 50 lb reported by adult clients and 20 lb seen in children. Not all clients gain weight, however, so the medication should not be avoided for this reason alone. The manufacturer recommends checking baseline weight, then repeating this at 2 weeks. If the client has gained 5 lb in 2 weeks, then it is likely that he or she will continue to gain weight and another medication may be considered. Olanzapine is also available in a rapid-acting intramuscular injection that is useful in emergency departments or inpatient treatment.

Clozapine (Clozaril®) has several small studies that indicate its efficacy in schizoaffective disorders (Dittman, Forsthoff, Thoma, & Grunze, 2002), but its use is limited by the strict FDA requirements for WBC monitoring (weekly for the first 6 months of treatment, then biweekly for 6 months, then monthly thereafter). Other side effects of clozapine are salivation, sedation, and weight gain. A small percentage of clients taking clozapine develop seizure disorders over time.

Risperidone (Risperdal®) is frequently utilized in child psychiatry as a mood stabilizing agent. It blocks dopamine release and seems to be effective in reducing agitation, anger outbursts, and the violent episodes seen in childhood-associated bipolar disorder with mixed mood presentations. It is FDA-approved for moodswings, irritability, and aggression associated with autistic disorder. Children may require a dose that is only one-third that of an adult's dose. This low dosing (less than 3mg/day) helps to minimize side effects that include tremors, weight gain, sedation, and the risk of extrapyramidal syndrome and tardive dyskinesia.

Risperidone is available in a dissolvable lozenge (Risperdal M-tab®) and in a long-acting intramuscular injection given every 2 weeks (Risperdal Consta®), which comes in three dosing strengths: 24, 37.5 and 50 mg.

Quetiapine (Seroquel®) is well studied and effective for bipolar disorder I and II as well as depression associated with bipolar disorder. Dosing for depression is 50% less than the recommended dosing for mania (300 mg versus 600 mg daily). Quetiapine has fairly significant initial sedation that tends to resolve in 2 to 4 weeks. It can also increase appetite and has been associated with weight gain and elevated triglyceride levels. Other side effects to quetiapine include sedation, nausea, headache, and GI upset. Quetiapine is often used off-label for a variety of problems, including anxiety, depression-associated insomnia, pain management, and as an adjunct treatment for children with attention deficit hyperactivity disorder that is associated with insomnia and aggression.

Ziprasidone (Geodon®) is an activating antipsychotic that is useful in the treatment of depression and bipolar disorder. Ziprasidone may precipitate agitation or hypomania in low doses because it has significant serotonin reuptake inhibition; however, when dosed rapidly, it is an effective bipolar medication. Ziprasidone has been shown to reduce triglyceride levels and weight gain in clients who were titrated off of other antipsychotic medications. Ziprasidone is available in a rapid-acting intramuscular injection that is useful in the emergency department. It tends to be more calming than sedating and can substitute for the oral titration to achieve therapeutic blood levels.

Aripiprazole (Abilify®) is approved for schizophrenia, bipolar disorder, and as an adjunct therapy for treatment-resistant depression. Aripiprazole is a dopamine agonist and replaces dopamine at the receptor sites (other antipsychotics works by antagonizing dopamine to block its release). Aripiprazole works gradually, achieving its maximum therapeutic potential in about 4 weeks. Dosing should start low and titrate to higher doses because extrapyramidal syndrome and akathisia can occur. Sedation and weight gain also may occur, but are generally less common than with olanzapine, quetiapine, or risperidone. Aripiprazole is also available in an orally disintegrating tablet and an intramuscular injection for emergency use.

Benzodiazepines

Benzodiazepines have potent antianxiety and antiepileptic properties. They are not used in epilepsy as primary agents because of problems with drug dependency, tolerance, and withdrawal. Short-acting agents (e.g., lorazepam) are useful in the emergency department for treating an agitated or manic client. Lorazepam (Ativan®) can be given orally, intramuscularly, or intravenously. Clonazepam (Klonopin®) is the best choice for maintenance care of the client with bipolar disorder, as an adjunctive treatment to antiepileptic or antipsychotic agents. Clonazepam has a long half-life, with treatment effects lasting 12 to 16 hours. Its side effects include sedation and dizziness or ataxia at higher doses. Clonazepam is a CNS depressant, and its sedation effects will be potentiated by other CNS depressants or medications metabolized by the enzyme cytochrome P450, such as fluoxetine and carbamazepine.

NURSING INTERVENTIONS DURING MANIA

Nursing care of the manic client can be very challenging. Protecting clients from inadvertently harming themselves or their reputations and protecting others from being physically or emotionally harmed by the clients are foremost; safety is a concern. Many clients with mania require hospitalization and clear nursing care plans that focus on behavior. Clients with mania have a tendency to be pushy, noisy, and intrusive and to test their limits continuously. Staff members need to maintain clear lines of communication with one another to prevent staff-splitting behaviors by the client. The nurse also needs to adopt a caring, but firm, approach and provide external structure for the client in the form of established routines, rules, and consistent behavior consequences. Clients with mania may forget to eat or bathe. It is up to the nurse to see that the client's basic needs are taken care of. It may be necessary to limit telephone calls to give family members a rest from constant demands by the client. Clients with mania suffer from distractibility and a loss of control. Reducing environmental stimuli, by providing private rooms, scheduling rest periods, allowing time for exercise, and limiting contact with other clients, may be helpful. Insomnia is a major problem for clients with mania. Administering bedtime sedatives and as needed medications throughout the night, keeping lights and noise levels low, and requiring that the client remain in the room during the night, not at the nurse's station talking with staff or on the phone is helpful. Staff should be cautious not to trigger aggression in a client who is manic. Impulse control is extremely poor, and even an apparently minor comment may cause the client to begin escalating. When signs of increasing tension are seen (pacing, clenched fists, raised voice, darting eye contact), the client should be offered an as needed medication (usually a benzodiazepine) and asked to wait quietly in the room until the medicine has worked. Inpatient nursing staff who regularly work with clients who are manic should be trained in seclusion and restraint policies and procedures and have adequate staffing backup, should it be necessary to utilize restraints (four to six persons).

CASE STUDY: BIPOLAR I DISORDER

Pablo is a 22-year-old man who has completed 2 years of fine arts study in a major university. Always creative, he started to find himself unable to stop painting or sketching until well into the night. Eventually, he found himself able to stay up for more than 48 hours with little effort. His friends commented that he always seemed to be "on a natural high" and he was "fun to be around." Pablo was very productive in his painting, but he started to miss classes as he began to think that there was nothing they could teach him that he didn't already know. After a few weeks, Pablo's irregular hours and poor eating habits caused him to look thin and tired. His energy level became more frenetic and agitated, and his friends stopped visiting because he had become irritable and short-tempered. In addition, they were tired of hearing about his "genius talent." One day, when Pablo had been awake for 4 consecutive days, he called his parents to tell them about the "great opportunity" he would have if they would buy him a plane ticket to Paris. He was certain that the Louvre would hang his paintings and give him a private showing on the spot. After all, he felt he was "channeling the spirit and soul of Van Gogh." When his parents questioned this, Pablo became agitated saying he would get the money somehow and no one could stop him. Subsequently, Pablo was arrested for attempted robbery of a convenience store. The arresting officer put in his report that "the perpetrator was shouting obscenities and appeared to be talking to someone he kept calling 'Vince'." Pablo was admitted to a secure psychiatric facility on an immediate detention order. He initially required four-way restraints and chemical sedation. He was started on Depakote ER® (valproic acid) and titrated to 2,500 mg/day. Additionally, he was prescribed Zyprexa® (olanzapine) 20 mg at bedtime and was given as needed doses of Ativan® (lorazepam). After 7 days as an inpatient, he was discharged to his parents' home for further recuperation.

Questions

1. What are the symptoms of mania in this client?

2. What serum laboratory monitoring should be done based on the medications prescribed?

3. When doing patient education, what should the client be told about his medications?

Discussion

Mania is characterized by an increase in energy, severe insomnia, and grandiosity. Signs of psychosis that may evolve during a manic state include delusions and hallucinations, both of which the client in this study was demonstrating. Valproic acid and olanzapine are metabolized by the liver and can cause weight gain. Olanzapine has been associated with hyperglycemia. Serum liver enzymes, lipids (cholesterol and triglycerides), fasting blood sugars, and hemoglobin A1c (if blood sugars are elevated) should be done at baseline and periodically thereafter. Patient education might include advising the client to take the medications at bedtime, maintaining a regular exercise routine, eating healthful meals, and complying with appointments.

NURSING CARE PLAN: CLIENT WITH BIPOLAR DISORDER

Problem Listing

• Altered mood states: agitation, excitability

• Altered thoughts: delusions of grandeur, ideas of reference, auditory hallucinations

• Inadequate sleep

• Poor nutrition

• Knowledge deficit regarding the illness or medications

• Potential for harm to self or others

Priority Nursing Diagnosis

Potential for harm to self or others related to altered thoughts (grandiosity, ideas of reference), as evidenced by extreme agitation and irrational behaviors.

Long-term Goal

Client will no longer demonstrate evidence of psychosis.

Short-term Objectives

1. Client will not harm self during the hospital stay.

2. Client will not harm others (staff, visitors) during the hospital stay.

3. Client will demonstrate compliance with recommended medication treatment.

Nursing Interventions

1. Nurse will administer as needed medications at the first sign of increasing agitation.

2. Nurse will educate the client in relaxation techniques to help in reducing anxiety.

3. Seclusion and restraints will be utilized by staff in a judicious manner and only when absolutely necessary.

4. Staff will adapt a non-confrontational, supportive approach with client to minimize potential misperceptions due to altered thoughts.

5. Staff will keep the client in a private room until all risk of assaultive behavior has passed.

6. Staff may elect to restrict visitors if client's behavior is inappropriate.

ADVANCED PRACTICE NURSING: THE TEXAS MEDICATION ALGORITHM PROJECT

The treatment of depression in a client with bipolar disorder was covered in Chapter 9; however, it is very important that clients with bipolar disorder do not take an antidepressant alone because of the risk of precipitating a manic episode. The Texas Medication Algorithm Project (TMAP) published guidelines in 2008 for treating acute mania and mixed symptoms in bipolar patients (Suehs et al., 2008).

Initial treatment for mania or hypomania (as evidenced by euphoria) should begin with monotherapy, using valproic acid, lithium, aripiprazole, quetiapine, risperidone, or ziprasidone. Initial treatment for mixed states (as evidenced by irritability and mood lability) can begin with monotherapy using valproic acid, aripiprazole, risperidone, or ziprasidone. The TMAP does not recommend olanzapine first-line because of its weight gain and hyperglycemia potential. If ineffective, the APRN should switch to a different monotherapy treatment from a different class of medication and may consider olanzapine. For clients who are still non-responders, adding a second agent from a different classification is recommended (e.g., valproic acid and quetiapine; lithium and olanzapine). For clients who continue to be unresponsive to treatment, the APRN may add off-label products, such as oxcarbazepine (Trileptal®), or more risky (in terms of drug-to-drug interaction) products such as carbamazepine (Tegretol®). Finally, clients who are persistently manic, despite several combination drug trials at therapeutic dosages over an adequate period of time, may be considered for clozapine therapy or referred for ECT (Suehs et al., 2008).

SUMMARY

Clients with bipolar disorder can be challenging to manage, whether in outpatient care or in the hospital. Many individuals present during depression stages only, and it may not be until they demonstrate irrational behavior, which comes to the attention of family members or authorities, that the mania is recognized. Bipolar I disorder is characterized by distinct episodes of extreme energy (or irritability), grandiosity, and insomnia and may also include the psychotic symptoms of hallucinations or delusions. Bipolar II disorder and cyclothymic disorder have less intense manic symptoms and no psychosis. Childhood bipolar disorder is clearly problematic, but experts have not come to a consensus yet on its recognition or treatment. Medications are almost always needed to stabilize the mood swings in clients with bipolar disorders. Mood stabilizers include lithium, several antiepileptics, the new-generation (or atypical) antipsychotics, and clonazepam. Polypharmacy may be needed in treatment-resistant clients. Nursing care of the hospitalized client with mania should focus on safety issues, protection of the client's privacy (due to his or her irrational behaviors), promoting sleep and good nutrition, and patient and family education.

EXAM QUESTIONS

CHAPTER 10
Questions 58-64

Note: Choose the one option that BEST answers each question.

58. Symptoms of bipolar I disorder include

    a. alternating episodes of depression with mania that may be accompanied by psychosis.

    b. manic and baseline episodes with no history of depression.

    c. depressed episodes alternated with periods of hypomania.

    d. chronically hypomanic and depressed episodes that last over 2 years.

59. Symptoms of bipolar II disorder include

    a. alternating episodes of depression with mania that may be accompanied by psychosis.

    b. manic and baseline episodes with no history of depression.

    c. depressed episodes alternated with some periods of hypomania.

    d. chronically depressed episodes that last over 2 years.

60. Bipolar disorder in childhood can be expressed as

    a. occasional temper tantrums requiring time-outs.

    b. frequent explosive and violent anger outbursts.

    c. poor focus, decreased attention span, and an inability to concentrate.

    d. problems achieving developmental milestones.

61. People who take lithium should have which laboratory studies monitored annually?

    a. Liver function tests

    b. Blood ureanitrogen, creatinine, and thyroid stimulating hormone

    c. Fasting blood sugar and hemoglobin A1c

    d. Cholesterol and triglycerides

62. An antiepileptic medication that is approved for use as a primary mood stabilizer is

    a. Valproic acid (Depakote ER®).

    b. Fluoxetine (Prozac).

    c. Topiramate (Topamax®).

    d. Phenytoin (Dilantin®).

63. Side effects of mood stabilizers may include

    a. sedation and appetite changes.

    b. depression and suicidal ideation.

    c. anger outbursts and irritability.

    d. restlessness and insomnia.

64. Symptoms that tell the nurse that a client with mania is escalating and may require prn medication include

    a. remaining socially isolated and refusing to participate in activities.

    b. increased lethargy, distractability, and sadness.

    c. narrow focus, withdrawn, and flat affect.

    d. pacing, clenched fists, a raised voice, and darting eye contact.

151

CHAPTER 11

ANXIETY DISORDERS

CHAPTER OBJECTIVE

At the end of this chapter the reader will be able to discuss symptoms of an anxiety disorder and relevant treatment, including therapy and medications.

LEARNING OBJECTIVES

At the end of this chapter, the reader will be able to

1. describe the symptoms of anxiety.

2. differentiate various types of anxiety disorders.

3. discuss treatment for anxiety disorders, including therapy and medications.

INTRODUCTION

Anxiety is a healthy, adaptive response that has a protective function in preventing an individual from harm. Anxiety stops us from engaging in high-risk activities and it helps us to think more clearly in emergency situations. It is only when anxiety becomes maladaptive that it becomes a problem. Anxiety, often described by individuals as "worry" or "nervousness" is probably the most common complaint heard in a mental health or medical setting. Anxiety frequently accompanies other psychiatric problems, such as depression or trauma.

Approximately 18% of the adult population experiences an anxiety disorder in a given year. This can be broken down into generalized anxiety (6.8%), panic disorder (1%), obsessive-compulsive disorder (3.5%), PTSD (3.1%), and specific phobias such as social anxiety (8.7%). Many anxiety disorders overlap with one another (NIMH, 2008).

This chapter will be examining some of the types of anxiety disorders and their medical and non-medical treatments. Nursing care of the anxious client will be discussed and a case study provided.

GENERAL ADAPTATION SYNDROME

Hans Selye (1956) recognized that human beings respond to stress in characteristic ways regardless of the stressor experienced. He classified these changes into three distinct stages that he called the "General Adaptation Syndrome: Alarm, Resistance, and Exhaustion" (Keltner, Schwecke, & Bolstrom, 2007). In the alarm stage, a client develops a heightened awareness of the stressor and mobilizes resources to cope with it. Clear biological changes occur in the body to prepare the person for fight or flight. These changes include discharges of norepinephrine and epinephrine, increased thyroid hormone and corticosteroid levels, a release of endogenous opiates, and diversion of blood from the organs to the skeletal muscles. During an alarm response, clients perceive an increased level of anxiety and other changes that are designed to prepare the person to deal with the stressor. Table 11-1 provides an overview of anxiety responses at the mild, moderate, severe, and panic levels and associates these with emotional, cognitive, and behavioral experiences of the client. If the stressor continues without resolution, the client moves into the next stage of resistance. During the resistance stage, the use of coping and defense mechanisms begin and physical symptoms may begin to develop. Chronically elevated epinephrine levels can lead to hypertension. Corticosteroids and gastric secretions are irritating to the gastric lining and may lead to ulcers or colitis. Headaches are common complaints, as are muscle aches or tension (particularly in the neck and back) and chronic pain. The third stage, called exhaustion, occurs when stressors persist over a long period of time and the client loses the ability to cope by utilizing normal mechanisms. Thinking becomes illogical. Sensory misperceptions may occur. Clients may become suicidal or violent, or they may shut down completely. Chronic and persistent anxiety early in life can lead to personality disorders or other dysfunctional ways of dealing with life later on. Exhaustion is a contributing factor to battered women's syndrome and domestic violence.

The *DSM-IV-TR* recognizes and describes more than 12 different types of anxiety disorders. For the purposes of this course, the following disorders will be reviewed: generalized anxiety disorder, panic disorder (with and without agoraphobia), social anxiety disorder, specific phobias, PTSD,

TABLE 11-1: OVERVIEW OF LEVELS OF ANXIETY			
Level of Anxiety	**Physical and Behavioral Changes**	**Emotional Changes**	**Cognitive Changes**
Mild	Increased heart rate & blood pressure, Muscle tension Blood shunts to skeletal muscles Frequent urination	Excitement Mild fear Pupil dilation	Increased alertness Improved concentration Increased awareness of surroundings
Moderate	Further increases in heart rate & blood pressure Need to pace; feelings of restlessness Body and muscle aches	Sense of foreboding (something about to happen)	Racing thoughts Trouble staying focused
Severe	Increased respiratory rates Hyperventilation Tremors, especially in hands GI upset: nausea, vomiting GI pain and diarrhea	Fearful, anxious or nervous, sense of dread	Flight-of-ideas Inability to focus or concentrate Inability to listen well to others Decreased decision-making ability
Panic	Wildly erratic vital signs Attempts to run away or flee Aggression or striking out Whole body tremors Suicidal or self-injurious Immobilization	Overt fears: fear of dying and fear of injury	Irrationality Illogical thoughts Disorganized May be delusional

obsessive-compulsive disorder, and pediatric autoimmune neuropsychiatric disorder associated streptococcal infections (PANDAS).

GENERALIZED ANXIETY DISORDER

A generalized anxiety disorder (GAD) occurs when a person experiences chronic and persistent anxiety, without a specific focus or cause, over a period of at least 6 months. Associated with muscle tension, there may be problems with trembling, feeling shaky inside, and muscle aches or soreness. Sweating, nausea, and diarrhea are common and an exaggerated startle response may occur. Children with GAD tend to be overly perfectionistic about the quality of their schoolwork, and they worry about criticism from teachers or other authority figures. They may have excessive concerns about punctuality or worry about catastrophic events or adult responsibilities such as paying the bills. They seek out constant reassurance from others, and they may complain of vague stomach aches or headaches. Table 11-2 provides the *DSM-IV-TR* criteria for diagnosing GAD.

To meet the criteria for GAD, there cannot be a specific focus or worry such as seen in phobic disorders or clear cause as identified in PTSD. The symptoms must significantly interfere with the client's functioning in the community.

Therapy for GAD

Cognitive behavior therapy, supportive therapy, and psychoanalysis are helpful in treating GAD. Learned patterns from childhood may have a significant impact on the development of the disorder. For example, a child who is bullied and threatened by siblings and criticized by parents, may grow into an adult who is always tense and waiting for someone to bully, intimidate, or criticize him or her. This can become a self-fulfilling prophecy if that person chooses a spouse or employer who is domineering or abusive.

TABLE 11-2: *DSM-IV-TR* **CRITERIA FOR GENERALIZED ANXIETY DISORDER**

1. Excessive anxiety and worry about a number of different things, more days than not, for at least 6 months; and

2. The client finds it difficult to control the worry.

3. Three or more of the following symptoms are present (only one is required in children):
   a. restlessness or feeling keyed up or on edge
   b. easily fatigued
   c. difficulty concentrating
   d. irritability
   e. muscle tension
   f. sleep disturbance (usually delayed onset or restlessness).

(American Psychiatric Association, 2000)

Counseling can help a client to uncover some of the coping techniques, defense mechanisms, and learned beliefs. Hopefully, change can occur as a result of improved awareness and insight. The therapist also needs to teach new tools and coping strategies to compensate for losing the more dysfunctional ones.

Relaxation Techniques and Guided Imagery

Educating the client in relaxation breathing and guided imagery is useful for reducing anxiety levels from severe or panic states to mild or moderate ones. During guided imagery, the client is asked to imagine a calm, peaceful, and safe place: What can be seen there? Smelled? Heard? Who else might be there? When the client is able to imagine being in a safe place, then he or she can be taught to allow fears to enter in and be confronted or thrown away. Relaxation breathing is a systematic exercise of alternatively tensing and relaxing muscles, in association with slow deep breaths, until the sensation of tension is drained away. Relaxation breathing and guided imagery can be rehearsed in the office setting and utilized in any number of other settings when tension is building.

Exercise

The importance of exercise in treating GAD cannot be overemphasized. The physiological responses associated with anxiety prepare the body for fight or flight. Physical exertion (difficult enough to cause an increase in heart rate and mild shortness of breath) will trick the body into believing that the survival response was initiated, leading to a draining away of tension and anxiety. Exercise can be a brisk walk or a jog, weight lifting, or a martial arts class. Exercise "prescriptions" should be tailored to the client and take into consideration any pre-existing medical conditions.

MEDICATION INTERVENTIONS FOR ANXIETY

Four categories of medications are commonly prescribed for treating GAD: benzodiazepines, nonbenzodiazepine anxiolytics, antidepressants, and antihistamines. Other medications may be given including antiepileptics (e.g., gabapentin) or new-generation antipsychotics (e.g., quetiapine), but their use is less frequent and usually occurs only after other drugs have been tried. Of the medications available, current practice is to utilize SSRIs as first-line treatment for all anxiety disorders and supplement them with other agents as necessary.

All of the SSRIs are highly effective in treating anxiety and most are FDA-approved for anxiety disorders as well as depression. Fluvoxamine (Luvox®) has a specific indication for obsessive-compulsive disorder. The relationship between serotonin, norepinephrine, and anxiety symptoms is pronounced and these medications are clearly superior in reducing the overall experience of anxiety. Tricyclic antidepressants (TCAs) have also been used quite effectively in treating anxiety for

years, but their use is limited by their extensive side effect profile and cardiac conduction problems. Clomipramine (Anafranil®) is a TCA that is approved specifically for the treatment of obsessive-compulsive disorders. Sertraline (Zoloft®) is also approved to treat obsessive-compulsive disorder in children older than 6 years of age. A detailed discussion of both SSRIs and TCAs is provided in Chapter 9.

Benzodiazepines are medications that work by enhancing the effects of the neurotransmitter gamma-aminobutyric acid (GABA). The action of GABA is to open chloride channels at the cellular level in the brain, which makes a neuron less responsive to other neurotransmitters, such as serotonin, norepinephrine, and dopamine. The overall effect is a slowing down of neuron firing. Benzodiazepines contribute to this brain-inhibition effect and slow down excitability, agitation, nervousness, and (often) alertness, attention span, concentration, and decision-making abilities. Some clients experience a paradoxical reaction to benzodiazepines (particularly diazepam and chlordiazepoxide) and may become more, instead of less, agitated. Different types of benzodiazepines are covered more thoroughly in Chapter 7. Medications most commonly used to treat anxiety include alprazolam (Xanax®), lorazepam (Ativan®), diazepam (Valium®), and clonazepam (Klonopin®). Benzodiazepines have the distinct disadvantage of being habituating; tolerance quickly develops and more of the drug is needed to achieve the desired effect. When the client runs out of medications, withdrawal symptoms occur. Withdrawal to benzodiazepines is characterized by anxiety, restlessness, and panic attacks. The longer-acting agents (clonazepam and diazepam) are not as difficult to manage as the shorter-acting ones (alprazolam and lorazepam). Withdrawal symptoms can develop within 8 hours of the last dose of alprazolam and 12 hours with lorazepam. A client who takes alprazolam three to four times a day over 1 to 2 weeks (long enough to become habituated to it), will wake up feeling anxious and in panic simply because of medication withdrawal effects.

One nonbenzodiazepine anxiolytic medication is approved for use in anxiety disorders. Buspirone (Buspar®) acts as a serotonin enhancer in the brain and has no activity on GABA. Buspar® is mildly sedating but it has no addictive properties, so habituation is not an issue. Unfortunately, Buspar® can take 2 to 4 weeks or longer to be fully effective and most clients want anxiety relief more rapidly (benzodiazepines are effective within 30 minutes or less following a single dose). Buspar® dosing is usually three to four times a day, making it less convenient to take.

Other medications are used "off-label" to treat anxiety. One of these is tiagabine (Gabitril®). Gabitril® is an antiepileptic agent that seems to mimic or enhance the activity of a subtype of GABA. Gabitril® is not a benzodiazepine and it has no addictive properties. Some clients report significant anxiety relief with Gabitril®, although it tends to be activating in other clients, causing them to feel restless or agitated. Gabitril® may also have some usefulness in bipolar disorders, particularly in bipolar II disorder. Side effects to Gabitril® include dizziness, drowsiness, and unsteady gait. Several of the antiepileptics have anxiolytic properties, particularly gabapentin (Neurontin®). A non-opioid pain medication approved for fibromyalgia disorder and peripheral neuropathy (and as an adjunct treatment for epilepsy) may also be useful. This medication, pregabalin (Lyrica®), acts to inhibit the excitatory neurons that affect glutamate in the brain. Glutamate works the opposite of GABA, by turning on excitability instead of inhibiting it.

Antihistamines can provide assistance in the short-term treatment of anxiety. They are added to preoperative medications (hydroxyzine) to help reduce anxiety in the healthcare setting. Their anxiolytic properties are primarily through the side effect of sedation, which is perceived as calming to the client. Diphenhydramine (Benadryl®) is more useful in adults because many children may have a paradoxical reaction to it. Cyproheptadine (Periactin®) is an antihistamine with a mild serotonin activity that is helpful as an adjunct treatment for children with insomnia and mood disorders. Hydroxyzine (Vistaril®, Atarax®) is useful in adults and children as a calming agent or at bedtime sleep-enhancing medication. Antihistamines are relatively safe (Benadryl® is sold over the counter) and low in side effects.

PANIC DISORDER

Panic Attacks

Panic attacks can occur without warning. They consist of a discrete period of intense fear or discomfort in the absence of any real danger. Table 11-3 provides the *DSM-IV-TR* criteria for a panic

TABLE 11-3: CRITERIA FOR A PANIC ATTACK
The *DSM-IV-TR* criteria for a panic attack require four or more of the following symptoms:
1. Palpitations, pounding heart, or increased heart rate
2. Sweating
3. Trembling or shaking
4. Shortness of breath or "smothering" sensation
5. Choking sensation
6. Chest pain or tightness
7. Nausea or abdominal distress
8. Feeling dizzy, lightheaded, faint, or unsteady
9. Feelings of unreality or detachment
10. Fear of losing control or going crazy
11. Fear of dying
12. Numbness or tingling sensations
13. Chills or hot flushing
(American Psychiatric Association, 2000)

attack. A panic attack may occur in association with another anxiety or psychiatric disorder or by itself. A trigger for the attack may not be apparent. Children may experience panic attack symptoms when asked to give a presentation in school or when facing a fearful situation such as a blood draw. Symptoms should, however, be differentiated from specific phobias such as a fear of needles. Clients usually present for initial treatment in an emergency department where they receive ECGs, blood testing, and other services, before being given sedatives and sent home. Panic disorder can be associated with suicide risk because of the intensity of the discomfort experienced. Panic attacks can occur once, weekly, monthly, or several times a day. They will usually persist from 30 minutes to 4 hours at a time.

Panic Disorder

A panic disorder develops when there is a presence of recurrent panic attacks that are followed by a persistent worry about having additional attacks a worry about the implications of the attack (e.g., losing control or "going crazy"), or when there is a significant change in the client's behavior related to the attacks. A fear of recurrent attacks may eventually cause the client to be afraid to leave the house or be "caught" out in public. Agoraphobia occurs when the client changes behaviors to avoid situations where a panic attack might prove to be embarrassing or from which escape may be difficult. For some clients, agoraphobia may be limited to an avoidance of long trips from home or extended bus rides. Other clients have more severe symptoms including the inability to leave one's own property or even to go outside of the house, without having a panic attack or experiencing overwhelming anticipatory anxiety.

Panic disorder, with and without agoraphobia, is treated with a combination of exposure therapy and medications. Exposure therapy consists of supporting the client in making steps toward panic-inducing situations (e.g., going outside),

while providing a great deal of reassurance and relaxation training. "Flooding" occurs when the client is thrust suddenly into a panic-inducing situation and not allowed to escape. Flooding can be emotionally traumatic, especially for a child, so its use is not routinely recommended. Panic symptoms can be alleviated by benzodiazepines, but they will do nothing to prevent reoccurrence. The best medical treatment for panic disorder continues to be SSRI medications on a daily basis for adults and children. Benzodiazepines may be used as supplemental, as needed drugs during panic-inducing situations. With treatment, panic symptoms may remit entirely or they may only be reduced to a more manageable level.

SOCIAL ANXIETY DISORDER

A social anxiety disorder is diagnosed when there is a persistent fear of social or performance situations in which humiliation or embarrassment may occur. Adults and most adolescents will recognize that their fears are unfounded (children typically do not yet have this level of cognitive awareness), but they are unable to prevent severe anxiety symptoms or panic attacks. Exposure to the social situation invariably provokes the anxiety (in children this may be expressed as immobilization freezing, crying, tantrums, or shrinking away). Because of the anxiety symptoms, the client will make inordinate efforts to avoid the precipitant, which can include such situations as isolated public speaking engagements, social situations such as parties, and places full of people (e.g., grocery store).

Treatment for social anxiety disorder consists of SSRI medications, when the disorder is disabling to day-to-day living, and intermittent benzodiazepines, when there is only rare exposure. Propanolol (Inderal®) can be prescribed for adult clients who must present research or perform in other public speaking venues. Inderal®, along with other beta adrenergic blockers, decreases tremors and heart rate (elevations of which occur with moderate anxiety) and provides clients with a sense that they are more in control. Inderal® does not produce the cognitive clouding and sense of mild euphoria as does a benzodiazepine (side effects to be avoided when speaking in front of a crowd). Nonmedical treatment consists of coaching clients to mentally rehearse the situation beforehand, while imagining themselves as being charming, witty, and well-liked by the audience.

SPECIFIC PHOBIAS

The essential feature of a specific phobia is a persistent, intense, and irrational fear of a specific object, circumstance, or situation. Many types of specific phobias exist (agoraphobia, claustrophobia, hydrophobia) but they are all classified into five basic types:

1. *Animal type:* fears are cued by animals (e.g., dogs, snakes) or by insects (e.g., spiders). Animal phobias typically have a childhood onset.

2. *Natural environment type:* fear is cued by natural occurrences, such as storms, lightning, tornadoes, or earthquakes. These disorders also frequently onset in childhood.

3. *Blood-injection-injury type:* fear is cued by seeing blood or an injury or by receiving an injection or invasive procedure. This type is highly familial and is often accompanied by a vasovagal response (fainting).

4. *Situational type:* fear is cued by specific situations, such as being in an airplane, a tunnel, a bridge, an elevator, enclosed places, or heights. This type tends to onset either in childhood or in the mid-20s and is similar to a panic disorder.

5. *Other type:* fear is cued by any other stimuli, which may include such things as a fear of

choking or vomiting, a fear of contracting an illness, a fear of falling down, or children's fears of loud sounds or clowns.

Treatment of a specific phobia (if treatment is necessary) is to gradually expose the client to the feared object or situation after educating him or her to relaxation techniques and guided imagery. Exposure may start out with simply talking about the object or situation, then move on to looking at pictures (or drawing pictures), then to watching video, and eventually to field trips for direct exposure. Medications are only necessary when exposure to the feared object or situation is unavoidable (e.g., airline travel), in which case benzodiazepines are the best options. Children with severe blood-injection-injury phobias may benefit from low doses of lorazepam prior to dental work or other necessary procedures. Diazepam is commonly used, but it can produce paradoxical reactions or agitation in young children and some adults.

POSTTRAUMATIC STRESS DISORDER

Posttraumatic stress disorder (PTSD) and acute stress disorder occur in response to extreme stressors that involve personal experiences of events with actual or threatened death or serious injury, witnessing an event that involves death or serious injury, or learning about unexpected or violent death, serious harm, or threat of death or injury to a family member or close friend. The client responds with feelings of intense fear, helplessness, or horror (children may express agitation or disorganized behaviors). In acute stress disorder, the symptoms from the trauma occur immediately and last from 2 days to 4 weeks. After this time period, the client may meet the criteria for PTSD. With an acute stress disorder, three or more of the following symptoms must be experienced to make the diagnosis:

1. A sense of numbing, detachment, or an absence of emotional responses

2. Feeling dazed or unaware of one's surroundings

3. Derealization (feeling as though in a dream)

4. Depersonalization (feeling as though outside of oneself)

5. Dissociative amnesia (can't remember parts or all of the trauma).

There must also be a persistent re-experiencing of the trauma through recurrent images, dreams, thoughts, or flashbacks. Clients will avoid stimuli that arouse recollections of the trauma and exhibit symptoms of increased arousal states, such as insomnia, irritability, poor concentration, exaggerated startle, restlessness, and hypervigilance.

PTSD is more persistent and long lasting. It can occur immediately following the trauma or memories can be repressed, with symptoms occurring years later. Clients with PTSD may describe guilty feelings about their experience (especially if others were injured or killed and they were not). Avoidance behaviors can lead to marital conflicts, work conflicts, or interpersonal problems. Severe cases may report auditory hallucinations or paranoia. Impulsive and self-destructive behaviors are associated with traumas related to physical or sexual abuse. Somatic complaints may be frequent. *DSM-IV-TR* criteria for PTSD are listed in Table 11-4.

Treatment for acute stress disorder and PTSD usually involves intensive therapy. The therapist must first establish trust with the client. Psychoanalysis may be beneficial to help the client to uncover forgotten aspects of the trauma; a trained therapist may use hypnosis cautiously. Eye movement desensitization and reprocessing (EMDR) is a relatively new type of therapy for trauma and PTSD. EMDR postulates that troubling emotional experiences are trapped in the nervous system. The therapist uses tactile stimulation and active promoting of rapid right and left eye movements, while encouraging the client to remember and talk about the traumatic event. Rapid eye movements (which occur naturally during dreaming)

are thought to speed the client's healing process. The Web site http://www.emdr.com/efficacy.htm cites a good deal of research into EMDR supporting it as an evidence-based practice.

For traumas that involve large groups of people (e.g., a school shooting), it may be beneficial to set up small group discussions. When the client is ready, talking about the trauma is the first step to healing. It may take years for the client to be able to discuss particularly horrendous experiences. Symptoms of anxiety, panic, and major depression typically emerge as memories are uncovered and discussed. Antidepressant medication use is usually beneficial: SSRIs are preferred for their low side-effect profiles and safety in overdosage. Assessing for suicidal or homicidal thoughts at different phases of recovery is essential. Alcohol and other substance abuse risk is high in individuals with acute stress disorder or PTSD. It may be helpful to provide education to the client regarding typical responses that others experience following a trauma. Because it serves to let clients know that they are not alone. Active listening and other therapeutic communication skills are more important than offering advice or expressing one's own opinions. Clients who have been traumatized need to be listened to and not lectured.

OBSESSIVE-COMPULSIVE DISORDER

The essential characteristics of an obsessive-compulsive disorder (OCD) are recurrent obsessions (intrusive thoughts) or compulsions (ritualistic behaviors) that cause marked distress to the client, are usually unwanted, and are severe enough to be time consuming. The intrusive thoughts associated with obsessions may seem to come out of nowhere. They are not delusional in nature, because the client understands that they are irrational or illogical. Children with OCD may not recognize that their thoughts or actions are excessive or unrea-

TABLE 11-4: CRITERIA FOR POSTTRAUMATIC STRESS DISORDER

1. The client was exposed to a traumatic event where

   a. there was actual or threatened death or serious injury or assault to the self or others; and

   b. the client's response involved intense fear, helplessness, or horror (agitated or disorganized behavior in children).

2. The traumatic event is persistently re-experienced in one or more of the following:

   a. recurrent memories of the event including images, thoughts or perceptions (children may reenact themes of the trauma through play)

   b. recurrent distressing dreams of the event (children may have vague, frightening dreams)

   c. feeling as if the event were reoccurring (e.g., flashbacks) (children may reenact portions of the event such as molesting younger children)

   d. intense emotional distress in response to internal or external cues symbolic of the event

   e. physical reactions to those internal or external cues

3. Persistent avoidance of anything related to the trauma, and a sense of numbing as indicated by three or more of the following:

   a. avoids thoughts, feelings, or conversations related to the trauma

   b. avoids activities, places, or people that arouse memories

   c. unable to recall important aspects of the trauma

   d. diminished interest in activities

   e. feelings of detachment or estrangement

   f. restricted range of affect

   g. lack of a sense of a future

4. Persistent symptoms of increased arousal with two or more of the following:

   a. difficulty falling or staying asleep

   b. irritability or outbursts of anger

   c. difficulty concentrating

   d. hypervigilance (always on guard)

   e. exaggerated startle responses

5. Duration of the symptoms in criteria 2, 3, and 4 lasting more than 1 month

6. The disturbance causing clinically significant impairments in functioning

(American Psychiatric Association, 2000)

sonable. Common obsessions include fears of germ or disease contamination, repeated worry or doubt, a need to have things in order, sexual imagery or, occasionally, aggressive or horrible acts. Individuals with obsessions initially attempt to ignore or suppress the thoughts, but almost always find that the behaviors provide some temporary relief from anxiety (defense mechanism of undoing). The compulsive behaviors may have some logical association with the obsession (e.g., washing hands with a germ fear or praying over aggressive thoughts) or they may not. The most common compulsive behaviors include counting, checking, cleaning or washing, ordering, demanding assurances, or repeating actions. Panic attacks are associated with OCD when clients feel that they may not be able to carry out compulsions. Compulsive behaviors can take hours and be quite disabling for the client; for example, a client may feel the need to shower in a certain way every day. If the client deviates from the steps in any way, he or she must start over at the beginning.

Consequences of OCD are impaired relationships with others, family and marital discord, work or school conflicts and, possibly, an inability to live life as fully and normally as possible. Skin conditions and infections can result in individuals with germ or contamination fears. OCD has a familial association and may have some genetic basis.

The most effective medication treatments for OCD are SSRI medications. The TCA, Anafranil® (clomipramine), is also effective; however, because of side-effect risks, the SSRIs should be first-line treatment. Luvox® is specifically indicated for OCD, but all of the medications in this class are effective. SNRI's, such as duloxetine (Cymbalta®), venlafaxine XR (Effexor XR®), and desvenlafaxine (Pristiq®), are also useful. Wellbutrin SR® is less useful because it has prominent dopaminergic activity, rather than serotonin.

Exposure therapy is also indicated in treatment of OCD. For example, clients with a fear of contamination may be asked initially to simply touch a desktop or watch the therapist eat food off of the desktop. They can then progress to touching money, doorknobs and, eventually, to shaking hands, all the while suppressing the compulsive urge to constantly wash their hands and using relaxation breathing to minimize or reduce their anxiety levels. Cognitive behavior techniques are also beneficial in helping the client to rehearse the association between his thoughts, feelings, and behavioral responses.

PANDAS

PANDAS is the acronym for pediatric autoimmune neuropsychiatric disorders associated with streptococcial infection. The primary two dis-

orders seen in PANDAS are OCD and tic disorders. In a study at the University of Rochester Medical Center, 12 children were identified with new onset PANDAS. They found that the mean age at presentation was 7 and there was a 4 to 1 ratio of males to females. All of these children developed a rapid onset of OCD or tic disorder following a strep throat infection; parents could identify the exact day the symptoms began. Prior to this date, there was no evidence of any neuropsychiatric disorders in any of the children. In these children, 75% of the compulsions were germ-related and more than half also had urinary urgency and frequency without infection. The children were treated with broad-spectrum antibiotics for 10 days and the OCD symptoms resolved in 14 days. Six of the children relapsed and again had positive throat cultures for Group A strep. Recommendations of the study were that if a parent calls with reports of a sudden onset of strange behaviors in a child and the child has had a recent sore throat or fever, then PANDAS should be considered and the child should be placed on a course of antibiotics. Currently it is not known if PANDAS is predictive of a later onset OCD or tic disorder (Hughes, 2002). For the reader interested in this disorder, Dr. Miroslav Kovacevic of Chicago, IL publishes an online resource that is replete with symptom clusters of PANDAS seen in his neuropsychiatric patients as well as real-life case studies of children that he has treated (http://www.web pediatrics.com/pandas.html).

NURSING INTERVENTIONS WITH THE ANXIOUS CLIENT

Clients with anxiety are commonly encountered in inpatient, outpatient, and general medical practice offices. Nurses can help by obtaining thorough histories that include symptoms and precipitating events. Anxiety disorders that can be tied to specific objects or events (e.g., PTSD, phobias, social anxiety) are sometimes easier to manage than are GAD and OCD. Pediatric nurses should be aware of PANDAS and ask parents about recent colds, fevers, or sore throats. Client education is beneficial because many clients with an anxiety disorder fear they are going crazy. Providing reassurance that they have a relatively common medical condition may help to alleviate some of those fears. Talking with clients and their families about the fight or flight response sets the groundwork for relaxation and guided imagery training and developing an exercise plan. Nurses can also advocate for the client with the prescribing practitioner. As tempting as the immediate relief provided by benzodiazepines may be, they should be prescribed judiciously. Most clients should be started on an SSRI or TCA prescription (including children) and be provided limited benzodiazepines for as needed usage only. In the primary care setting, clients with anxiety disorders need to be referred to counselors, particularly ones who specialize in cognitive behavior therapy techniques or have extra training in the treatment of PTSD. Nurses can help to facilitate these referrals and explain to the client and family the rationales for therapy. Hospitalized clients frequently have anxiety (in both the mental health and general medical populations). Implementing relaxation techniques and providing as needed medications will help. Establishing a rapport with the client is essential. Spending a little extra time actively listening to the client's concerns is as valuable for a client with anxiety, as is catheter care to the postoperative client.

CASE STUDY: GENERALIZED ANXIETY DISORDER

Casey is a 16-year-old girl who is being seen in the pediatrician's office for complaints of stomach aches nearly every day at school. She has been going to the nurse's office frequently and asking the health aid to call her mother. Occasionally, she also requests an acetaminophen tablet for headaches. Casey was an honor roll student her freshman year, but this year her grades have dropped to a B or C average. During her appointment, she tells the nurse that she is worried that she won't be able to get into college with such poor grades. A college student was recently abducted while out riding her bicycle in Casey's hometown; she was later found murdered. Casey has been asking her mother to carry a cellular phone when she goes out jogging in the evenings and she calls her every 15 minutes. When her mother doesn't return promptly in 45 minutes, Casey calls her cellular phone in a panic. One time she called 911 to report her mother as missing when the cellular phone batteries went dead. At home, Casey has reported trouble falling asleep at night before 1:00 a.m., and then she has vague nightmares of being chased by vampires and zombies. She feels tired during the day at school. Casey's parents divorced 14 years previously, but she has a stable home life at both her mother's and her father's homes. Lately she hasn't wanted to go out with friends or leave home very often, unless her mother leaves with her (even then she really wants to remain at home). Medically, Casey is healthy. She has no allergies or history of any medical problems. She does not take any medications. She was a full-term infant and met all of her developmental milestones on target. There is a positive history of anxiety and depression on her mother's side of the family, but none presently. The pediatrician diagnoses Casey with gastritis secondary to a generalized anxiety disorder. After consulting with the parents, she prescribes sertraline (Zoloft®) 50 mg once daily plus Zantac® 150 mg at bedtime.

Questions

1. Children may have anxiety symptoms that are similar to or different from those experienced by adults. What anxiety symptoms is this child exhibiting?

2. What medical condition might be related to a sudden onset of an anxiety disorder?

3. Sertraline (Zoloft®) is from which category of medications?

Discussion

Children with anxiety disorders often demonstrate gastrointestinal complaints and separation fears. A generalized anxiety disorder has no one specific fear; but is an overall worry about many aspects of life. Children often worry about their parents' health and well-being. PANDAS (pediatric auto-immune neurologic disorders associated with streptococcal infections) can be the cause of a sudden onset of an anxiety disorder, most often obsessive-compulsive disorders. Obtaining medical histories of children should include inquiring about any recent strep infections. Sertraline is an SSRI that is highly effective for anxiety disorders. Its use is approved for OCD treatment in individuals 6 years of age or older..

NURSING CARE PLAN: GENERALIZED ANXIETY DISORDER

Problem Listing

- Stomach aches
- Nonspecific worries
- Feelings of being unsafe
- Feelings that her family is unsafe
- Headaches
- Social isolation
- Sleep disturbance

Priority Nursing Diagnosis

Anxiety related to perceived threats to integrity of self and family as evidenced by persistent worries, stomach aches, and a drop in academic performance.

Long-term Goal

Client will have anxiety reduced to a level that no longer interferes with her functioning.

Short-term Objectives

1. Client will report no stomach aches.

2. Client will stop calling her mother every 15 minutes while jogging.

3. Client will bring her grades back to the previous A to B average.

Nursing Interventions

1. Establish a sense of rapport and trust with the client by utilizing the active listening techniques of open-ended questions, clarifying, validating, and reflecting feelings.

2. Remain nonjudgmental and noncritical of the client.

3. Teach the client relaxation breathing to be utilized in times of stress. Practice these techniques until the client has mastered them.

4. Talk the client through a guided imagery session and teach her how to utilize guided imagery when alone.

5. Consult with parents regarding client's need for reassurance and support.

6. Provide medication education for SSRIs.

7. Assist the client in developing a plan for completing homework in a timely manner.

8. Ask the client to keep a daily journal of thoughts and feelings and how they impacted behavior for that day.

9. Encourage client to resume social activities with peers.

ADVANCED PRACTICE NURSING: MANAGING ANXIETY PHARMACOLOGICALLY

Complaints of anxiety or nervousness are among the top three emotional symptoms presented by clients in both medical and psychiatric settings (the other two are depression and insomnia). Anxiety management can be very challenging for the nurse clinician. Therapy is always advisable, but some clients are unable to access affordable services or they resist opening up to their fears. The APRN who is trained in therapeutic interventions, such as CBT, psychoanalysis, or EMDR, may elect to provide this along with medication management. Clients want immediate relief; however, the most effective medications (benzodiazepines) also cause habituation, tolerance, and dependency. Withdrawal from these medications is highly uncomfortable for the client and may provoke increased anxiety and panic, hypertension, tachycardia, and seizures. The Texas Medication Algorithm Project did not specifically address the treatment of anxiety disorders, and no consistent, evidence-based practice recommendations currently exist. This leaves the nurse prescriber to make decisions on anxiety treatment independently, which can be frustrating. Some practices maintain protocols to guide the prescriber, but most do not. Figure 11-1 presents an algorithm used by the author in outpatient

FIGURE 11-1: ANXIETY TREATMENT ALGORITHM

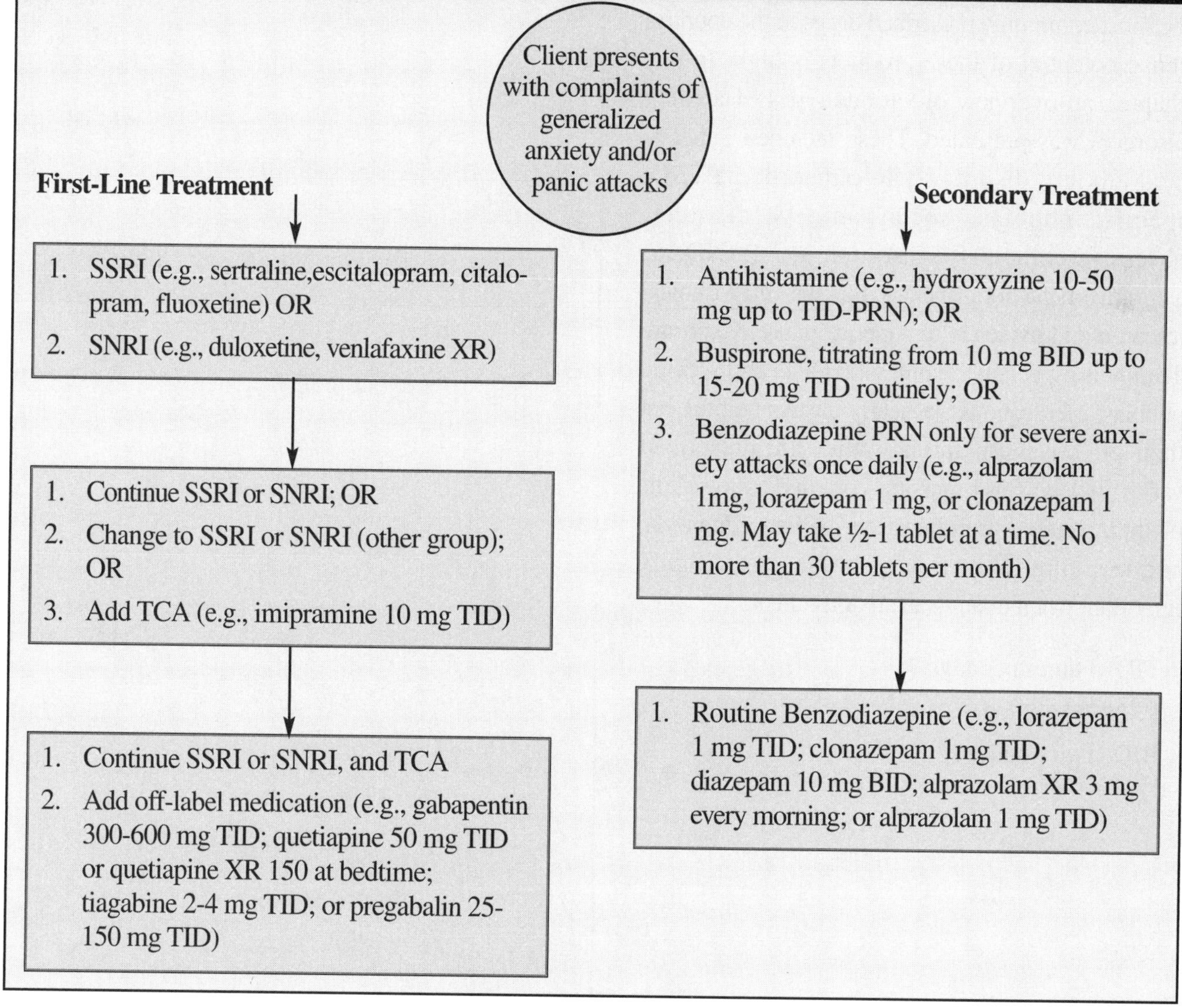

Client presents with complaints of generalized anxiety and/or panic attacks

First-Line Treatment

1. SSRI (e.g., sertraline, escitalopram, citalopram, fluoxetine) OR
2. SNRI (e.g., duloxetine, venlafaxine XR)

↓

1. Continue SSRI or SNRI; OR
2. Change to SSRI or SNRI (other group); OR
3. Add TCA (e.g., imipramine 10 mg TID)

↓

1. Continue SSRI or SNRI, and TCA
2. Add off-label medication (e.g., gabapentin 300-600 mg TID; quetiapine 50 mg TID or quetiapine XR 150 at bedtime; tiagabine 2-4 mg TID; or pregabalin 25-150 mg TID)

Secondary Treatment

1. Antihistamine (e.g., hydroxyzine 10-50 mg up to TID-PRN); OR
2. Buspirone, titrating from 10 mg BID up to 15-20 mg TID routinely; OR
3. Benzodiazepine PRN only for severe anxiety attacks once daily (e.g., alprazolam 1mg, lorazepam 1 mg, or clonazepam 1 mg. May take ½-1 tablet at a time. No more than 30 tablets per month)

↓

1. Routine Benzodiazepine (e.g., lorazepam 1 mg TID; clonazepam 1mg TID; diazepam 10 mg BID; alprazolam XR 3 mg every morning; or alprazolam 1 mg TID)

practice that has been very useful. It is also helpful to educate the client in anxiety management, using concepts of prevention and rescue medication (similar to asthma treatment). SSRIs, SNRIs, buspirone, and a TCA are the medications to be used routinely to prevent anxiety and panic attacks; whereas, benzodiazepines and antihistamines are used to rescue the client when the errant attack occurs.

SUMMARY

Anxiety disorders are one of the more common and challenging psychiatric and mental health problems encountered. They occur in all clients (male and female), in all age groups, and across the socioeconomic spectrum. Anxiolytics are some of the most commonly prescribed drugs in the country; abuse potential of these products is high. In this chapter, an overview of various types of anxiety disorders was presented. These included generalized anxiety disorder, panic disorder, PTSD, specific phobias, social anxiety disorder, obsessive-compulsive disorder, and PANDAS. Cognitive-behavioral therapy has the most clinical research and evidence to support its use. Exposure therapy is especially helpful with OCD and specific phobias. Medications are nearly always helpful, but their effectiveness and how they are prescribed varies widely. Basic nursing communication skills of therapeutic communication, patient education, and teaching relaxation techniques are highly important when treating an anxious client.

TID: 3 times per day

PRN: As needed

BID: Twice daily

EXAM QUESTIONS

CHAPTER 11
Questions 65-71

Note: Choose the one option that BEST answers each question.

65. Symptoms of generalized anxiety disorder include

    a. having a specific focus of fear.

    b. muscle tension.

    c. vomiting.

    d. blurred vision.

66. Helping a client to imagine sitting on a beach, listening to the waves, and feeling the warm sun is called

    a. cognitive behavior therapy.

    b. interpersonal therapy.

    c. behavior modification.

    d. guided imagery.

67. First-line medication treatment for anxiety disorders should include

    a. a benzodiazepine.

    b. an antipsychotic.

    c. an SSRI.

    d. an MAO inhibitor.

68. The usefulness of benzodiazepines is limited by

    a. their potential for habituation and dependency.

    b. a high risk of toxicity.

    c. the development of extrapyramidal syndrome symptoms.

    d. a lack of efficacy in anxiety disorders.

69. *Eugene presents to the emergency department complaining of shortness of breath, trembling, feeling numb in his face and hands, and a sensation of choking. He thought he was having a heart attack.*

The most likely cause of this client's symptoms is

    a. a dissociative episode.

    b. claustrophobia.

    c. a psychotic break.

    d. a panic attack.

70. Posttraumatic stress disorder symptoms may include

    a. problems being in a room full of people.

    b. repetitive and nonproductive behaviors.

    c. generalized fears of a variety of events or situations.

    d. flashbacks and nightmares of the traumatic experience.

71. Repetitively checking to see that the windows are closed, the range is turned off, and the doors are locked is an example of

    a. generalized anxiety disorder.

    b. obsessive-compulsive disorder.

    c. posttraumatic stress disorder.

    d. panic disorder.

CHAPTER 12

EATING, SLEEPING, AND SOMATOFORM DISORDERS

CHAPTER OBJECTIVE

At the end of this chapter, the reader will be able to recognize mental health disorders that are expressed by poor nutrition, medical complaints, or sleep problems.

LEARNING OBJECTIVES

By the completion of the chapter, the reader will be able to

1. describe symptoms of anorexia nervosa and bulimia.

2. differentiate somatoform disorders from other medical conditions.

3. discuss relevant treatment for disorders involving health, nutrition, and sleep problems.

INTRODUCTION

In this chapter, psychiatric disorders that relate to medical or physical health conditions are explored. These are divided into three broad groups: eating disorders, somatoform disorders, and sleep disorders. The primary eating disorders that will be addressed are anorexia nervosa and bulimia. It should be noted that anorexia is a term that describes a lack of eating, which can be caused by many medical conditions (e.g., metastatic cancer), and it is only considered a psychiatric issue when there is no medical condition causing the symp-

tom. "Soma" means "of the body" and it is widely used in mental health care to describe bodily complaints (see Chapter 3 discussion on somatic delusions). Somatoform disorders describe conditions that consist of numerous physical complaints (somatization), a persistent belief that one is ill (hypochondriasis), sensory or motor dysfunctions without medical cause (conversion disorder), and the persistent belief that there is something gravely wrong with one's body (body dysmorphic disorder). Chronic pain disorders are often seen in mental health settings for their secondary problems of depression, fatigue, and hopelessness. Finally, several sleep disorders will be discussed, including primary insomnia, hypersomnia, obstructive sleep apnea, and circadian rhythm sleep disorders.

EATING DISORDERS

The *DSM-IV-TR* recognizes two types of eating disorders: anorexia nervosa and bulimia nervosa. Both are characterized by severe disturbances in eating behavior, often accompanied by body perception distortions. Eating disorders often begin in mid to late adolescence, following a stressful life event. Severe cases may require hospitalization. Mortality related to anorexia nervosa is slightly more than 5% of diagnosed clients (the lifetime prevalence for anorexia nervosa is about 0.5%). Approximately 90% of all clients are female. Causes of eating disorders are still unknown; however, contributing factors include sociocultural pressures, family dynamics and possibly, biological issues. Images presented in the fashion or entertainment industry often portray the ideal body type as one with little to no fat. This sends a message to young women that they are flawed if they are unable to obtain this appearance. A character-type often seen in anorexia nervosa is a young woman with obsessive, perfectionistic tendencies; overly rigid or anxious coping responses; and enmeshed or controlling parents. There can be a familial component to the disorder as well, with food and eating behaviors assuming an inappropriate overly important role in the family's interactions with one another.

Anorexia Nervosa

The essential feature of anorexia nervosa is a refusal to gain or maintain weight, accomplished primarily through starvation. Diagnostic criteria for anorexia nervosa include the following:

1. Refusal to maintain body weight at a minimally normal weight for age and height, or failure to make expected weight gains

2. Intense fear of gaining weight or becoming fat (even when underweight)

3. Disturbances in the way body shape or weight is experienced (i.e., undue influence on self-esteem, self-valuation, or denial of the seriousness of the problem)

4. Amenorrhea (in postmenarcheal clients), or the absence of at least three menstrual cycles

Subtypes of anorexia nervosa include restricting (absence of self-induced vomiting or misuse of laxatives, diuretics, or enemas) and binge eating and purging (presence of regular binge-eating or purging during an episode of anorexia).

Seriously underweight clients may manifest depression, irritability, insomnia, and social withdrawal. There may be concerns about eating in public, feelings of inadequacy, or an apparent lack of emotional expression. There is usually an obsession about food, which may take the form of hoarding. Clients with a binge eating and purging subtype are more likely to have a personality disorder or to abuse substances. Other self-destructive behaviors may present, such as sexual promiscuity, self-mutilation, or suicide attempts. Relationships with family and peers can become strained and marked by conflict.

Physical findings associated with anorexia nervosa are attributable to starvation. In addition to amenorrhea, there are complaints of constipation, abdominal pain, cold intolerance, fatigue, and lethargy. Low blood pressure and body temperature and bradycardia may be found. Dry hair and skin and hair loss are common. Some clients develop lanugo, which is a fine, downy body hair similar to that seen in newborn infants. Peripheral edema, bruising or petechiae, enlarged parotid (salivary) glands, and a yellowing of the skin may occur. Clients who induce vomiting may have tooth enamel erosion or tooth loss. Later findings can include dehydration, osteoporosis, impaired renal function, cardiac arrhythmias, and congestive heart failure.

Bulimia Nervosa

In bulimia nervosa, binge eating and purging behaviors are seen, but without the severe dietary restrictions found in anorexia nervosa. The client's self-perception and evaluation are excessively influenced by body shape and weight.

A binge is defined as eating an excessive amount of food in a short period of time – usually less than 2 hours. Binge foods typically are high-calorie, sugary foods, such as ice cream or cake. Clients who binge are typically ashamed of the behavior and attempt to hide it. Binges are often precipitated by emotional stress and are followed by feelings of self-criticism, guilt, and depression. A sense of lack of control usually accompanies the binging.

Purging occurs in response to feelings of shame and guilt. The most common form of purging is self-induced vomiting (80% to 90%). The immediate gains from vomiting include relief from physical discomfort due to excessive intake and a reduced fear of gaining weight. Other purging behaviors include the misuse of laxatives (30%), diuretics, or enemas. Excess exercising with the express purpose of purging calories is also a form of bulimia nervosa. Use of diet pills, diet aids, or even thyroid hormone supplements can also occur.

Medical complications due to binging may include significant and permanent tooth enamel loss, dental cavities, calluses or scars of the back of the hand, menstrual irregularities, bowel problems (with chronic laxative use), fluid and electrolyte imbalances, esophageal tears, gastric rupture, and cardiac arrhythmias. Low weight does not often occur – in fact, most clients with bulimia nervosa maintain their body weight.

NURSING INTERVENTIONS FOR THE CLIENT WITH AN EATING DISORDER

Nurses will usually encounter clients with anorexia nervosa in an inpatient setting. Clients with bulimia nervosa rarely require hospital care. Nurses need to work diligently to avoid seeming judgmental of the client. Active listening, combined with consistent behavioral limitations helps to provide a sense of security and support. Staff should de-emphasize weighing the client more than necessary because it may promote control issues. Instead, the nurse should focus on the feelings associated with eating (or binging and purging) and the associated consequences. Helping a client to develop awareness of the link between behavior and feelings may help to change the behavior in a positive manner. Calorie counts are usually necessary to determine actual food intake. The monitoring of electrolyte, cal-

cium, and magnesium levels is important. Intravenous fluids or feeding tubes with liquid supplements may be needed for severe starvation. Observing for signs of purging is usually recommended. Encouraging light activity and providing diet education help to promote a healthy lifestyle. Support or therapy groups can be powerful tools as young adults and adolescents tend to be peer-oriented and the feedback from others is invaluable. Staff should expect the client to experience a good deal of anxiety with any weight gain. Positive reinforcement for even small gains is extremely important.

Medication Interventions

There are no medications specifically indicated for the treatment of eating disorders. Commonly, vitamin and mineral supplementation is provided. Antidepressant medications are useful in helping to treat associated depression, mood swings, and anxiety symptoms. Anxiolytics may be used on an as needed basis.

CASE STUDY: ANOREXIA NERVOSA

Brittany is an attractive, petite cheerleader in the 8th grade. She wants to make the high school squad next year, but some of her friends tell her that the competition is really hard and she has to be perfect to get selected. Brittany goes through a growth spurt the summer before high school and she grows to 5'7" and puts on 10 lb, bringing her weight up to 135 lb. One of the boys from her school sees her at the mall, and says, "Hey, have you been eating all summer or what?" Brittany becomes determined to lose weight. She starts to skip breakfast, then lunch. Soon she is eating once a day. She tells her family that she is going to be a vegetarian "because meat is gross." She starts exercising 2 to 3 hours every evening. Her weight starts to come off and she starts to get compliments from her friends. At 120 lb her mother suggests that she looks a little thin, but Brittany only sees fat around her thighs and stomach. Soon she is only eating a little lettuce (no dressing) and an apple for the day. Her weight continues to drop and she notices some of her hair falling out in the shower. Although she is still exercising, she stops going out with friends because she is too tired. At 105 lb her menstrual cycles cease. By now, her parents are very concerned and they take her to a pediatrician. He tells them it's "just a phase, a lot of girls go through," so they try not to worry. By Christmas, Brittany weighs only 90 lb and she looks emaciated. She tells her best friend, Jennie, that she "just needs to lose a little more." At 84 lb Brittany faints at school and is rushed to the hospital. She is admitted to the intensive care unit for premature ventricular contractions and starvation syndrome. A psychiatric referral is made as well. Once stabilized, she is referred to an eating disorder specialist who meets with her and her family once a week to help Brittany develop some understanding of the disorder and set a reasonable goal weight for maintenance.

Questions

1. What are some of the environmental pressures experienced by this client that may have contributed to her anorexia?

2. Describe the relationship between anorexia nervosa and cardiac disorders.

3. Would therapy or medications be more effective for this client?

Discussion

Anorexia nervosa often has its onset during adolescence, especially in girls. Such pressures as attention from the opposite sex and a desire to look like fashion models seen on television and in magazines can contribute to the development of the disorder. Some teens also have perfectionistic tendencies and perceive others to be hypercritical of them. Severe anorexia leads to cardiac arrhythmias

due to electrolyte imbalances; congestive heart failure may even occur. Therapy is always indicated for the client as well as the family. Medications are of limited usefulness, although antidepressants are commonly prescribed to treat underlying depression and anxiety symptoms.

NURSING CARE PLAN: CLIENT WITH ANOREXIA NERVOSA

Problem Listing

*   Calorie intake less than body requirements
*   Cardiac arrhythmia
*   Amenorrhea
*   Distorted body perception
*   Low self-esteem

Priority Nursing Diagnosis

Alteration in nutrition, less than body requirements, related to self-induced eating disorder, as evidenced by a body weight of 84 lb with a height of 5'7."

Long-term Goal

Client will return to a body weight of 115 lb or above.

Short-term Objectives

1. Client will gain 1 to 2 pounds every week.

2. Client will eat a combination of carbohydrates, fats, and proteins.

3. Client will identify three positive qualities about self not related to physical appearance or weight.

4. Client will verbalize an understanding of the diet plan.

Nursing Interventions

1. Daily calorie count – instruct the family and client for home usage.

2. Monitor fluid intake and electrolyte balance.

3. Educate the client about healthy food choices.

4. Provide support and encouragement with rewards for healthy weight gain.

5. Refer the client to appropriate therapy (individual and group) and support services in the community.

SOMATOFORM DISORDERS

The common features of the somatoform disorders are the occurrence of physical symptoms in the absence of a diagnosed medical condition or substance abuse problem. The symptoms must cause clinically significant distress or functional impairment. Somatoform disorders are often encountered in general medical practices and may account for numerous unnecessary tests, X-rays, hospitalizations, and surgeries every year. Five types of somatoform disorders are discussed here: somatization disorder, conversion disorder, pain disorder, hypochondriasis, and body dysmorphic disorder.

Somatization Disorder

A somatization disorder is one in which there is a pattern of recurring, multiple physical complaints that result in significant functional impairment or medical intervention (including medications). Symptoms occur before 30 years of age, and continue for years. Somatization disorders are seen more often in women and they have a familial tendency. The men in these families tend to have a greater occurrence of substance dependence and antisocial personality disorder. Making the diagnosis of a somatization disorder requires ruling out all other medical causes, which may include such disorders such as hypothyroidism, lupus erythematosus, arthritis, multiple sclerosis, and Lyme disease. *DSM-IV-TR* diagnostic criteria for somatization disorder are presented in Table 12-1.

Conversion Disorder

The essential features of a conversion disorder are the presence of symptoms that affect motor or sensory function and that suggest a neurological disorder or other medical condition. To diagnose a conversion disorder, one must first rule out any actual medical conditions. Voluntary motor or sensory functions might include such symptoms as paralysis, blindness, deafness, seizures, weakness or falling, loss of touch or pain sensation, or impaired coordination. Conversion symptoms are often inconsistent and do not follow expected neurological pathways (e.g., a paralyzed arm will move during sleep). Electromyelograms and electroencephalograms (EEGs) are normal. Psychologically, the conversion symptoms may be reflective of an underlying trauma or distress (e.g., the man who witnesses a murder may become blind). Although the client may receive secondary gains from the symptoms, in the form of increased attention and nurturance, it is important to note that these symptoms are not faked – that is, they are real to the client and quite distressful. Culturally sanctioned symptoms, such as visions as a part of religious rituals, are not considered to be conversion symptoms. Subtypes of conversion disorders include motor symptom or deficit (loss of voluntary muscle controls), sensory symptom or deficit (loss of touch, pain, eyesight, or hearing.), seizures or convulsions, and mixed presentation.

Pain Disorder

In a pain disorder, the pain must be the predominant focus of the client and it must cause clinically significant distress or interference with social, occupational, or other important areas of functioning. The pain is not intentionally produced or faked (as in factitious disorder and malingering), nor is it associated with psychosis, anxiety, or a depressive disorder. There may be accompanying medical conditions, but the pain must be the predominant concern and demonstrate chronicity in

TABLE 12-1: DIAGNOSTIC CRITERIA FOR A SOMATIZATION DISORDER

1. A history of many physical complaints over several years, resulting in treatment being sought or significant functional impairment

2. Each of the following criteria must be met:

    a. four pain symptoms (e.g., headaches, joint pain, backaches)

    b. two gastrointestinal (GI) symptoms (e.g., nausea, gas, bloating, heartburn, vomiting, constipation, diarrhea)

    c. one sexual symptom (e.g., irregular menses, pain with intercourse, erectile dysfunction)

    d. one pseudo-neurological symptom (e.g., impaired balance, weakness, trouble swallowing, numbness or tingling of extremities, double vision, blindness, fainting, paralysis)

3. Either (a) or (b)

    a. No medical cause found for the symptoms in criterion 2.

    b. In the presence of an actual medical condition, the symptoms or functioning of the client worsening more than what could be reasonably expected.

4. The symptoms not intentionally produced or feigned (as in factitious disorder or malingering)

An undifferentiated somatoform disorder may also occur when only one or two symptoms are present and they persist for 6 months or longer. These symptoms may include such complaints as chronic fatigue, loss of appetite, GI problems or urinary tract diorders.

(American Psychiatric Association, 2000)

nature. Psychological factors have an important role in the onset, severity, exacerbation, or maintenance of the pain.

A chronic widespread pain disorder called fibromyalgia, which is thought to have autoimmune causes, is often seen in psychiatric settings. This disorder occurs in women 20 times greater than in men and may have some relationship to estrogen (onset is often around the time of menopause, whether natural or surgically induced via hysterectomy with oophorectomy). Not all clients with fibromyalgia have accompanying anxiety, depression, or insomnia, but a great number of them do. This has led to stigmatization in the medical world that fibromyalgia is a hypochondriacally induced disorder (see following discussion on hypochondriasis); in fact, fibromyalgia is more similar to a connective tissue and joint disorder than any psychiatric problem. In PET scan trials done at the University of Alabama, the brain's perception threshold of pain was significantly lower in fibromyalgia patients than in controls, in the limbic portion of the brain (part of the brain thought to be associated with emotional arousal).

Hypochondriasis

A client with hypochondriasis is preoccupied with fears of having or developing a medical disorder. In many cases, personality traits exist where clients have a lifelong pattern of focusing on body symptoms and seeking medical advice. Clients with hypochondriasis may have intrusive thoughts and compulsive behaviors. Hypochondriasis differs from an OCD subtype in that, with OCD a client fears getting a disease, whereas in hypochondriasis, the client believes to have some, as yet undiagnosed, disease. *DSM-IV-TR* criteria include:

1. Preoccupation with a fear of having a serious disease based on bodily symptoms.

2. The preoccupation persists despite medical evaluation and reassurance.

3. The belief does not meet the criteria of being a delusion.

4. The belief causes clinically significant distress in various areas of functioning.

5. The duration is at least 6 months.

6. The preoccupation cannot be better accounted for by generalized anxiety disorder, OCD, panic disorder, major depression, or another psychiatric or substance abuse disorder.

Body Dysmorphic Disorder

A preoccupation with a defect in physical appearance is known as body dysmorphic disorder. The defect is either not present or is so slight that the amount of preoccupation seen is extreme. There must be significant distress and impairment of functioning. Complaints seen may take the form of imagined flaws of the face or head (e.g., hair thinning, acne, wrinkles, vascular markings, swelling, or asymmetry) or other preoccupations such as the shape or size of body parts (e.g., eyes, ears, breasts, or penis). Any body part, or more than one, may be a focus. Because of severe embarrassment over the perceived flaw, clients may view themselves as ugly and feel unloveable. Thoughts about the defect may become significantly intrusive and negative, to the point that self-mutilation or suicide can occur. The client may try to hide the defect with clothing, beards, or hairstyles. Insight is often poor and some clients reach the point of becoming delusional. Clients with this disorder also often believe that everyone else is talking about the defect and feeling either disgust or pity for them. Clients may quit jobs or school or stop going out of the house altogether. Clients with body dysmorphic disorder may go to extremes to try and alter the defect including steroid use with body building, plastic surgery, implants, or even self-surgery. Body dysmorphic disorder tends to be equally prevalent in men and women and is higher in association with anxiety and depressive disorders. In cosmetic and dermatology settings, prevalence rates are as high as 6% to 15% (American Psychiatric Association, 2000).

NURSING INTERVENTIONS FOR THE CLIENT WITH A SOMATOFORM DISORDER

It is important for the nurse to realize that, unlike factitious disorders (in which clients fabricate symptoms) or malingering (in which clients lie about symptoms), clients with a somatoform disorder are in a great deal of distress. They truly believe that there is a medical problem and no one can, or will, help them. The best approach for the nurse is to provide support and compassion to the client. Frequently, healthcare providers are frustrated with clients who have no clear diagnosis and seem to be attention seeking, and they tend to shun them or disregard their complaints. A more helpful approach is to provide the client with nurturance and reassurance in order to forge a more collaborative relationship. Refocusing the client on strengths and abilities, rather than on liabilities, helps to promote self-esteem. Assisting the client in identifying coping strategies provides a sense of control for the client. Clients may be resistant to therapy because they believe the problem to be medical and not psychological. The nurse can encourage the client to see a counselor, in addition to any medical testing, on the rationale that the stress experienced by the medical symptoms certainly warrants additional support. A therapist can help the client identify the purpose that the symptoms serve and to reframe or discover other ways to get emotional needs of love and belonging met in the absence of an illness.

CASE STUDY: SOMATIZATION DISORDER

Bertha is a 45-year-old divorced woman who has been going to physicians since she was 22 years old. Her ex-husband was abusive and an alcoholic. She suffers from chronic fatigue, headaches, diarrhea (or sometimes constipation), pain in her legs, funny tingling feelings in her feet, hot flashes, and dizziness. At age 25 she had a total abdominal hysterectomy for irregular cycles. Persistent abdominal pain resulted in an exploratory laparoscopy at age 27. Bertha also had a cholecystectomy and incidental appendectomy for small gallstones when she was 32. When her surgical wound became infected and separated, she had to have a mesh placed. At home, she "takes to her bed" frequently with migraine headaches. Bertha "threw out her back" carrying groceries one day last year and she takes prescription pain medications several times a day. Most of her family won't visit anymore because they have grown tired of hearing her persistent complaining and tales of medical treatments gone awry. The rheumatologist put Bertha on nonsteroidal anti-inflammatory medications for her joint pain, the surgeon gave her antacids for her "heartburn," and her family doctor gives her hormone replacement plus sleeping pills (for her chronic insomnia). Bertha is increasingly depressed and doesn't understand why no one can tell her what is wrong with her. Her son came to visit her and found her unconscious with numerous empty pain pill bottles lying on the table. She was rushed to the hospital, admitted to the intensive care unit, and then transferred to the inpatient psychiatric unit for depression and personality disorder when she was medically stable.

Questions

1. What symptoms does this client present that suggest a somatization disorder?

2. Could any of her symptoms be attributed to a true medical disorder?

3. What kind of therapeutic approach might be helpful for this client?

Discussion

This client presents with headaches, joint pain, pain in her legs, and abdominal pain (4 pain symptoms). She also has heartburn and diarrhea (2 GI

symptoms), hot flashes (sexual symptom), and numbness and tingling in her feet (neurological symptom). Medical disorders should be initially ruled out because diabetes can cause numbness and tingling, arthritis can cause joint pain, and so forth. The challenge is that many of these medical disorders are subjective and not objectively measured. Therapy for this client would consist of a supportive (not confrontational) approach, exploration into past abuse issues, and redirection during sessions away from medical preoccupation and toward problem-solving life issues, exploring her emotional responses, and encouraging empowerment.

NURSING CARE PLAN: CLIENT WITH SOMATIZATION DISORDER

Problem Listing

- Chronic pain – headaches, backaches, abdominal pain, joint pain

- GI symptoms – diarrhea, constipation, heartburn

- Sexual symptoms – hot flashes, surgically-induced menopause

- Neurological symptoms – weakness, numbness, and tingling extremities

- Psychological symptoms – depression, suicide attempt, low self-esteem

- Social problems – family rejection, no diversional activities, unemployed, children grown and more independent

Priority Nursing Diagnosis

Chronic low self-esteem related to long-standing reliance on others to meet her emotional needs as evidenced by the development of numerous physical ailments that require frequent medical evaluation.

Long-term Goal

Client will develop supportive relationships in the community to meet her needs for support and reassurance.

Short-term Objectives

1. Client will identify two activities that she can do on a weekly basis (may include volunteer work).

2. Client will be able to list at least three positive attributes.

3. Client will be able to have a 30-minute conversation with another adult and not discuss any physical complaints.

4. Client will report improved relationships with the three children.

Nursing Interventions

1. Assist the client in identifying community resources and volunteer opportunities.

2. Support the client in finding and listing three positive attributes.

3. Gently redirect the client away from physical complaints during conversations and toward social or life events.

4. Provide a nonjudgmental, caring approach.

5. Refer for family therapy for the client and her children.

SLEEP DISORDERS

Sleep disorders, or dyssomnias, are primary disorders of initiating or maintaining sleep or of excessive sleepiness. The *DSM-IV-TR* recognizes several types: primary insomnia, primary hypersomnia, narcolepsy, breathing-related sleep disorder, and circadian rhythm sleep disorder. Each of these will be discussed individually along with recommended treatment. Dyssomnia disorder, not otherwise specified, is used for sleep disorders that do not fit into another, more specific category.

Primary Insomnia

Primary insomnia is a complaint of difficulty in initiating or maintaining sleep that lasts at least 1 month. There must be impairment in social, occupational, or other important areas of functioning as a result. The insomnia cannot be better accounted for by a substance abuse problem. Some clients claim to sleep, but feel that their sleep is not restful or restorative. Primary insomnia is often a combination of hyperarousal (due to physical, cognitive, or emotional concerns) and negative conditioning. The anxiety over chronic sleep problems may contribute to the development of a cycle in which the anticipation of insomnia compounds the sleeping problem. Maladaptive sleep habits (e.g., daytime napping, following an erratic sleep schedule) can worsen the symptoms. Chronic insomnia may lead to fatigue, poor concentration, decreased attention to details, and moodiness (irritability or lability). "Short sleepers" are differentiated from insomnia, in that the client requires less sleep to feel restful.

Nursing Interventions for Primary Insomnia

Combining medication intervention with sleep pattern restructuring is the most effective means of treating primary insomnia. Nursing interventions that may be useful are identified in Table 12-2 and medications that are commonly utilized are detailed in Table 12-3.

Primary Hypersomnia

Hypersomnia refers to excessive sleepiness for at least 1 month. Symptoms include either prolonged sleep or daytime sleep episodes occurring almost daily. The sleepiness must interfere with functioning in some manner, and it cannot be caused by another mental disorder or substance use. Clients with primary hypersomnia may sleep 8 to 12 hours, have difficulty waking up, and still feel sleepy during the day. Unintentional sleep episodes typically occur in low-stimulation situations, such as driving long distances, reading, attending lectures, or watching television. Episodes come on

TABLE 12-2: NURSING INTERVENTIONS FOR PRIMARY INSOMNIA

1. Eliminate or significantly reduce caffeine (no more than two caffeine beverages daily, no caffeine after 5:00 p.m.).

2. Eliminate or significantly reduce alcohol intake (may interfere with rapid eye movement sleep stages).

3. Set the alarm clock and get up at the same time every day.

4. Eliminate daytime napping.

5. Perform light exercises daily – but not within 2 hours of bedtime.

6. Have a light snack in the evening – avoid heavy foods within 2 hours of bedtime.

7. Sleep with the lights off and curtains or shades drawn.

8. Keep the room temperature comfortably warm in the winter, and cool in the summer.

9. Consider use of "white noise" (electric fan, water fountain, sound machine).

10. Avoid television or talk radio.

11 Go to bed at the same time. Read or listen to acoustic music. If not asleep in 20 minutes, try as needed medications.

12. Do not use the bedroom for working, studying, or performing other mentally challenging activities.

gradually rather than abruptly and may be quite embarrassing for the client. Often, primary hypersomnia is associated with mild to moderate depression.

Narcolepsy

Narcolepsy involves repeated, irresistible attacks of refreshing sleep, cataplexy, and recurrent intrusions of rapid eye movement (REM) sleep into the transition period between sleep and wakefulness. The sleep attacks must occur daily over a period of at least 3 months. One or both of the following must also occur: cataplexy (episodes of sudden, bilateral loss of muscle tone that last for seconds to minutes) or intrusive REM sleep with paralysis of voluntary muscles or dreamlike hallucinations. As with most other conditions, the presence of substance use or another medical or psychiatric condition must be ruled out. Narcolepsy episodes can be dramatic and occur in the middle of an activity or conversation. Episodes typically last 10 to 20 minutes and may occur up to 6 times per day. Clients vary in their ability to fight off the sleep attacks. The symptom of cataplexy is often triggered by a strong emotion (laughter, anger, surprise) and may be mild (slight drooping of the eyelids) or dramatic (fall to the ground). Motor

control is always regained. The symptoms of sleep paralysis (being aware of surroundings but unable to move) and hallucinatory dreams are thought to be due to REM sleep intrusions.

Research into narcolepsy and cataplexy at the Stanford Medical School Center for Narcolepsy, has identified some significant genetic markers for the disorder (http://med.stanford.edu/school/Psychiatry/narcolepsy). Additionally, sleep studies have identified a correlation between REM sleep abnormalities and the occurrence of the disorder.

Treatment for narcolepsy and cataplexy involves medications. Stimulant-type medications are indicated for the sleep attacks. These include:

• Methylphenidate (Ritalin®, Ritalin SR®, Metadate CD®, Concerta®)

• Methamphetamine HCl (Desoxyn®)

• Dexamphetamine (Dexedrine®, Dextrostat®)

• Dexamphetamine-salts (Adderall®, Adderall XR®)

• Modafinil (Provigil®) and armodafinil (Nuvigil®).

Side effects of stimulant medications include insomnia, jitteriness, tachycardia, decreased appetite, and irritability. The symptoms of abnormal REM sleep (cataplexy, sleep-wake hallucinations,

TABLE 12-3: MEDICATIONS FOR INSOMNIA			
Category	**Generic Name**	**Trade Name**	**Comments**
Antihistamine	diphenhydramine	Benadryl®, Tylenol PM®	Safe, gentle agent
	cyproheptadine	Periactin®	Useful for children
Alternative	melatonin	Melatonex®	Hormone produced in response to sunlight Bizarre dreams may occur
	ramelteon	Rozerem®	Melatonin receptor binding Designed for nightly use (not PRN)
Benzodiazepine	temazepam	Restoril®	Potential for dependency
	flurazepam	Dalmane®	Potential for dependency
	triazolam	Halcion®	Potential for dependency & psychosis
Benzodiazepine-like	zaleplon	Sonata®	Potential for habituation
	zolpidem	Ambien®	Potential for habituation
	eszopiclone	Lunesta®	Can cause metallic taste
Miscellaneous	trazodone	Desyrel®	Mild antidepressant. Extremely sedating
	chloral hydrate	Noctec®	Good for 1 to 2 nights only

and sleep-paralysis) are better treated with antidepressant medications. Side effects of antidepressants are specific to the type of antidepressant. A thorough discussion of antidepressants appears in Chapter 9.

Breathing-related Sleep Disorder

Breathing-related sleep disorders, also known as *sleep apnea* are problems in sleep on an as needed basis associated with abnormalities of ventilation and respiration. The most common presenting complaint is excess daytime sleepiness, which occurs because of frequent wakening during the night, as the client attempts to breathe normally. Breathing-related sleep disorder consists of three subtypes: obstructive sleep apnea (usually seen in overweight individuals and in children with enlarged adenoids and tonsils), central sleep apnea (cessation of breathing during sleep, without obstruction), and central alveolar hypoventilation syndrome (waking occurs because of low oxygenation, usually secondary to morbid obesity). Clients may complain of chest pain, choking, suffocation feelings, or anxiety. Clients with obstructive prob-

lems typically snore loudly, may have difficulty awakening, and report headaches. Dry mouth and thirst lead clients to excessive fluid intake, resulting in nocturia – compounding the problem of interrupted sleep. The daytime sleepiness can lead to mood changes, poor concentration, memory problems, irritability, and personality changes. Children with a breathing-related sleep disorder may present as extremely hyperactive or aggressive, with poor attention spans and concentration, leading to an initial diagnosis of attention deficit hyperactivity disorder.

Treatment for breathing-related sleep disorders involves identifying the cause through sleep studies and physical exams. Surgery to remove tonsils and adenoids may be recommended. Weight loss will reduce both obstructive and hypoventilation types. Often, a continuous positive airway pressure (CPAP) machine is prescribed. The CPAP is a device that consists of an airway mask that is worn by the client during sleep, which provides either room air or a mixture of air plus oxygen in a small, continuously pressurized system. This serves to hyper-oxygenate the alveoli of the lungs to keep blood levels of oxygen within a normal range. The medication modafinil (Provigil®) is approved for fatigue associated with obstructive sleep apnea. Provigil® is classified as a pro-histamine. It appears to work by activating the waking part of the brain's sleep-wake cycle without interfering with normal sleep patterns. Provigil® is taken every morning or twice daily at 200 to 400 mg daily.

Circadian Rhythm Sleep Disorder

Formerly referred to as a sleep-wake schedule disorder, circadian rhythm disorder is a persistent or recurrent pattern of sleep disturbance that is relative to a discrepancy between a client's sleep-wake urges and the ability to follow those patterns based on societal expectations. Four subtypes exist: delayed sleep phase (normal sleep at socially unacceptable hours; e.g., 4:00 a.m. to 12:00 p.m.), jet lag (sleep requirements for a new time zone), shift work (adjusting to a night-shift schedule or a variable shift schedule), and unspecified (any others, including an advanced sleep phase, in which the individual falls asleep early, and then wakens early; e.g., 6:00 p.m. to 2:00 a.m.). Familial patterns have been identified for both delayed sleep and advanced sleep subtypes. Treatment consists of following sleep hygiene recommendations and utilizing sleep aids at the designated hour of sleep. Jet lag is frequently treated with melatonin supplements or Rozerem® at bedtime (melatonin is a hormone secreted normally by the body in response to daylight hours, and it may be associated with seasonal affective disorder). Modafinil (Provigil®) is also approved by the FDA to treat daytime fatigue associated with shift-work sleep disorder.

ADVANCED PRACTICE NURSING: COMORBID MEDICAL AND PSYCHIATRIC CONDITIONS

Treating a client with numerous medical problems can be a challenge for the psychiatric APRN, and adding the psychosocial issue of a lack of healthcare insurance or other resources makes this even more so. Graduate education in psychiatric nursing teaches us to always rule out medical conditions first, which is further reinforced in the psychiatric world by the *DSM-IV-TR*. How does one approach the treatment of depression, anxiety, insomnia, pain, or other conditions when the client lacks resources to diagnose or manage these conditions? Partnering with a community health clinic, rural health clinic or federally-qualified healthcare center is a cost-effective means of obtaining diagnostic lab work and other tests. Two common medical conditions that present with comorbid psychiatric symptoms are diabetes (mood instability, nervousness, tremors, fatigue) and hypothyroidism (fatigue, depressed moods, hypersomnia), both of which are diagnosed based on simple blood tests. Fibromyalgia is also seen with increasing frequency (but is not as easy to diagnose), as are all chronic pain disorders (fatigue, depressed moods, hopelessness, social isolation). Best practice guidelines dictate that the APRN should always practice with the best interests of the client in mind. For example, refusing to prescribe an antidepressant because the client has not yet had a thyroid stimulating hormone level drawn may lead to worsening depression and suicide. A better approach is to contract with the client and develop a plan of care (treatment plan) that realistically incorporates the basic medical care necessary, where this care will be received and from whom, and the basic psychiatric care indicated. Sometimes "good enough" care has to be implemented until the client reaches a point where he or she can take advantage of other resources in the community. To apply this to the preceding example: The APRN performs in a more ethically and humane manner by starting the potentially hypothyroid client on an SSRI, while waiting for lab tests to be done, and then seeing the client on a more frequent basis for short visits to assess response and provide support and encouragement, until the client can afford to initiate more formal therapy.

SUMMARY

Anorexia nervosa and bulimia are eating disorders that affect many young women (and some men) each year. Without treatment for the client and the family, anorexia can be lethal because of cardiac arrhythmias. Somatoform disorders are comprised of a family of psychiatric problems that have some relationship to, or arise out of, medical problems. In somatization disorder, numerous pain, abdominal, reproductive, and neurological complaints persist, each of which is not particularly disabling or problematic when alone. Clients with somatization disorder often end up unable to work or get healthcare insurance and tend to fall through the cracks. In conversion disorder, the client has a specific sensory or motor condition that is real to the client, but has no basis in reality. Pseudoseizures are a good example of a conversion disorder. A client with pseudoseizures will drop to the ground and appear to be having a seizure (usually a tonic-clonic type) but his or her EEG at that time will be completely normal. To further complicate this, a client may have real seizures (detectable on EEG) and have pseudoseizures that occur in times of emotional distress. Hypochondriasis occurs when clients are preoccupied with having a disease and seek out numerous tests to try to find it, to the point of significant distress to the client and his or her family. Clients with body dysmorphic disorder believe that there is something seriously wrong with their bodies or body parts. They may never feel good enough (as in the case of body builders) and may abuse their bodies trying to achieve some idealistic goal. In extreme cases, people have had numerous cosmetic surgeries to correct their flaws, sometimes resulting in actual body deformities. Chronic pain is usually managed by medical practitioners, but clients with chronic pain will often present in mental health settings because of persistent depression, fatigue, and hopelessness associated with the pain. Sleep disorders are commonplace in the mental health field and every nurse should be comfortable in identifying and developing care plans to manage them. Numerous sleep hygiene techniques can be tried, in conjunction with (or preceding) sleeping pills.

EXAM QUESTIONS

CHAPTER 12
Questions 72-77

Note: Choose the one option that BEST answers each question.

72. Diagnostic criteria for anorexia nervosa include

    a. self-induced vomiting.

    b. disturbances in the way body shape or weight is experienced.

    c. a dysfunctional family system.

    d. a weight loss of 20%.

73. Bulimia is characterized by

    a. restricting intake to the point of starvation.

    b. eating more calories than required.

    c. self-mutilating behaviors.

    d. eating an excessive amount of food, and then trying to purge it.

74. Diagnostic criteria for somatization disorder include

    a. two pain symptoms and several psycho-neurological symptoms.

    b. at least four GI symptoms that are accompanied by pain.

    c. a sexual abuse history that is accompanied by seizures.

    d. four pain symptoms, two GI symptoms, one sexual symptom, and one pseudo-neurological symptom.

75. A client with hypochondriasis has

    a. an obsession with cleanliness and germ prevention.

    b. a preoccupation of having a medical disorder.

    c. a belief that a body part is defective.

    d. numerous drug-seeking behaviors.

76. The best nursing approach for the client with a somatoform disorder is to

    a. be confrontive and set firm limits.

    b. be supportive and compassionate.

    c. avoid becoming overly attached.

    d. maintain a technological focus.

77. An important nursing intervention for primary insomnia would be to

    a. set the alarm clock to get up at the same time every day.

    b. encourage liberal use of bedtime sedatives.

    c. tell the client to stay in bed "as long as it takes to fall asleep."

    d. advise the client to stop working night shifts.

CHAPTER 13

DOMESTIC VIOLENCE, DISSOCIATION, AND PERSONALITY DISORDERS

CHAPTER OBJECTIVE

At the end of this chapter, the reader will be able to discuss problems associated with domestic violence and how they relate to the development of dissociative and personality disorders.

LEARNING OBJECTIVES

Upon completing this chapter, the reader will be able to

1. describe the power and control wheel and how it relates to domestic violence.

2. recognize the various expressions of a personality disorder.

3. discuss nursing management for clients who have personality disorders.

INTRODUCTION

This chapter will deal with some of the psychosocial stressors that lead to emotional and mental health disturbances in adulthood. Violence permeates every aspect of our society. Personal violence (rape, childhood sexual abuse) can have profound effects on emotional and, sometimes, physical development. Family violence (domestic violence, intimate partner violence) has far-reaching effects on the experience of the individual in a family system and has the consequence of causing repeated patterns of dysfunction when children in a violent family grow up to marry and have children of their own. Environmental violence (natural and manmade disasters, war) will be discussed more completely in Chapter 14. Violence exposure is associated with illnesses, such as PTSD and personality disorders, which will be examined here in more depth.

VIOLENCE AND TRAUMA

Violence permeates our society. Rape and sexual assault occur most commonly to women between 16 and 19 years of age, but may be underreported as much as 30% of the time. Over 85% of domestic violence victims are females, with over 5.3 million women abused and over 1200 women killed each year by an intimate partner in the United States (American Bar Association, n.d.). The American Institute on Domestic Violence (2001) reports that health-related costs to society as a result of domestic violence exceed $5.8 billion annually, of which nearly $4 billion is attributed to direct medical and mental health care, and $1.8 billion to lost productivity and earnings. Domestic violence occurs in every culture, country, and age group, affecting people from all socioeconomic, educational, and religious backgrounds. In the United States, 30% to 50% of women who are murdered are killed when they attempt to leave a domestic violence situation (http://www.aidv-usa.com/statistics.htm). Stressors, such as loss of job or income, physical illnesses, depression, birth of children, and relocation, may contribute to violence within the home. Alcohol abuse is a significant contributor to domestic violence. Ritual abuse, torture, and cult-related mind control are still present and usually affect children or young men and women. Perhaps, the most devastating abuse of all does not occur in response to terrorism or outside forces but is within the home itself. A family history of violence, abuse (physical or emotional), neglect, or sexual molestation can emotionally and psychologically cripple a person, leading to years of dysfunctional relationships, acting-out behaviors, substance dependence, and depression.

INTIMATE PARTNER ABUSE

Intimate partner violence is abuse that occurs between two people in a relationship. It includes emotional, physical, and sexual abuse as well as intimidating or threatening behavior. It can lead to lost work, low self-esteem, eating disorders, depression, and suicide. Victims of intimate partner violence are more likely to engage in harmful health behaviors, such as smoking, drug or alcohol abuse, or risky sexual behaviors (Centers for Disease Control and Prevention [CDC], 2006). Most portrayals of intimate partner abuse involve the male as perpetrator, and more than 90% of the time, this is the case. Partner-abuse victims tend to conceal their situations. Fear, shame, and guilt play a major role in perpetuating the abuse. Some women who are abused do not feel they can financially support themselves and their children. A vast number of women are also intelligent or well educated and still find themselves in abusive relationships. To understand how this can occur, as well as why a woman would remain in an abusive relationship, it is helpful to look at the Power and Control Wheel developed by the Domestic Abuse Intervention Project in Duluth, Minnesota (Domestic Abuse Intervention Project, 2003).

Before any physical violence occurs, numerous small steps condition the couple and lead them toward a path of abuse. The Power and Control Wheel (Figure 13-1) divides abuse into parts, each of which has increasingly oppressive and controlling behaviors, leading eventually to physical or sexual assault.

A partner to the Power and Control Wheel is the Equality Wheel (Figure 13-2). The Equality Wheel addresses each of the areas of intimidation, threats, and abuse outlined in the Power and Control Wheel, but presents the clients with healthier options: "Using emotional abuse" is replaced by "Respect;" "Minimizing, denying, and blaming" is replaced by "Honesty and accountability;" and "Negotiation and fairness" are taught as alternatives to "Using coercion and threats."

The effects of being in a domestic abuse situation on the female partner are a learned hopelessness and helplessness, resignation, and a feeling of "giving up." During the early stages of abuse, the male partner is often extremely apologetic and genuinely remorseful. He may promise "it will never happen again" and purchase gifts for his intimate partner. After this honeymoon phase, the violence tends to escalate in frequency and intensity. Women stay in abusive relationships for a variety of reasons: they feel at fault; they still love their partner; they were raised to be submissive; they have no family willing to help; they are financially dependent; they are afraid of being alone; they are protecting the image of the family; or they have low self-esteem. Stopping this cycle usually requires legal intervention. Long-term consequences of chronic partner abuse (if survived) lead to a phenomenon known as battered woman's syndrome, which is similar to the PTSD discussed in Chapter 11. Victims report nightmares, flashbacks, hyperarousal states, recurrent fear, chronic anxiety, emotional detachment or numbness, insomnia, guilt feelings, low self-esteem, depression, and difficulty concentrating. It is important to recognize

FIGURE 13-1: THE POWER AND CONTROL WHEEL

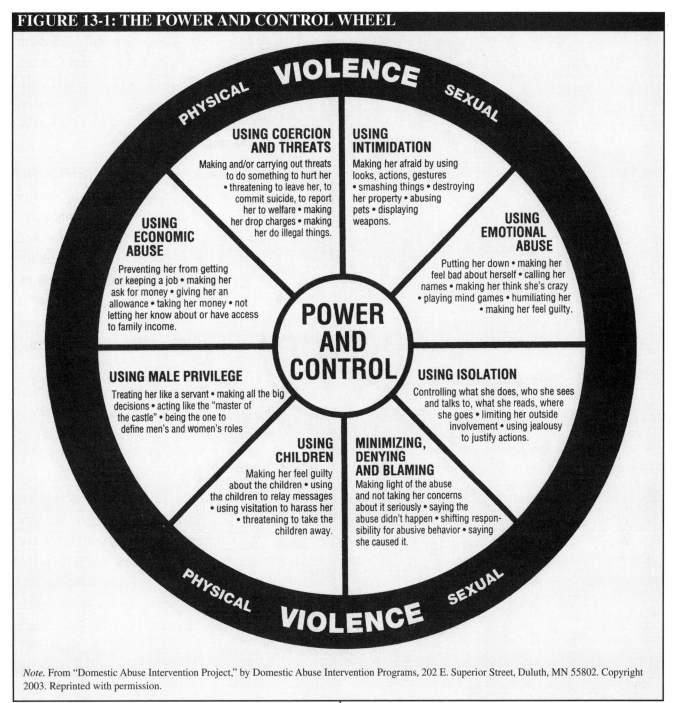

Note. From "Domestic Abuse Intervention Project," by Domestic Abuse Intervention Programs, 202 E. Superior Street, Duluth, MN 55802. Copyright 2003. Reprinted with permission.

that the symptoms are a result of the trauma and to work with the victim toward recovery.

Domestic Violence Interventions

The Duluth Domestic Abuse Intervention Project recognizes domestic violence as a societal, not individual, problem. Intervention is geared toward changing the community's response to violence by providing protection for the victim and using the legal system to change the behaviors of the abuser. When perpetrators are convicted, they are given the option of attending psychoeducational groups, instead of prison, to develop better insight into their behaviors and learn new tools to cope with life. Failing to complete the classes results in a revocation of probation and incarceration. Safety of the victim is always foremost and child visitations may be restricted (or supervised).

Nurses can provide valuable assistance as well. Abused women and their partners are frequently

FIGURE 13-2: THE EQUALITY WHEEL

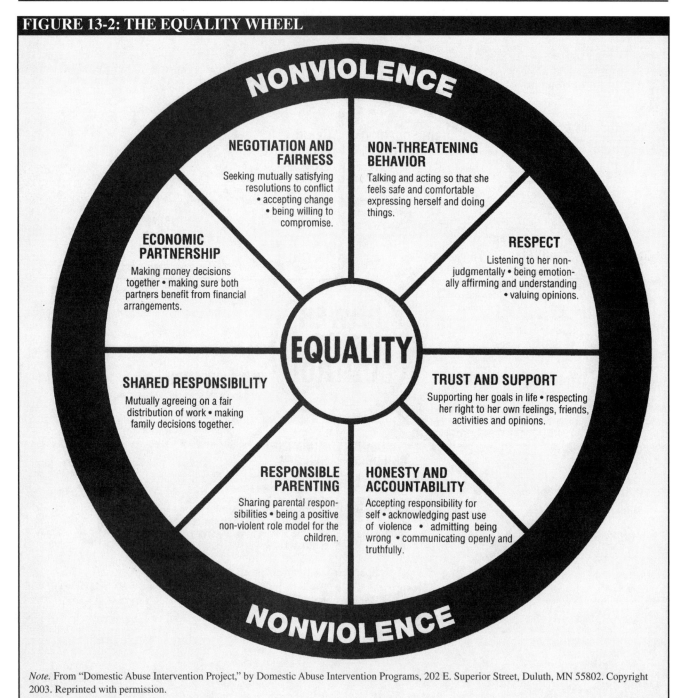

Note. From "Domestic Abuse Intervention Project," by Domestic Abuse Intervention Programs, 202 E. Superior Street, Duluth, MN 55802. Copyright 2003. Reprinted with permission.

encountered in emergency department settings or community office settings. It is important to remain nonjudgmental and supportive while performing physical assessments to determine the extent of the abuse. Safety is of utmost importance. Unlike with children or elderly clients, there is no government institution for reporting domestic abuse. At the time of this printing, six states now require reporting of intimate partner violence: California, Rhode Island, Kentucky, Colorado, New Hampshire, and New Mexico (Iavicoli, 2005). Of these, only California requires reporting, despite the wishes of the victim, and levies fines on clinicians of up to $1000 or 6 months in prison for failure to comply (Rodriquez, McLoughlin, Nah, & Campbell, 2001). Letting the victim know the options for shelter and treatment, by providing phone numbers and addresses for crisis centers or emergency housing, is essential.

CHILDHOOD SEXUAL ABUSE

The number of clients sexually abused as children is not known. Estimates have gone as high as 20% for girls and 7% for boys in some reports. It is likely that males underreport abuse because of embarrassment and shame. Abuse may include incest (relatives as perpetrators), fondling, intercourse, voyeurism, or exhibitionism. Victims come from every economic and social background and cultural and ethnic group. Childhood sexual abuse perpetrators are often trusted adults, teenagers, or older children. The relationship is usually thought of (initially) as supportive, trusting, or loving. There is always an imbalance in power – the perpetrator is able to persuade or coerce the victim through threats, intimidation, or fear. Children may be told that their parents or siblings will be killed or that they will be "taken away" if they tell anyone about the abuse. Substance use contributes to the occurrence of sexual abuse. The child who is abused may have serious conflicting feelings – there may be physical pain, fear, and confusion that is intermingled with a feeling of being "special" or "the favorite." Behaviors that may indicate a child or an adolescent is being abused are listed in Table 13-1. Children who grow up with sexual abuse often have difficulty in discriminating emotional love from control and sex and may end up with abusive partners as adults. Trust issues are significant in the adult client who has survived childhood abuse. PTSD (covered in Chapter 11) is frequently seen in adult survivors. Symptoms of PTSD are what will commonly lead the client to therapy. There has usually been a history of avoidance, unstable relationships, emotional numbing, or self-destructive behaviors (including substance dependence) prior to presentation. Repression, a selective amnesia in which events that become too overwhelming for the client to deal with are buried in the subconscious and forgotten, can occur. Repression is not the same as suppression,

in which memories are painful but easily retrieved. In true repression, the client has no recollection of the events and attempting to recover the traumatic memories can result in anxiety, panic attacks, or dissociation, which is a mental separation from reality that is similar to psy-

TABLE 13-1: BEHAVIORS INDICATIVE OF CHILDHOOD SEXUAL ABUSE	
Child	**Adolescent**
• Sleep disturbances	• Acting-out
• Nightmares	• Truancy
• Refusal to sleep in own bed	• Runaway
• Eating disorders	• Sexual promiscuity
• Enuresis	• Violent behaviors
• Encopresis	• Anger and rage
• Blood-stained underwear	• Depression
• Recurrent urinary tract infections	• Guilt
• Vaginal yeast infections	• Anxiety
• Refusal to bathe	• Substance abuse
• Bedwetting	• Prostitution
• Anxiety symptoms	• Early pregnancy
• Anger	• Early marriage
• Irritability	• Perpetrating against others
• Depressive symptoms	• Self-mutilation
• Aggression in play	• Suicidal behaviors
• Sexualized play activities	• Regression
• Masturbation	• Depersonalization
• Poor impulse control	• Dissociation
• Self-destructive behaviors	• Impaired relationships
• Perpetrating against younger children	

chosis. During dissociative episodes, clients may not know where they are and may attempt to reenact abusive situations. Fear and panic are intense. The client can become agitated and violent toward others, requiring emergency intervention. Dissociative disorders will be discussed in more depth in the following section.

Nursing management of the sexually-abused child or adolescent is geared toward the symptoms and needs of the client. Support and maintaining safety is foremost. The healthcare provider must report any suspicion of abuse (sexual or physical) by calling the appropriate agencies, usually the Child Protective Service division of the Office of Family and Children. Reporting abuse is a federal law. Choosing not to report can result in legal action and loss of any professional licenses. Child Protective Services obtains the information (which should include name of victim, suspected circumstances, address where the victim can be found, and relevant phone numbers) and immediately sends an investigator to interview the child. If the case is found to be substantiated (meaning there is significant evidence), then the child and siblings are taken into custody and placed in foster care. Child Protective Services can obtain emergency "child in need of services" status, which makes the county agency the legal guardian of the child. The suspected perpetrator may be arrested. The non-perpetrating parent can also be arrested for "failure to protect" if there is evidence that the parent had knowledge of the abuse and did nothing to prevent it. Other interventions might include allowing the child to stay at home, but ordering the suspected adult to leave while an investigation is underway, or allowing the child to stay with grandparents or other relatives. If the case is unsubstantiated, Child Protective Services files it with no other action. Adolescents may present a difficult situation. Age 16 is considered to be the "age of consent" for adolescents to engage in sexual activity. Child Protective Services will rarely intervene after a child reaches this age unless other factors are present, such as a mental handicap of the child, a vast discrepancy in age between child and perpetrator (e.g., a 16-year-old girl having relations with a 30-year-old man), or if the alleged perpetrator is a family member.

Nursing care of the adult client who has been sexually abused combines providing empathy and support with assessing the client for any self-harm ideas or actions. Sometimes, self-injurious behavior occurs in a person who has been repressing anger about abuse, possibly as a displacement mechanism, resulting from the lack of ability to directly address the abuser. Directly asking about abuse during a nursing assessment is important because the client may not be forthcoming. Examples of questions the nurse can ask include: "Were you ever molested as a child?" or "What's the worst thing that's ever happened to you in your life?" Assessing for memory lapses helps to determine if repression and dissociation are present. Teaching relaxation and stress management techniques to use during anxiety or panic attacks may be helpful. Making referrals to appropriate therapists or support groups (that specialize in sexual abuse trauma) is necessary. Medications are usually indicated based on the symptoms presented. Anxiolytics may be needed for the anxiety and panic, antidepressants may be needed for depression, and antipsychotics for dissociation. Monitoring for substance abuse or dependence and providing safe detoxification services are appropriate, when indicated.

DISSOCIATIVE DISORDERS

The primary feature of a dissociative disorder is a disruption in the functions of consciousness, memory, identity, or perception. Dissociative disorders can onset rapidly or more insidiously. They may persist for a short time or on a chronic basis. The *DSM-IV-TR* recognizes five dissociative disorders, which include dissociative disorder, not otherwise specified. The following four will be discussed: dissociative amnesia, dissociative fugue, dissociative identity disorder (formerly known as multiple personality disorder), and depersonalization disorder.

Dissociative Amnesia

The predominant concern of dissociative amnesia is an inability to recall important personal information. The memories lost are usually of a traumatic or highly stressful situation, the extent of memory loss is too great to be explained by forgetfulness. Localized amnesia refers to an inability to recall events in a specific time period, such as with an automobile accident. In selective amnesia, generalities are remembered, but specifics may not be (e.g., violent combat experiences). Localized and selective amnesia are relatively common. Less common (but sensationalized on television and in movies) are generalized, continuous, and systematized amnesia. In generalized amnesia, clients cannot remember any of their life's events and may present for emergency care in a frightened state. Continuous amnesia refers to an inability to recall events from a specific time up to the present. It is ongoing and the client may not remember what occurred the day before. Finally, in systematized amnesia, certain groups or characteristics (such as family members) cannot be remembered. Clients experiencing an amnesia disorder frequently experience depression, anxiety, depersonalization, trance-like states, and age regression. Impaired social relationships occur. The client may be more suggestible to hypnosis in therapy settings than individuals with other diagnoses.

Dissociative Fugue

A dissociative fugue state is characterized by sudden, unexpected travel away from one's home or customary activities, accompanied by an inability to remember some or all of one's past. There is usually confusion regarding identity, and the client may assume a new identity. The period of travel may be only hours or as long as months. During a fugue, the client does not appear to be suffering from any clinical abnormalities, such as depression or psychosis. Although rare, if a new identity is assumed, it is usually a more outgoing and uninhibited type than the baseline personality. After the fugue state ends, traumatic events may be recalled (or selective amnesia may be present) and the client can experience depression, anxiety, grief, guilt, shame, and other forms of psychological distress. Certain cultural groups have "running" syndromes that are seen as a sudden onset of a high level of activity, a trancelike state, potentially dangerous running behaviors, and ultimate exhaustion, sleep, and amnesia (Appendix A).

Dissociative Identity Disorder

Perhaps one of the most popularized, and most rare, forms of psychiatric disturbance is the dissociative identity disorder, formerly known as multiple personality disorder. In a dissociative identity disorder, two or more distinct identities or personality states are present that recurrently take control of a client's behavior. Important personal information may be forgotten. In children, the symptoms cannot be attributed to imaginary playmates or other fantasy play. Each personality state may be experienced as if it has a separate personal history, self-image, and even age. Often, the individual personalities assume different aspects of a "whole" person (i.e., one is aggressive, one is playful and impulsive, one is studious and responsible, one is promiscuous) and will emerge at times when his or her particular "talents" are needed. The client with this disorder will experience frequent memory gaps of personal history. Usually, the client will not have knowledge or awareness of the other personality states, although the other personalities may "know" each other. Transitions or "switching" usually occur at times of psychological stress. Behavioral manifestations include rapid blinking, facial changes, disrupted thoughts, mannerism changes, or voice changes.

Fifty percent of reported cases have 10 or fewer personality states; although up to 100 have been documented (American Psychiatric Association, 2000).

Clients with dissociative identity disorder frequently report a history of severe physical, emotional, and sexual abuse starting early in childhood. They may demonstrate a number of PTSD symptoms (nightmares, flashbacks, depression, or hypervigilance), suicidal or self-mutilation behaviors, or aggression. Relationships with others are often dysfunctional. Eating disorders, sexual disorders, and other problems also may be present. Clients with this disorder commonly report migraine headaches and other stress-related physical problems. Different personality states may also have different physical responses, such as pain tolerance or conversion disorders (e.g., blindness).

Depersonalization Disorder

A depersonalization disorder is a persistent or recurrent experience of feeling detached from (or observing) one's own body or mental processes. The client may report feeling as if in a dream state. During the depersonalization experience, reality orientation remains intact and the client can respond to others. Age of onset is about 16, and the client usually reports another, more distressful symptom, such as panic attacks or depression. Depersonalization symptoms are usually precipitated by severe stress, and they develop in nearly one-third of individuals exposed to life-threatening danger (e.g., auto accidents, military combat, or victim of a crime). The client may report a sensation of being out of control of his or her body or thoughts. A lack of emotional response and sensory anesthesia can occur (feeling numb all over). Depersonalization experiences are common and a diagnosis should be made only if the symptoms cause a marked impairment in functioning.

TREATMENT OF DISSOCIATIVE DISORDERS

Therapy for a dissociative disorder usually takes a long time and may involve some form of hypnosis by a trained hypnotherapist. Establishing trust between the caregiver and client is essential. Ultimately, the client's mental state is extremely fragile during a dissociative disorder. Recovering memories can be painful, especially if the forgotten events were particularly traumatic. Providing a secure, safe environment during these episodes is necessary to prevent the client from potentially causing self-harm or harming others. The goal in dissociative identity disorders is eventual reintegration of the client. Clinician opinions vary on how to address or converse with the other personality states. In general, the nurse should not promote further splitting of the client by encouraging communication with altered states. Medications are not specifically indicated for dissociative disorders; however, clients may be treated for concomitant anxiety, panic attacks, or depression. Antipsychotics are sometimes prescribed.

PERSONALITY DISORDERS

Personality disorders are classified by the *DSM-IV-TR* as "Axis II" disorders. This means that they are not usually the primary focus of treatment; rather, they are traits or characteristics of the client that tend to be dysfunctional and counterproductive for fitting into society. Personality disorders tend to be culture-specific. A client with a personality disorder may not feel that anything is wrong; in fact, often the client believes that the problems in social relationships lie in other people. General diagnostic criteria for a personality disorder are presented in Table 13-2.

Causes for personality disorders were traditionally thought to be based in childhood experiences and learned behaviors in the family. Newer biological

TABLE 13-2: *DSM-IV-TR* **CRITERIA FOR A PERSONALITY DISORDER**
1. A pattern of behavior that deviates markedly from the expectations of the client's culture that is manifested in two or more of the following areas:
a. cognition – ways of perceiving and interpreting self, other people, and events
b. affectivity – range, intensity, lability, and appropriateness of emotional responses
c. interpersonal functioning
d. impulse control.
2. The pattern is inflexible and pervasive across a broad range of situations.
3. The pattern leads to clinically significant distress.
4. The pattern is stable and of long duration (at least to adolescence or early adulthood).
5. The pattern cannot be accounted for by another mental disorder (e.g., paranoid symptoms in schizophrenia).
6. The pattern cannot be due to the direct effects of alcohol or drugs.
(American Psychiatric Association, 2000)

theories, based on twin studies and longitudinal family studies, suggest that some personality traits may be inherited (Keltner et al., 2007). The *DSM-IV-TR* recognizes 10 distinct personality disorders, with an 11th diagnosis of personality disorder, not otherwise specified. Personality disorders are further divided into subtypes or clusters as demonstrated in Table 13-3. An overview of these disorders follows.

Paranoid Personality Disorder

A paranoid personality disorder is seen in a client who demonstrates a pattern of pervasive distrust and suspiciousness of others. Paranoia due to alcohol, drugs, or a major disturbance, such as schizophrenia or dementia, must be ruled out. Four or more of the following symptoms must be present:

1. suspects (without basis) that others are exploiting or deceiving him or her;

2. has unjustified doubts about the loyalty or trustworthiness of friends or family;

3. is reluctant to confide in others for fear the information will be used against him or her;

4. reads hidden messages into benign remarks or events;

5. persistently bears grudges;

6. perceives character or reputation attacks, and is quick to anger or retaliate; or

7. has recurrent, unjustified suspicions regarding fidelity of spouse or partner.

TABLE 13-3: SUBTYPE CLUSTERS OF PERSONALITY DISORDERS
Cluster A
Characterized by distinctly odd or eccentric behaviors
1. Paranoid
2. Schizoid
3. Schizotypal
Cluster B
Characterized by overly dramatic, emotional, or erratic behaviors
1. Antisocial
2. Borderline
3. Histrionic
4. Narcissistic
Cluster C
Characterized by chronically anxious or fearful behaviors
1. Avoidant
2. Dependent
3. Obsessive-compulsive

Clients with paranoid personalities can be unpleasant, if not frightening, to live with. Always vigilant to insults and quick to react, this type of person can become agitated and violent with little provocation.

Schizoid Personality Disorder

Individuals with schizoid personality disorders often seem indifferent to the approval or opinions of others and they have a detachment from social relationships. These clients seem to lack a desire for intimacy or relationships with others. They are not bothered by insults or criticism or buoyed up by praise or rewards. The person with a schizoid personality may demonstrate a limited range of emotional expression and affect. To make this diagnosis, at least four of the following must be seen:

1. neither desires nor enjoys close relationships (including family),

2. chooses solitary activities,

3. has little interest in sexual activities with another person,

4. takes pleasure in very few activities,

5. lacks close friends or confidants,

6. appears indifferent to praise or criticism, or

7. shows emotional coldness, flattening, or detachment.

Goals may be vague and clients with schizoid personality disorder may seem to drift through life with little aim or direction.

Schizotypal Personality Disorder

In contrast to a schizoid personality disorder, the client with a schizotypal personality disorder demonstrates a pervasive pattern of social and interpersonal deficits that is marked by discomfort and a reduced capacity for relationships and accompanied by cognitive distortions or behavior eccentricities. Superstitions, unusual beliefs, or preoccupation with paranormal experiences may be seen. Thoughts may contain a magical component. Dress or mannerisms may be described as "odd." Diagnostic criteria require at least five of the following:

1. ideas of reference (not delusions),

2. odd beliefs or magical thinking that influences behavior,

3. unusual perceptual experiences,

4. odd thinking and speech,

5. suspiciousness or paranoid ideation,

6. inappropriate affect,

7. behavior or appearance that is odd or eccentric,

8. lack of close friends or confidants, or

9. excessive social anxiety (associated with paranoid fears).

Clients diagnosed with a schizotypal personality disorder occasionally will progress to developing more traditional symptoms indicative of schizophrenia.

Antisocial Personality Disorder

Also known as a sociopath, an individual with an antisocial personality disorder lacks the ability to have empathy for others and persistently violates the rights of others. The disorder may begin in childhood when it is diagnosed as a conduct disorder. Clients with antisocial personality are often charismatic criminals who may feel special entitlements are owed them by society. Diagnostic criteria for an antisocial personality disorder must include at least three of the following elements and must occur by 15 years of age (but cannot be diagnosed prior to 18 years of age):

1. failure to conform to social norms with respect to obeying the law,

2. deceitfulness (lying, using aliases, conning others for profit),

3. impulsivity or failing to plan ahead,

4. irritability and aggressiveness (repeated physical fights or assaults),

5. reckless disregard for the safety of others or self,

6. irresponsibility in work behaviors or financial obligations, or

7. lack of remorse or rationalizing that others "deserve it."

Clients with antisocial personalities are frequently seen in the prison system. Currently, there are no good psychological treatments to change these character traits and the protection of society may be warranted.

Borderline Personality Disorder

Clients with borderline personality disorders demonstrate a pervasive pattern of unstable and erratic relationships. They tend to view the world in terms of "black or white," and they make dramatic efforts to avoid perceived abandonment by others. Gender-identity and other identity issues may be present. Their emotions and behaviors may be extremely labile and unpredictable. Suicide gestures, self-mutilation, and substance abuse problems are frequent. To make a diagnosis of borderline personality disorder, at least five of the following criteria must be met:

1. frantic efforts to avoid real or imagined abandonment;

2. a pattern of unstable and intense interpersonal relationships demonstrating extremes of idealization and devaluation;

3. unstable self-image or sense of self (identity disturbance);

4. impulsivity in at least two areas that are self-destructive (e.g., reckless driving, dangerous sexual practices, eating disorders);

5. suicidal behaviors, gestures or threats, or self-mutilating behaviors;

6. marked mood instability;

7. chronic feelings of emptiness;

8. inappropriate or uncontrollable anger; or

9. transient, stress-induced paranoia, or dissociative episodes.

Clients with borderline personality disorder can be the most difficult of all psychiatric clients. They will go to great lengths to engineer discord among staff members and attempt to split staff into disagreements over aspects of treatment planning, such as therapy needs, discharge planning, and milieu management.

Histrionic Personality Disorder

Attention-seeking behaviors and excessive emotionality are the hallmarks of a histrionic personality disorder. Clients with this personality type tend toward manipulation of others and crave excitement or stimulation. They may enact a role of victim in interpersonal relationships. At least five of the following *DSM-IV-TR* criteria must be met to diagnose a histrionic personality disorder:

1. discomfort in situations in which they are not the center of attention,

2. interactions are often characterized by seductive or provocative behaviors,

3. displays rapidly shifting and shallow emotions,

4. uses physical appearance to draw attention to self,

5. speech is excessively impressionistic and lacking in detail,

6. exaggerated emotions or theatrical or dramatized emotions,

7. easily influenced by others or circumstances (suggestible), or

8. considers relationships more intimate than they really are.

Although emotional reactivity is seen, clients with histrionic personalities often lack the depth of character necessary to sustain long-term relationships. This personality type may be encountered more often in the entertainment industry.

Narcissistic Personality Disorder

The primary features of a narcissistic personality disorder are a need for admiration, persistent grandiosity, and a lack of empathy for others. Clients with this disorder have an exaggerated sense of self-importance and accomplishments. They feel that they are superior to others and should only associate with similar, "gifted" individuals. Criteria to meet the diagnosis of narcissistic personality disorder must include at least five of the following:

1. an exaggerated or grandiose sense of self-importance,

2. preoccupation with fantasies of power, wealth, success, and beauty,

3. belief of being special and unique and should only associate with others who also are gifted or of high-status,

4. excessive self-admiration,

5. a sense of entitlement (owed things by others),

6. exploitative in interpersonal relationships,

7. lacks empathy (unwilling to recognize the feelings and needs of others),

8. envious of others or believes that others are envious of him or her, or

9. arrogant, haughty behaviors or attitudes.

Many highly successful clients display traits that could be considered narcissistic; however, it is only when these traits become maladaptive, inflexible, and cause impairment in important areas of functioning that the diagnosis of a personality disorder applies.

Avoidant Personality Disorder

Clients with avoidant personality disorder display a pattern of social inhibitions, feelings of inadequacy, and hypersensitivity to criticism. They may avoid work or school activities for fear of embarrassment, rejection, or disapproval. Intimate relationships are difficult for these clients. *DSM-IV-TR* diagnostic criteria for this disorder must include at least four of the following:

1. avoids activities that involve significant interpersonal contact for fear of criticism, disapproval, or rejection;

2. is unwilling to become involved with people unless certain that he or she will be liked;

3. shows restraint in relationships for fear of shame or ridicule;

4. is preoccupied with being criticized or rejected;

5. feels inadequate and is inhibited in new situations;

6. views self as inferior, socially inept, or unappealing; or

7. is reluctant to take personal risks or engage in new activities because they might be embarrassing.

Avoidant behaviors often begin in childhood with extreme shyness, a tendency to isolate, and fears of strangers or new situations. Behaviors will worsen during adolescence (rather than dissipate, as in most people), but there is some evidence that the disorder may become less pronounced with aging.

Dependent Personality Disorder

Individuals with dependent personality disorder demonstrate a pervasive need to be taken care of that leads to clinging and submissive behaviors. These behaviors are designed to elicit caretaking by others. They arise from a self-perception of being unable to function without the help of others. Diagnostic criteria for a dependent personality disorder must include at least five of the following:

1. difficulty making everyday decisions without excess advice and reassurance,

2. needs others to take responsibility for most major areas of his or her life,

3. difficulty expressing disagreement with others (fears loss of support or approval),

4. difficulty doing things alone (due to a lack of self-confidence),

5. goes to excessive lengths to obtain nurturance and support from others,

6. feels uncomfortable or helpless when alone,

7. urgently seeks another relationship when one relationship ends, or

8. is unrealistically preoccupied with fears of being left to take care of self.

Clients who have a dependent personality disorder may jump into relationships rapidly. They sometimes find themselves in abusive situations from which they are unable to leave because of their extreme fear of being responsible for self-care.

Obsessive-Compulsive Personality Disorder

In contrast to an obsessive-compulsive disorder (OCD), clients with obsessive-compulsive personalities have a preoccupation with orderliness, perfectionism, and mental and interpersonal control at the expense of flexibility, openness, or efficiency. *DSM-IV-TR* criteria for obsessive compulsive personality disorder must include at least four of the following:

1. preoccupation with details, rules, lists, order, schedules, or organization;

2. perfectionism that interferes with task completion;

3. excess devotion to work and productivity, to the exclusion of friendships and recreational activities;

4. over-conscientious, scrupulous, and inflexible about issues such as ethics, values, or morality;

5. unable to discard worn-out or worthless objects – even those without sentimental value;

6. reluctant to delegate tasks or work to others;

7. miserly-spending style toward self and others (money is viewed as something to be hoarded for catastrophes); or

8. shows rigidity and stubbornness.

Clients who have obsessive-compulsive personality traits can be especially adaptive in certain situations. It is only when the need for control and orderliness become more important than the task or relationship that a personality disorder is diagnosed.

NURSING INTERVENTIONS FOR THE CLIENT WITH A PERSONALITY DISORDER

Nursing approaches vary when a personality disorder is identified, depending on the specific needs and concerns of the client. For clients with Cluster-A disorders (paranoid, schizoid, and schizotypal personality disorders), establishing trust and being truthful are important. It is not helpful to challenge ideas or beliefs. Allowing distance from other clients and not attempting to force social interactions can limit the client's anxiety. With clients demonstrating Cluster-B disorders (antisocial, borderline, histrionic, and narcissistic personality disorders), consistency and a firmer approach may be necessary. There should be a greater emphasis on routines and established rules of the healthcare setting. The nurse should avoid getting pulled into histrionics or staff-splitting behaviors. Positive reinforcement should be provided for socially-acceptable behaviors, whereas overly dramatic or destructive behaviors should be ignored as much as is safely possible. Cluster-C disorders (dependent, avoidant, and obsessive compulsive personality disorders) may require additional nurturance and support by the nurse. Teaching assertiveness skills and relaxation techniques can be helpful. Therapy that focuses on cognitive behavior restructuring should be recommended. Allowing and encouraging the client to make decisions and develop treatment goals can increase a sense of self-control and empowerment.

CASE STUDY: BORDERLINE PERSONALITY DISORDER

*D*anny is a 32-year-old man with a history of over 10 psychiatric hospitalizations for superficial cuts to his wrists, overdoses, or suicidal threats. He has also been in jail twice: once for a DUI charge and once for domestic violence. Danny has been in the hospital four times in the past 6 months alone. One year ago, Danny's third wife left him after only 18 months of marriage and filed a restraining order to prevent him from contacting her. Upon examination, Danny tells the nurse that, "life isn't worth living unless you have someone to love you." He also states that "I don't know what I'll do if you make me leave the hospital again." Danny goes on to report that the staff on the previous shift "wouldn't listen to me" and that one of the technicians had threatened to "beat me up if I didn't straighten up and quit lying." Danny feels that the social worker is the only one who really understands him. Since the divorce, Danny has been homeless and staying in shelters. He isn't working "because my ex-wife screwed that up for me" and he has no insurance or source of income. He states his family abused him as a child and "I won't have anything to do with them." The nurse finds that he has a history of unstable relationships, some of them heterosexual and some of them with same-sex partners. Danny also tends to downplay his substance abuse history stating, "It's really not a problem. I just drink when I'm depressed." Danny's primary admission diagnosis is adjustment disorder with depressed mood, but he is also diagnosed with a borderline personality disorder.*

Questions

1. How is this client demonstrating the "black or white" thinking that is characteristic of persons with borderline personality disorders?

2. What would be an appropriate response to this client's complaints that a technician on another shift had threatened to harm him?

Discussion

Individuals who have borderline personality disorders have a lot of difficulty in life with ambiguity and "gray" areas. This is demonstrated in this client by his "all or none" thinking about love and his relationships with others. Clients with this personality type also tend to manipulate other people into situations in which they feel stuck with their choices. In this case, the client has reported that a staff person threatened him. The appropriate response would be to discuss this openly in the treatment team meetings, support the staff member, and not allow the client's accusations to create conflict in the team (which serves to deflect time and energy away from his own issues and ties up time and energy in employee relations).

NURSING CARE PLAN: CLIENT WITH BORDERLINE PERSONALITY DISORDER

Problem Listing

- Potential for harm to self or to others
- Poor coping strategies to deal with life stressors
- Lack of housing, income, other resources
- Impaired social interactions

Priority Nursing Diagnosis

Potential for harm to self related to impulsivity, as evidenced by a history of previous attempts when under severe psychosocial stress.

Long-term Goal

Client will identify and utilize more effective means of dealing with stressors, other than harming himself.

Short-term Objectives

1. Client will verbally and in writing contract with staff not to harm himself during the hospital stay.

2. Client will verbalize self-harm urges to staff prior to acting on them.

Nursing Interventions

1. Staff will perform 15-minute safety checks to assess client's well-being.

2. Staff will assist the client in listing five activities to perform to prevent harming himself (for example, journaling, exercising, or calling support hotlines).

3. Staff will assist the client in identifying the precipitants to self-harm behaviors as well as thought processes (cognitive interpretations) of events that led up to those feelings.

ADVANCED PRACTICE NURSING: WORKING WITH TRAUMATIZED CLIENTS

APRNs who work in psychiatric or mental health settings encounter traumatized clients on a regular basis. Personal experiences of trauma (physical or sexual abuse, domestic violence exposure, death of family members) may be expressed as an acute stress reaction, or much later in the delayed symptoms of PTSD. Clients who have been traumatized need to be handled gently by the nurse clinician so as not to worsen their symptoms. The nurse clinician should understand that when painful memories surface and are open for discussions, the client may go into an anxiety-related fight or flight mode. Behaviors seen may include missing appointments or dropping out of treatment, angry outbursts, increasing depression, increased substance abuse, self-injurious behaviors, and suicidal thoughts.

Particular attention should be paid to the controversial issue of recovered memories, which refers to the client's delayed recollection of traumatic events that occurred years earlier but had been repressed (see Defense Mechanisms in Chapter 3). Clients who are in therapy may be vulnerable and open to suggestions. Several cases have been documented in which clinicians uncovered sexual abuse memories that later were disproved, but not before causing considerable emotional and, sometimes, legal and financial harm to the accused. Children are especially vulnerable to suggestions about the past because of their desire to please adults and immature cognitive development. Clinicians should use open-ended questions and encourage expression, without suggesting specific details, as much as possible.

SUMMARY

In this chapter, personal experiences of violence inside and outside of the home have been examined and placed into a societal context. The Power and Control Wheel provided a look at the escalating cycle of violence: from threats and coercion to blaming and isolation to physical intimidation and assault. The Equality Wheel conversely provides behaviors that prevent violence, including respect, trust, honesty, shared responsibility, and partnership. Successful interventions in domestic (or intimate partner) violence have included psychoeducational groups in lieu of incarceration, with safety for the victim foremost. Childhood sexual abuse is a particularly egregious act in our society and has far-reaching consequences for the individual. Children who are sexually abused may develop a poor concept of the difference between parental and romantic love and have poor interpersonal boundaries as a result. Sometimes, these children engage in behaviors as adolescents or adults that are overly promiscuous, overly rigid, or otherwise dysfunctional. One of these dysfunctional patterns is the tendency to perpetrate abuse against children (once an adult) or to marry partners who abuse children, thus perpetuating the cycle.

Personality disorders are character traits that are currently thought to be inherent in an individual; however, borderline personality disorders are closely related to perceived emotional neglect and abandonment during early childhood (prior to 5 years of age). Working with clients who have personality disorders can be frustrating for the nurse because these individuals don't seem to want to follow the rules or be compliant. Staff splitting is common and angry feelings may result. These reactions by staff members further serve to perpetuate perceived feelings of rejection in the client (especially with borderline personality disorders). A strong team approach and trust in other staff persons is essential in these situations.

EXAM QUESTIONS

CHAPTER 13
Questions 78-83

Note: Choose the one option that BEST answers each question.

78. The Power and Control Wheel

    a. divides abuse into different types of controlling behaviors.

    b. demonstrates how domestic violence can lead to death.

    c. explains why men become abusive in relationships.

    d. puts the emphasis of responsibility on the woman.

79. The effects of a domestic abuse situation on the partner-victim are

    a. a learned hopelessness and helplessness.

    b. abnormal relationships with children.

    c. increased societal costs for incarcerations.

    d. increased feelings of self-control and assertiveness.

80. In childhood sexual abuse

    a. the child may be a willing partner.

    b. the perpetrator is always from a lower-class home environment.

    c. the non-perpetrating parent is protected from prosecution.

    d. there is always an imbalance of power between the perpetrator and victim.

81. Clients who have borderline personality disorder

    a. are anxious and fearful.

    b. attempt to split staff into disagreements.

    c. are preoccupied with lists and rules.

    d. are odd or eccentric.

82. Nursing care of Cluster-B personality disorders (antisocial, borderline, histrionic, and narcissistic) should focus on

    a. nurturance and unconditional positive regard.

    b. consistency of routines, rules, and responses to client behaviors.

    c. teaching assertiveness and relaxation techniques.

    d. providing as needed medications for complaints of anxiety.

83. Nursing care that helps the client to set goals, make independent decisions, and learn assertiveness skills is useful for the individual with

    a. dependent or avoidant personality disorders.

    b. borderline or histrionic personality disorders.

    c. antisocial or narcissistic personality disorders.

    d. paranoid or schizoid personality disorders.

CHAPTER 14

NATURAL AND MANMADE DISASTERS

CHAPTER OBJECTIVE

At the completion of this chapter, the reader will be able to discuss natural and manmade disasters and the expected and pathological psychological effects they can cause in survivors.

LEARNING OBJECTIVES

At the end of this chapter, the reader will be able to

1. Discuss types of natural and manmade disasters

2. Relate models of stress and adaptation to the disaster experience.

3. Describe psychopathology that may result from exposure to a disaster or trauma event.

4. Discuss the application of psychological first aid.

INTRODUCTION

Disasters, both natural and manmade, occur throughout the world every year. The toll on human lives is tremendous with deaths, injuries, property loss, and destruction as immediate effects and homelessness, violence, disease, and other costs to society coming shortly thereafter. In the United States, two significant disasters have occurred in the past 10 years: the terrorist attacks in Washington, D.C. and New York City in 2001 and the devastation of flooding from Hurricane Katrina across the mid-Southern states (particularly New Orleans, LA) in 2005. However, the American Red Cross responds to hundreds of national disasters (e.g., floods, fires, ice storms) and thousands of local disasters (e.g., house fires) annually. The Federal Emergency Management Agency (FEMA) has a role in designating national disasters and emergencies. In 2008, FEMA designated 71 disasters (55 and 49 in 2007 and 2006 respectively) (Federal Emergency Management Agency [FEMA], 2009). Worldwide, an average of 62,000 people are killed annually due to a disaster (American Red Cross, 2009).

This chapter will be examining the differences between a natural disaster and a manmade disaster and will provide some examples of each throughout the past several centuries. Human response to disasters will be discussed with several psychological models provided to aide in understanding normal reactions to extreme situations. Pathological responses following a disaster will be examined, including depersonalization and dissociation, acute stress disorder, PTSD, major depression, suicide, and substance abuse. Therapeutic intervention is presented with an emphasis on the immediate emergency techniques of psychological first aid, which is practiced by the Red Cross and taught by the Veteran's Administration in their disaster mental health treatment courses.

NATURAL DISASTERS

Natural disasters occur as a result of two things: a natural occurrence or hazard and a vulnerable population. Blizzards, floods, tornadoes, earthquakes, ice storms, hurricanes, wildfires, and other occrrences are only disastrous when they take a toll on human beings, resulting in property destruction, injury, illness, and death. The degree of harm incurred is directly proportional to the extent of the disaster; for example, one damaged house with no deaths is not as disastrous as are 10,000 damaged or destroyed homes, 8000 injured, and 500 dead. One might argue, though, that to the one individual who lost the home, the effects are just as traumatic. Pandemics, such as the Spanish Flu or Bubonic Plague can also be classified as natural disasters because their origins are rooted in natural events. Hurricane Katrina in 2005 was the most significant natural disaster to occur in recent memory in the United States. Damage occurred from the Category 5 hurricane as well as from the ruptured levees and extensive flooding throughout the southern United States. A lesser known natural disaster is a limnic eruption. Limnic eruptions result from large quantities of carbon dioxide at the bottom of a lake that erupt, pulling oxygen out of the surrounding air and suffocating any living animal or person in the vicinity. Two of these known events are recorded, both near Cameroon Africa: 1984 at Lake Monoun causing 37 deaths and in 1986 at Lake Nyos killing 1700 to 1800 persons, though others are suspected. There are too many natural disasters every year in the United States and other countries to describe them all; however, Table 14-1 provides an overview of some of the more notable natural disasters in terms of magnitude and destruction across the world.

MANMADE DISASTERS

Manmade disasters are events that are a direct result of human activity. These would include acts of war, terrorism, bombings, industrial events (mass power outages, structural collapses, mining collapses), fires from arson, nuclear fallout and radiation poisoning, chemical spills, transportation disasters (airplane and railroad crashes), and space disasters. The terrorist attacks on September 11, 2001 are in recent memory for the United States. Three airplanes were used as suicide bombing devices by Al-Qaeda terrorists and were flown into the Pentagon in Washington, DC, and into the two World Trade Center towers, killing thousands. A fourth plane was thought to be headed for either the White House or the U.S. Capital Building, but it was diverted by heroic passengers and crew and crashed into the countryside in Somerset, PA, killing only those on the plane. Between 1950 and 2006, over 1800 airline disasters were recorded worldwide. Of these, 53% were attributed to pilot error, 21% to mechanical failure, 11% to weather, 6% to sabotage or attack, and the remainder to miscellaneous other causes. Table 14-2 provides other examples of manmade disasters that have involved the United States over the past two centuries. Events such as oil spills are environmental disasters, but will not be covered in this chapter because they do not generally cause death or injury to humans and are secondarily traumatic (loss of property, loss of occupation, emotional distress).

SOCIETAL RESPONSES TO DISASTER

The American Red Cross, International Red Cross, and Red Crescent

The American Red Cross (ARC) was founded in 1881 by Clara Barton. The ARC offers domestic disaster relief services by providing basic needs following a disaster that include emergency shelter, food, clothing, medications, and health care. They

TABLE 14-1: HISTORY OF NATURAL DISASTERS

Year	Event	Location	Death Toll	Additional Information
2008	Earthquake	Sichuan China	68,000	8.0 Richter Scale
2005	Earthquake	Pakistan	79,000	7.6-7.7 Richter Scale
2005	Hurricane Katrina	Southern U.S.A.	1836	Category 3 Hurricane/levee failure
2004	Earthquake + Tsunami	Indian Ocean	229,000	9.3 Richter Scale
2003	Heat Wave	Europe	52,000	100°F-104°F for weeks
1999	Mud Slide	Vargas, Venezuela	20,006	27 miles at 3' deep
1989	Tornado	Bangladesh	1300	50 miles long, 1 mile wide
1975	Banquiao Dam Flood	Henan Province	90,000-230,000	41.7" of rain in 1 day
1972	Blizzard	Iran	4000	Over 1 week duration
1970	Cyclone + Storm Surge	Bangladesh	200,000-400,000	115 mph winds
1931	Floods	Central China	2-4 million	Yellow River, Yangtzee River, Huai River
1918-20	Pandemic Spanish Flu	Worldwide	20-100 million	2 years duration
1910	Avalanche	Wellington, WA	96	More than 11' of snow in 9 days
1906	Earthquake	San Francisco, CA	3000+	7.8 Richter Scale
1900	Hurricane	Galveston, TX	8000+	Category 4 Storm
1888	Flood from Dam Break	Johnstown, PA	2200	20 million tons of water
1887	Yellow River Flood	China	900,000-2 million	50,000 sq miles
1876-78	Drought + Famine	India	25,250,000	257,000 sq miles, 2 years
1871	Wildfire	Peshtigo, WI	1200-2500	1875 sq miles
1815	Volcanic Eruption	Indonesia	92,000	9.8' deep ash deposits
1631	Volcanic Eruption	Italy	10,000-25,000	Mt Vesuvius, Pompeii
1556	Earthquake	Shaanxi Province	830,000	520 mile wide area
526	Earthquake	Antioch, Turkey	250,000	Turkey and part of Syria

do not provide rescue services, but they do feed and assist rescue workers during an operation. Rescue workers, also called first responders, are made up of police, fire department, ambulance crews and, sometimes, the National Guard. In addition to its disaster services, the ARC is also charged to serve as a link between military families and soldiers for compassionate notification and in facilitating visits home. The ARC also provides educational services for communities, collects and processes lifesaving blood, and participates in international relief and development operations. Completely funded by volunteer donations, the ARC does not receive federal or state funds. The ARC has over 700 local chapters. After a disaster, the ARC system is activated locally, then regionally, and then nationally in an ever-enlarging circle. The ARC employs around 35,000 people, but has a

TABLE 14-2: SELECT MANMADE DISASTERS INVOLVING THE UNITED STATES

Year	Event	Causative Factor	Location	Death Toll
2010	Oil Spill	Drilling rig explosion	Gulf of Mexico	11
2006	Sago Mine	Mine collapse	West Virginia	12
2001	Terrorist Attack	Al-Qaeda Terrorists	Washington DC, New York	3017
1993	Terrorist Attack	Car Bomb	World Trade Center, NY	6
1992	Riots/Civil Unrest	Rodney King Verdict	Los Angeles, CA	53
1991	Persian Gulf War	–	Persian Gulf	100,000
1983	Space Shuttle	Structural failure	Challenger	7
1981	Space Shuttle	Structural failure	Columbia	7
1981	Hyatt Walkway	Structural collapse	Kansas City, MO	114
1950-53	Korean War	–	Korea	2.5-3.5 million
1967	Silver Bridge	Structural failure	Ohio and West Virginia	46
1959-75	Vietnam War	–	Vietnam	2.3-3.8 million
1945	Nuclear Bomb	WWII – U.S.A.	Hiroshima	140,000
1945	Nuclear Bomb	WWII – U.S.A.	Nagasaki	80,000
1939-45	World War II	–	Europe, Japan, etc.	60-72 million
1914-18	World War I	–	Europe	20 million
1918	Train Wreck	Direct collision	Nashville, TN	101
1907	Monongah Mine	Explosion	West Virginia	362
1871	Chicago Fire	Unknown	Chicago, IL	200-300
1861-65	Civil War	Secessionism/slavery	Southern United States	620,000

volunteer pool of over half a million. Volunteers are well-trained and can be activated to open emergency shelters in fewer than 24 hours after the onset of a disaster.

ARC disaster volunteers have pre-assigned roles for which they have been trained prior to deployment. Mental health workers are required to be licensed as a therapist, social worker, psychiatrist, or psychiatric nurse. Nurses must be licensed to practice in their home states. Client service workers are trained to perform social service activities and work closely with mental health and nursing staff persons. Specialized teams of all three specialties are created when disaster mortality is high. Table 14-3 describes the author's role on a Red Cross

Disaster Action Team while volunteering during the 9/11 disaster at the Pentagon site in Washington, DC.

The International Red Cross/Red Crescent (ICRC) exists to prevent or alleviate human suffering, to protect life and health, and ensure respect for the human being. International volunteers must remain impartial, neutral, and maintain their autonomy. The international organization exists outside of any religious affiliation (as does the ARC). One of the key roles of the ICRC is to visit with and evaluate prisoners of war for neglect, torture, or other violations of the international Geneva Convention, which is designed to protect prisoners. Another job of the ICRC is to respond to interna-

TABLE 14-3: EXAMPLE OF RED CROSS DISASTER TEAM ACTIONS

"I was assigned to work on a Disaster Action Team on September 14, 2001 in Washington, D.C. My team consisted of myself (a psychiatric clinical nurse specialist), a registered nurse with a background in community health, and a client services worker who was a retired businessman. My team was given the job of working with family members of survivors of the Pentagon explosion who were hospitalized in the intensive care burn unit at George Washington Hospital. We initially had 11 of the patients' families, but two of the patients died that first night. Our patients were critically ill and were under sedation. Our job was to meet with their families and ensure that they had a place to stay, clothes to wear, food to eat, transportation to the hospital, and basically whatever was needed to meet their own basic needs. As a mental health counselor, I spent time talking with the families and encouraging them to express their feelings. I also helped them to identify resources at home for long-term counseling if needed. One of the other teams helped families of the deceased find appropriate clothing and funeral homes, and the Red Cross paid for funerals for some of the indigent through 9/11 donated funds. I also had secondary clients, who were the hospital and fellow Red Cross volunteers. I helped them to talk about their feelings (anger, fear, sadness) and try to make some sense of it all."

tional disasters, ensuring that victims have food, clean water, and shelter. They are also involved in missing persons and land mine education. The ICRC employs 1400 persons worldwide and is very careful in their screening process. Multicultural experience and more than one language is an asset. The intra-denominational emblems of the ICRC are the red cross, red crescent, and a red crystal (Figure 14-1).

FIGURE 14-1: EMBLEMS OF THE INTERNATIONAL RED CROSS/RED CRESCENT

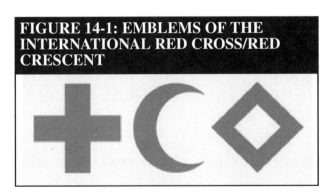

Federal Emergency Management Agency

FEMA is a component of the U.S. Department of Homeland Security. The primary mission of FEMA is to reduce the loss of life and property and protect the nation from all hazards, natural and manmade. FEMA comprises a comprehensive emergency management system of preparedness, protection, response, recovery, and mitigation. FEMA has approximately 2,600 full-time employees and about 4,000 stand-by employees who are ready

to deploy in times of a disaster. One of the main activities of FEMA is to provide financial assistance for housing and non-housing losses not covered by insurance. Housing needs include temporary housing, repair and replacement, and construction assistance. Non-housing losses may include disaster-related medical, dental, or funeral costs; clothing, household items, tools needed for one's job, or educational materials; primary heating fuels; cleaning items; replacement or repair of disaster-damaged vehicles; and moving and storage expenses. Disaster victims can apply for FEMA benefits online (http://www. fema.gov/assistance/ index.shtm).

Faith-Based Programs

Faith-based organizations are the primary long-term disaster assistance programs and are nearly always made up of volunteers with donated funding from members of the religious group. Pretty much every religious or faith-based organization has some type of disaster assistance. For purposes of illustration, a brief discussion of a few of these follows: The American Baptist Men's Disaster Relief Ministry aides in cleaning up disaster sites and doing construction tear-downs; The Mennonite Disaster Service focuses on clean up, repair, and rebuilding homes after a disaster; The American Jewish World Service places volunteers all over the world to assist in disaster and other human service needs; Catholic Charities USA work in disaster situations to provide emergency food, shelter, financial assistance, counseling, and other support; The Lutheran Disaster Response offers hardship grants to affected individuals, along with spiritual and emotional care; and the Society of St. Vincent de Paul, Inc. collects donations of clothing and other items and provides them at reduced or no cost to disaster victims through their thrift shops.

The Salvation Army is instrumental in disasters and has been named by the federal government as an officially recognized relief and disaster operation (along with FEMA and the ARC). In a disaster situation, the Salvation Army is on the scene early and provides support to rescue workers along with the ARC. They also provide spiritual guidance, counseling, material support, mobile feeding, sheltering, financial assistance, rebuilding assistance, and victim location, identification, and registration.

One will often find the Southern Baptist Convention's portable kitchens at every large disaster recovery site. Set up in closed fairgrounds, businesses, or parking lots, the Southern Baptists prepare large quantities of food to be distributed by other relief organizations such as the ARC. In 2008, the Southern Baptist Convention distributed 7,914,391 meals to disaster victims. Along with food preparation, they help with clean-up and clearing of debris and have a fairly extensive fleet of work automobiles. Other services they provide include short-term childcare, laundry and shower services, and home repair.

U.S. Veteran's Administration

The U.S. Veteran's Administration (VA) estimates that there are 25 million U.S. veterans currently alive and 70 million people eligible for VA benefits as a veteran, family member, or survivor of a veteran. This constitutes nearly a quarter of the nation's population. The VA provides a number of services, including healthcare programs, death and disability benefits for veterans and families, a debt management center, homeless assistance, business and vocational rehabilitation, educational grants and scholarships, and women veteran support. They also collaborate in services with faith-based organizations and provide disaster mental health and other trainings to the community.

MODELS OF STRESS AND ADAPTATION

Psychological and social models are a useful way for nurses to think about how an individual responds to a disaster situation. They can explain what appear to be maladaptive patterns of behavior and serve as a framework for developing a plan of care. This section will cover several relevant models and apply them to general disaster situations.

Selye's General Adaptation Syndrome

Psychologist Hans Selye (1956) described the general adaptation syndrome, an individual's response to a perceived danger or threat. The syndrome is made up of three stages: alarm, resistance and exhaustion. Chapter 11 provided a thorough discussion of the general adaption syndrome in relation to anxiety disorders. In disaster situations, the initial alarm phase is triggered at the time of the disaster. It is instrumental in insuring survival by causing the individual to quickly seek safety. Through certain chemical reactions (i.e., adrenalin release), the person is better able to ignore discomfort and pain and to perform what may at times seem like super-human feats to save himself and others. During the resistance phase, the individual is prepared to deal with chronic stressors such as homelessness caused by the disaster; coping and defense mechanisms become evident. However, over time the traumatized individual will become exhausted in the face of continued stress and illness, substance abuse, or depression may be the result.

Kübler-Ross's Cycle of Grief

Elisabeth Kübler-Ross (1969) described five stages of grief that are experienced by an individual following a loss such as a death in her seminal book, *On Death and Dying*. These stages are not meant to be sequential; instead, the person may move in and out of stages during the grief process. Although originally intended to describe the grief process, these stages of grief are very applicable to disaster situations as well.

Stage One: Denial. Denial is the conscious or unconscious refusal to deal with a loss. In disaster situations this may be evident when a person refuses to believe that his or her home is lost or that a loved one is missing and presumed dead. Behaviors seen include verbal refusals, refusing to listen to others, insisting that everything is fine (may even act as though nothing has happened), and insistence on returning to the disaster site repeatedly.

Stage Two: Anger. Anger can manifest in many ways. It may be seen as blaming others, threatening physical harm or lawsuits, verbal aggression, or even physical assault. Volunteers working in disaster recovery sites are often surprised to find that victims are irritable, moody, grouchy, demanding, and don't seem to be grateful for the services that they are receiving.

Stage Three: Bargaining. Bargaining can take a lot of different forms. In the traditional sense, individuals will ask God to bring back whatever is lost. Other forms of bargaining may be more covert; for example, victims of a disaster may try to negotiate more services or monies from relief organizations.

Stage Four: Depression. Sadness, regret, crying episodes and, in general, early acceptance of the loss can occur. Depression following a disaster is normal and expected, but may become dangerous if symptoms are not remitting or suicidal thoughts occur. Multiple research studies have reported a significant increase in suicides (up to 10%) after surviving natural disasters or experiencing manmade disasters or trauma, such as war.

Stage Five: Acceptance. In this phase, the individual comes to accept and internalize the loss. Victims of disasters will begin to make plans to relocate, rebuild, or move on.

Maslow's Hierarchy of Basic Needs

Abraham Maslow (1943) provided a theory of psychology based on what he called "basic human needs" that provides a useful framework for understanding victim responses in disaster situations. Maslow's hierarchy is built on a pyramid with the most important needs at the bottom. After these needs are met, other needs are presented in descending importance and necessity. The following description reviews Maslow's hierarchy of needs:

1. *Basic physiological needs:* food, water, air, sleep, freedom from pain, etc.; then

2. *Safety and security needs:* housing, safety of the body, family, and property; then

3. *Love and belonging needs:* intimacy, relationships with others, friendships; then

4. *Self-esteem needs:* respect by others, respect of self, achievement, accomplishments;

5. *Self-actualization:* creativity, problem-solving, imagination, producing.

Maslow's hierarchy can be directly applied to disaster situations as seen in Figure 14-2.

PSYCHOPATHOLOGICAL RESPONSES

Disorders related to trauma and other psychological disorders have been covered in numerous other chapters on anxiety, depression, substance abuse and alcoholism, and domestic violence exposure. Problems specific to disaster response and trauma are highlighted in the following discussion

FIGURE 14-2: APPLYING MASLOW'S HIERARCHY OF NEEDS TO DISASTER SITUATIONS

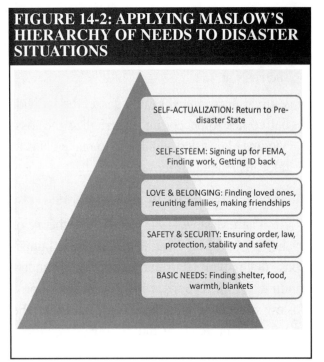

of information that was covered in previous chapters (the reader is encouraged to review Chapters 7, 8, 9, 11, and 13 for specific *DSM-IV-TR* criteria for these disorders).

Dissociation and Depersonalization

The primary feature of a dissociative disorder is a disruption in the functions of consciousness, memory, identity, or perception. Dissociative disorders can onset rapidly in response to a trauma, or begin more insidiously. In depersonalization disorders, the individual reports a persistent or recurrent experience of feeling detached from (or observing) one's own body or mental processes. The client may report feeling as if in a dream state. During this experience, reality orientation remains intact and the client can respond to others. Depersonalization symptoms are usually precipitated by severe stress and they develop in nearly one-third of clients exposed to life-threatening danger (e.g., auto accidents, military combat, or crime victims). The clients may report a sensation of being out of control of his or her body or thoughts. A lack of emotional response and sensory anesthesia can occur (feeling numb all over). Symptoms may persist for a short time or become chronic.

In a dissociative fugue, an individual leaves a specific location and becomes confused about his or her identity, sometimes assuming a new identity. Fugue states usually end, the person recalls the traumatic event, and then he or she may experience the event as if it had just occurred. Sometimes, a person may experience a dissociative amnesia, in which the event cannot be voluntarily recalled. In extreme cases, a person can become amnesic of his or her own identity (but this is rare). More commonly, certain aspects of the trauma cannot be remembered; for example, a man may remember what he was doing prior to the attack on the World Trade Center twin towers, but not be able to remember how he got out of the building or anything for the 2 hours afterward.

Acute Stress Disorder

Acute stress disorder occurs in response to an extreme stressor that involves personal experience of an event with actual or threatened death or serious injury of others. It may also occur from witnessing an event that involves death or serious injury or from learning about an unexpected or violent death, serious harm, or threat of death or injury to a family member or close friend. The person responds with feelings of intense fear, helplessness, or horror (children may express agitation or disorganized behaviors). Symptoms from the trauma occur immediately and last from 2 days to 4 weeks. Clients with an acute stress disorder may experience any of the following: a sense of numbing, detachment, or an absence of emotional responses; feeling dazed or unaware of one's surroundings; derealization (feeling as though in a dream); depersonalization (feeling as though outside of oneself); or dissociative amnesia (can't remember parts of or the entire trauma). Clients also re-experience the trauma through recurrent thoughts, dreams, images, or flashbacks and they avoid things that remind them of the event. Frequently, clients exhibit increased arousal states, including insomnia, irritability, poor concentration, exaggerated startle, restlessness, and hypervigilance. If unrelieved, acute stress disorder progresses to PTSD.

Posttraumatic Stress Disorder

PTSD is more persistent and longer lasting than acute stress disorder. It can occur immediately following the trauma or memories can be repressed and symptoms occur years later. Clients with PTSD may describe guilty feelings about their experiences (especially if others were injured or killed and they were not). Avoidance behaviors can lead to marital conflicts, work conflicts, or interpersonal problems. Environmental triggers, such as certain smells or sounds, may induce panic level anxiety attacks. Severe cases may report auditory hallucinations or paranoia. Impulsive and self-destructive behaviors are associated with traumas related to physical or sexual abuse. Somatic complaints may be frequent. Although the *DSM-IV-TR* lists PTSD as an anxiety disorder, it is, by definition, associated with one or more precipitating traumas. Existing PTSD from past traumas is exacerbated, triggered, or worsened with a new disaster exposure. The rates of new onset occurrences of PTSD following a disaster range from 29% to 36% (SAMSHA, 2005).

Major Depression and Suicide

Rates of depression and suicide increase significantly after a disaster or trauma experience; however, the nurse needs to remember that depression is the most common psychiatric disorder and many victims may have pre-morbid depressive disorders prior to the disaster experience, which may be worsened by their experiences. All victims of disasters should be considered for depression and treated appropriately with referrals for counseling and medications if needed. Reports of a new onset of major depression following a trauma range from 8% to 30% (SAMSHA, 2005).

Disaster and trauma exposure are major risk factors for suicide. Suicide occurs when an individual feels stuck or trapped in a situation or emotional state (i.e., depression), without having any hope for getting out of the situation. Suicide has become a crisis for the United States military; suicide rates for soldiers stationed in Iraq or Afghanistan are at an all time high. In 2008, 128 Army soldiers committed suicide. In 2007, 117 soldiers died of suicide and there were 934 nonfatal suicide attempts. In 2006, 102 soldiers took their own lives. Despite more attention on this problem, suicide rates appear to be on the increase. Demographically, suicides are more likely in young, Caucasian enlisted men. Most suicides occurred at the soldier's personal home, while he or she was on leave. The majority of deaths were by firearm (63%) and 60% of nonfatal attempts were by overdose. Approximately 44% of the soldiers had a history of some type of mood, anxiety, or substance use disorder. A failed marital or partner relationship was the social event most often associated with the completed suicides and 61% of these soldiers had served at least one tour of duty in Iraq or Afghanistan (only 8 soldiers had multiple deployments) (Levin, 2008).

Substance Abuse and Dependence

Alcohol use to deal with stress occurs in about 15% to 25% of victims and first responders following a disaster; however, new onset substance dependence disorder rates are lower, ranging from 1% to 8% (SAMSHA, 2005). In an informal study done in lower Manhattan after 9/11, respondents reported an increase in alcohol use by 24%, marijuana use by 3%, cigarette use by 9%, and "any" drug use by 28% (National Institute on Drug Abuse, 2009). Perhaps the most significant issue in regard to substance abuse is that the disinhibition that occurs from the effects of substances can lead to an increased number of suicide attempts and completions.

THERAPEUTIC INTERVENTIONS

Individuals who have experienced trauma and develop major depression, suicidal ideation, or PTSD should be referred to local mental health care providers for therapy. Most often, a combination of relaxation training, cognitive behavioral therapy (CBT), and medications will be helpful. One type of CBT is prolonged exposure therapy, in which the individual is asked during therapy to discuss, journal, and talk repeatedly about the trauma, while practicing relaxation and using reframing cognitive techniques under the support and guidance of the therapist.

Psychological First Aid

Psychological first aid (PFA) is an evidence-based treatment that is designed to provide short-term immediate intervention to assist victims of disasters. In PFA, the goal is not to develop more traditional, long-term relationships between the therapist and client (as in CBT). Instead, strategies are utilized to reduce the initial distress of the disaster and to foster short- and long-term adaptive functioning and coping skills. PFA is the counseling treatment of choice for mental health professionals who are dealing with the immediate aftermath of a disaster, and it is promoted by the ARC and the VA. The basic objectives of PFA are provided in Table 14-4. The overall goal of PFA is to reduce distress, assist with current needs, and promote adaptive functioning; however it is not to intentionally elicit details of traumatic experiences and losses. Asking for details about the trauma is not beneficial in helping the victim develop coping strategies and may worsen symptoms. PFA techniques offer suggestions for dealing with children, older adults, and disabled individuals and can be applied to group settings as well. Nurse clinicians who practice PFA must be calm, pleasant, and show compassion for the client. Being culturally sensitive and understanding the social environment

TABLE 14-4: GOALS AND OBJECTIVES OF PSYCHOLOGICAL FIRST AID

1. Establish connections with survivors of disasters
2. Enhance safety and provide physical and emotional comfort
3. Calm distraught or overwhelmed disaster survivors
4. Gather information to determine specific, immediate needs
5. Offer practical assistance and information for immediate needs
6. Connect survivors with social support networks, family, friends, and resources
7. Support adaptive coping and encourage the use of coping efforts
8. Provide information on psychological effects of disasters
9. Link the survivor to local mental health resources and organizations

is essential. Many disaster victims are indigent and lack resources prior to the disaster. Notoriously, lower cost housing is often placed in flood plains (e.g., the Ninth Ward in New Orleans) or in tornado prone areas such as mobile home parks. Poverty is also associated with higher pre-disaster mental health problems, domestic violence, and substance abuse problems, further complicating recovery following the event. PFA principles are also used when counseling disaster responders and volunteers.

Care Providers and Their Needs

People who choose to work in disaster areas are generally caring and have concern for their fellow human beings. They may be retirees who volunteer their time and skills, employees in the social service or medical field, or members of faith-based organizations. When a person is called to work after a disaster, the initial reaction is excitement and some apprehension. Once on duty, care providers are energetic and hard-working. They work long hours and sometimes forget to take breaks, eat healthy meals, get exercise, or relax.

Shelter work often requires the volunteers to sleep on the same portable cots that disaster victims sleep on and insomnia is a problem. Occasionally, disaster volunteers have preconceived ideas about their own roles in the disaster and are disappointed to find out that they are most needed to do menial tasks, such as answering phones or transporting other volunteers. Sometimes this disappointment leads to anger and job refusals. One of the roles of the disaster mental health worker is to ensure that fellow disaster workers and first responders are taking care of themselves. Additionally, care providers may not recognize signs of stress in themselves, which may be demonstrated as irritability, moodiness, or firm rigidity to rules. Sometimes, disaster mental health workers have to gently confront volunteers and other workers and encourage them to take a few steps back and look at themselves during this high stress time. Stress management techniques and approaches are highly valued when working with first responders and disaster aid workers. In the ARC system, nurses working in health services and mental health counselors are empowered to require ARC workers to take days off or to send home volunteers who are physically or emotionally unhealthy.

CASE STUDY: HURRICANE KATRINA AND THE RIVER CENTER SHELTER

*O*n August 28, 2005, 13-year-old Marcus spent the night with his best friend Johnny. Just before 10:00 pm, his mother called and said to stay indoors because a big storm was moving in that night. Marcus heard the storm moving in during the night and did what his mother said; it was very windy and he was scared. He woke up about 5 a.m. to voices calling him to "get up...we got to go." Sometime early that morning, the levees keeping back the Gulf of Mexico had broken through in places and the neighborhood was rapidly flood-

ing. Marcus refused to stay with Johnny's family and he ran for home. A few blocks away, he found himself wading in chest deep water. It smelled dank and fishy. "You can't go that way" some people told him. At one point, he was swept off of his feet and fell under the water's surface. Some people pulled him up and dragged him along with them to the Superdome in New Orleans. It took hours for them to get there and Marcus's family wasn't there. Shortly after they arrived, the flood waters rose further and trapped everyone in the Superdome. Marcus was there for 4 days. On the second day, the electricity shorted out and there was no air conditioning in the August Louisiana heat. The toilets backed up and no one could clean up. Someone brought in some bottled water, but there was very little food. Marcus saw some men beat up another man and he heard from some other kids that a few people had died and were pushed outside and covered with tarps. He didn't know what to do. He met a policeman who told him to come with him and they would try to find his family. Marcus rode with the policeman to Houston, TX (120 miles away) but his family wasn't there. He then went to Baton Rouge, LA and the policeman brought him to the River Center Shelter. Marcus was checked in and given something to eat. He wanted to shower and change clothes. He was assigned a Red Cross mental health counselor named Valerie to talk to. She helped him to find some clean clothes and, together, they started hunting for his family. At night, Marcus slept in a special area with 10 other "orphaned" children (children evacuated without a parent or guardian). Someone told him there were over 6000 people staying in the big shelter. On September 4th, he got to meet Will Smith and he saw Jesse Jackson visit the shelter. The next day John Travolta came to visit, but he didn't meet him. On September 9th, Valerie found out that Marcus's mother had been evacuated by helicopter to a shelter in Illinois along with his siblings. He didn't know where his father was. Valerie arranged for an Angel Flight for Marcus and he, along with some other shelter evacuees, left River Center that evening to reunite with their families.

(Figures 14-3 to 14-7: Photos of River Center Shelter)

Questions

1. What health hazard would a nurse working with Marcus be concerned about?

2. In regard to normal growth and development, what considerations should be made for this client?

3. What safety concerns are described in this example?

Discussion

Waterborne diseases are problematic after a flood. Cryptosporidiosis parasites, enteroviruses, E. coli bacteria, hepatitis A bacteria, leptospirosis bacteria (from animals), and methycillin-resistant staphylococcus are a few of the diseases found in flood waters that may invade if ingested. The risk of West Nile virus from mosquito bites is high because of the standing water. Tetanus can infect injuries and people exposed to flood waters should be given tetanus shots. As an adolescent, it is very important for Marcus to spend time with other children who are about his age and not to be isolated only with adults. The safety concerns for children following Hurricane Katrina are too numerous to list; being without parents, exposure to violence, the risk of abduction or abuse, and inadequate nutrition or proper sleeping quarters are just a few.

NURSING CARE PLAN: DISASTER RESPONSE

Problem Listing

- Exposure to potentially infectious flood waters

- Dehydration

- Inadequate nutrition

- Inadequate sleep

- Risk for violence exposure

- Fear of the unknown

- Lack of family contact or communication

Priority Nursing Diagnosis

Lack of primary support systems related to disaster evacuation, as evidenced by separation from family and lack of communication or contact with family members.

Long-term Goal

Client will be reunited with his family.

Short-term Objectives

1. Client will find out where his family is located.

2. Client will demonstrate effective coping strategies to manage daily life decisions.

3. Client will remain safe.

Nursing Interventions

1. Staff will assess client for any signs of illness or waterborne pathogens.

2. Staff will ensure client has safe sleeping arrangements.

3. Staff will provide adequate nutrition and fresh water to drink.

4. Staff will provide access to clean clothes and bathing water.

5. Staff will utilize resources available through the Red Cross and Salvation Army to locate client's family.

6. Staff will secure transportation for client to be reunited with his family.

7. Staff will implement principles of psychological first aid to provide comfort, educate, and inform the client and help him to develop coping skills appropriate to his developmental age.

FIGURE 14-3: THE RIVER CENTER SHELTER, BEFORE HURRICANE KATRINA, BATON ROUGE, LA, 2005

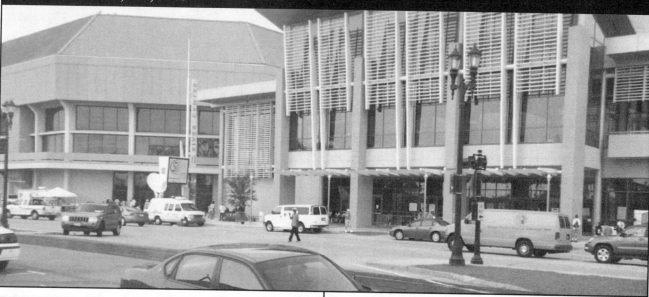

FIGURE 14-4: OUTSIDE RIVER CENTER SHELTER ONE WEEK AFTER HURRICANE KATRINA, BATON ROUGE, LA, 2005

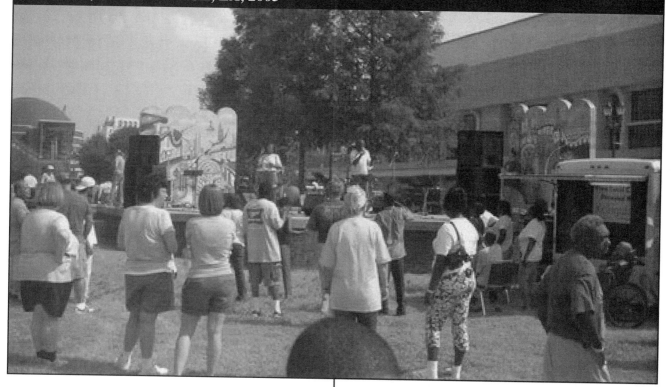

FIGURE 14-5: RIVER CENTER SHELTER FOLLOWING HURRICANE KATRINA, BATON ROUGE, LA, 2005

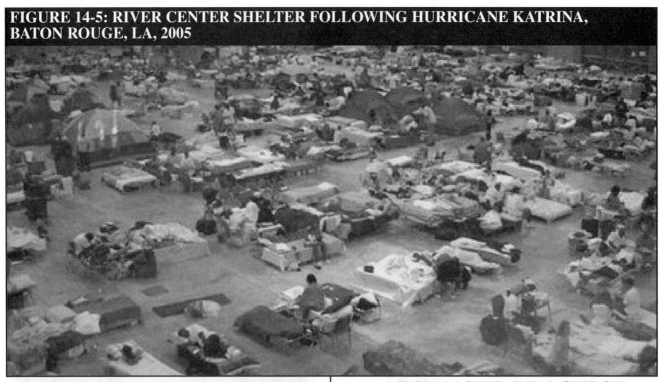

FIGURE 14-6: INSIDE THE RIVER CENTER SHELTER FOLLOWING HURRICANE KATRINA, BATON ROUGE, LA, 2005

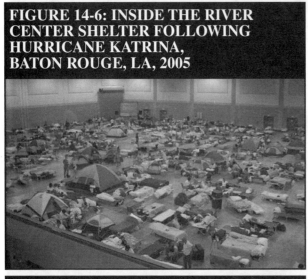

FIGURE 14-7: LETTERS FROM CHILDREN FOLLOWING HURRICANE KATRINA, 2005

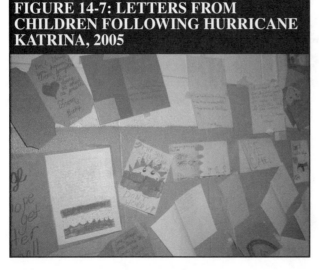

ADVANCED PRACTICE NURSING: THE UNIFORM EMERGENCY VOLUNTEER HEALTH PRACTITIONERS ACT AND THE GOOD SAMARITAN ACT

In 2006, legislation was drafted by the Uniform Law Commission to facilitate a better response to large disasters, by providing some safeguards for licensed practitioners who want to volunteer in those disasters. As of 2008, the Uniform Emergency Volunteer Health Practitioners Act had been introduced in 12 states and enacted in Indiana and New Mexico. Two key points are outlined in the act: 1) To protect public health, the act requires that volunteers must be registered with public or private systems that are capable of determining whether they have been properly licensed and are in good standing in their practice jurisdictions; and 2) To alleviate uncertainty and confusion, the types of services that may be provided by volunteers are limited to activities for which they are licensed, trained, and qualified to perform. Furthermore, volunteer health practitioners must adhere to restrictions imposed by the laws of host states, disaster response agencies and organizations, and host entities. For APRNs, this act may actually restrict practice in some disaster areas because states vary considerably on the language of "collaboration" versus "supervision;" on prescribing of controlled substances; and on the percent of prescription reviews required.

Good Samaritan laws are laws or acts that protect those who offer voluntary assistance in times of emergencies from liability. Specific statutes vary among states – some states only protect healthcare providers who are volunteering. All states only cover unpaid assistance. Some general principles to follow include obtaining consent from the victim when he or she is conscious and can give consent; to provide care that is reasonably careful; to call for help from others; not to act in ways that are wantonly negligent or reckless; and to provide the care immediately and at the site of the emergency. Disaster volunteer work is generally covered under Good Samaritan statues.

SUMMARY

Disaster work is demanding, physically exhausting, and extremely rewarding to healthcare providers. Natural disasters occur as a result of a natural occurrence, such as a storm, wildfire, or earthquake. Manmade disasters occur as a result of an act of man and include wars, terrorist attacks, industrial accidents, structural defects, and transportation accidents. The individual's response to a disaster, whether natural or manmade, is mediated by his or her pre-disaster social support networks, social resources such as income, and pre-existing physical and mental health care problems. Often, the poorest and most disenfranchised members of society are the ones most profoundly affected by a disaster. Normal psychological responses to disasters include depersonalization and, sometimes, dissociation to the immediate events. Acute stress reactions are also expected. Complicated or unresolved problems may lead to increases in substance abuse, depression, chronic PTSD, and suicide. Suicide rates in U.S. Army soldiers have increased every year and primarily occur after return home or during passes home. Suicide attempts in soldiers are more lethal because of the ownership of firearms and the training to be able to use them. Nonfatal suicide attempts are more often caused by overdoses. Disaster survivors who are experiencing suicidal thoughts, depression, or PTSD should be referred to professional, local mental health providers. Disaster response workers, including nurses, are taught psychological first aid (PFA), the goals of which are to support and encourage the victim and assist him or her in identifying coping strategies and dealing with the immediate problem at hand. The worker assisting a disaster survivor may only have one contact with that person, and PFA provides a guideline as to how to make that contact as meaningful as possible. Lastly, disaster aid workers and first responders don't function in a vacuum – they have needs and problems too. Aid workers can be so caught up in the disaster response that they forget to take care of themselves. Disaster mental health specialists have the added responsibility of ensuring that other aid personnel remain physically and mentally healthy and take time off for personal needs and relaxation during a disaster assignment.

EXAM QUESTIONS

CHAPTER 14
Questions 84-89

Note: Choose the one option that BEST answers each question.

84. A natural disaster occurring within the past 10 years was

    a. the terrorist attacks on the World Trade Center.

    b. the Johnstown floods in Pennsylvania.

    c. Hurricane Katrina in the southern U.S.A.

    d. the Exxon Valdez oil spill.

85. An example of a manmade disaster is

    a. a wildfire caused by lightning strikes.

    b. an earthquake.

    c. a flood.

    d. an airplane crash.

86. According to Maslow's hierarchy of needs, which of the following must come first?

    a. Love and belonging needs

    b. Basic needs for food, shelter, warmth

    c. Safety and security needs

    d. The need for self-actualization and creativity

87. An acute stress disorder is characterized by

    a. increased anger.

    b. hypersomnia.

    c. repeated panic attacks.

    d. intense fear or helplessness.

88. The primary feature of a dissociative disorder is

    a. a disruption in consciousness, memory, identity, or perception.

    b. losing blocks of time for days on end.

    c. demonstrating psychotic symptoms that are unrelated to stressful events.

    d. refusal to participate in social activities.

89. Objectives of psychological first aid include

    a. gathering information to determine specific, immediate needs.

    b. teaching the victim about his or her psychopathology.

    c. soliciting detailed information about the disaster experience.

    d. developing a long-term therapeutic relationship with the victim.

CHAPTER 15

CHILDHOOD DEVELOPMENTAL DISORDERS

CHAPTER OBJECTIVE

At the completion of this chapter, the reader will be able to discuss both normal childhood development and cognitive and emotional disorders that arise from disruptions in development.

LEARNING OBJECTIVES

At the end of this chapter, the reader will be able to

1. discuss normal childhood cognitive and emotional development.

2. describe effects of prenatal exposure to drugs and alcohol on the neonate and child.

3. identify the consequences of abuse and neglect for select childhood disorders.

4. differentiate mental retardation and developmental delay disorders.

INTRODUCTION

The treatment of childhood psychiatric disorders in conjunction with developmental delays is a challenging but rewarding specialty. It is important to have an understanding of normal and expected age-related changes in a child to better recognize and treat developmental disorders. In the specialty of psychiatric nursing, problems in emotional, moral, cognitive, and social development are frequently encountered. In this chapter, several conceptual frameworks with wide acceptance in the field will be utilized to better illustrate these important areas of development. Additionally, specific developmental delays will be reviewed including mental retardation, autism, Asperger's syndrome, and pervasive developmental delay. Child abuse, including prenatal drug and alcohol exposure, are discussed and the relationship between fetal alcohol syndrome and psychiatric and cognitive disorders is discussed. Reactive attachment disorders occur when children are prevented from developing normal, healthy attachments to their caregivers. Other developmental disorders, such as learning disabilities and bedwetting and soiling disorders are presented. Finally, a case study of a child with a developmental disorder and a nursing care plan are provided.

NORMAL CHILDHOOD DEVELOPMENT

Sigmund Freud was one of the first clinicians to put forth theories regarding emotional development. Considered somewhat quaint and outdated by many, Freud's theories have the important function of recognizing that needs, desires, and behaviors change as the client matures. Freud believed that changes occur in relationship to a biological drive for the survival and propagation of the species. An overview of his "Stages of Psycho-sexual

TABLE 15-1: FREUD'S STAGES OF PSYCHOSEXUAL DEVELOPMENT

Age of Child	Stage	Primary Focus	Discussion
0-18 months	Oral	Mouth	The subconscious "id" tries to reduce tension by encouraging the child to suck, bite, or chew.
18 months-3 years	Anal	Defecation	Society demands control over impulses and urges, resulting in the first conflict with parental figures.
3 years to 5-6 years	Phallic	Genital (penis)	Child becomes infatuated with opposite-sex parent and competitive (jealous) with same-sex parent. Fears of castration. Resolves conflict by identifying with same-sex parent and adopting socially-appropriate sex roles.
5-6 years to Puberty	Latency	Cognitive	Stormy periods lessen and energy is devoted to assimilating cultural values and social learning.
Puberty to Adulthood	Genital	Genitals	Energy is directed toward a peer of the opposite sex, resulting in mature, adult relationships with the goal of reproduction.

(Wolraich, 1996)

Development" is provided in Table 15-1. Stunted development under this model leads to emotional disorders and neuroses, which are similar to the personality disorders presented in Chapter 13.

In 1950, Erik Erikson developed a theory of emotional development that is still widely used in nursing and healthcare settings today. His eight stages are based on the client's interaction with society. Growth is accomplished through task completion – an inability to obtain a positive outcome at any level will result in a delay of emotional development that may persist late into adulthood. Erikson's "Eight Stages of Psychosocial Development" are covered in Table 15-2. Erikson postulated that if a client is unable to master a particular level (e.g., Trust versus Mistrust) due to poor interpersonal relationships (e.g., childhood sexual abuse), then the client is unable to ever fully develop emotionally or complete other developmental tasks (e.g., self-identity, industriousness, or intimacy).

Behavioral learning models are based on the premise that clients grow and learn subsequent to operant conditioning. The best-known behaviorists were Ivan Pavlov and his student B.F. Skinner.

Behaviorism states that behaviors that are reinforced positively will be repeated and eventually internalized. Behaviors that are punished or ignored will be extinguished. Acting in a particular way in order to stop a negative reinforcer (e.g., doing homework to stop your parents' nagging) will also cause behaviors to be learned. Operant conditioning principles are widely utilized in school settings, psychiatric hospitals, and in teaching behavior management techniques to parents.

Vicarious learning is an extension of the behavioral model in that clients can also learn through the process of imitation or modeling. Albert Bandura and R.H. Walters developed a "social learning model" in response to complaints that behaviorism was too passive and did not give credit to the client for being a part of the process. Modeling behaviors after others can help to explain why children grow to behave much like their parents or why adolescents choose to dress similarly to celebrity musicians or actors (imitation).

Jean Piaget's theory of cognitive development helps us to understand intellectual development. The model stresses that children take an active role

TABLE 15-2: ERIKSON'S 8 STAGES OF PSYCHOSOCIAL DEVELOPMENT

Age of Child	Stage	Primary Task	Result of Failure to Complete
0 to 1 year	Trust vs. Mistrust	The development of trust in others. Met by parental love and care taking behaviors.	An inability to develop trust in relationships.
1-3 years	Autonomy vs. Shame/doubt	Developing control of self, including bodily functions.	A sense of insecurity, anxiety, fearfulness.
3-5 years	Initiative vs. Guilt	Testing limits. Becoming independent of parents.	A lack of confidence, dependency on others.
5-11 years	Industry vs. Inferiority	Skill development. Rapid learning. Becoming flexible and adaptable.	Overly rigid. Low self-esteem.
11-18 years	Identity vs. Role confusion	Developing a sense of self and how one relates to others. Peer groups.	Confusion over ones place in society. Poor self-concept.
Young adulthood	Intimacy vs. Isolation	Developing love relationships. Learning compromise and giving.	Remaining self-centered. Problems with intimacy.
Adulthood	Generativity vs. Stagnation	Contributing to the greater society. Benefiting future generations.	A sense of hopelessness, or uselessness.
Late	Ego-integrity vs. Despair	Developing contentment and satisfaction with how life was lived.	Depression. Despair. Feeling of worthlessness.

(Wolraich, 1996)

in learning and adapting to their environments. It incorporates the concepts of assimilation and accommodation. Assimilation refers to adopting new ideas into existing cognition (e.g., learning that dachshunds, beagles, and terriers are all classes of dogs). Accommodation allows for the learning of new information (e.g., learning that cats are not dogs). Piaget's theory sees intelligence as a process whereby information is assimilated or accommodated at a greater or a lesser degree, depending on the client's existing cognitive abilities. The four stages of cognitive development postulated by Piaget are presented in Table 15-3. Summarized, they represent reflexive responses (birth to 2 years of age), early imagination and use of language (2 to 7 years of age), developing concrete ideas and rules (7 to 12 years of age), and thinking abstractly by using reasoning (12 years of age to adulthood). Not all clients will progress to the fourth, or "Formal Operational" stage. Mental retardation or otherbiological processes may keep a client thinking and reasoning at a level far below chronological expectations.

Lawrence Kohlberg's theory of moral development addresses the manner in which a client develops a sense of right and wrong. He theorized that there are three basic levels of moral reasoning (Table 15-4). Kohlberg's stages are not widely accepted, but they provide an important framework for understanding moral development, particularly in the area of criminal behaviors, frontal lobe injuries, and fetal alcohol syndrome.

TABLE 15-3: PIAGET'S STAGES OF COGNITIVE DEVELOPMENT

Age	Stage	Tasks	Comments
Birth to 2 years	Sensorimotor	Increasingly sophisticated responses to the environment.	Child develops symbolic thought representing early language.
2 years to 7 years	Pre-Operational	Trying to make sense of the world.	Thoughts are still rigid and errors in reasoning occur; imagination begins.
7 years to 12 years	Concrete Operational	Internalizing mental operations to learn ideas.	Logical reasoning; less egocentrism; more flexibility; better recognition of social interactions; role-playing.
12 years to Adult	Formal Operational	Applying hypotheses. Formulating ideas.	Abstract thinking begins; ability to use deductive reasoning begins; ability to draw conclusions and project into the future begins.

(Wolraich, 1996)

TABLE 15-4: KOHLBERG'S THEORY OF MORAL DEVELOPMENT

Level	Age	Principles
Preconventional	Substage 1: Birth to preschool age	Children do not consider the interests of others. Actions are based on the avoidance of punishment.
	Substage 2: Preschool to early adolescence	Children become more aware of others and develop ideas of fairness and social exchange.
Conventional	Substage 3: Adolescence	Adolescents begin to appreciate the moral codes of society and become aware of shared feelings and "being good." Requires some "Formal Operational" (Piaget) cognitive development.
	Substage 4: Adolescence	Shifting from relationships between individuals to relationships within groups. Recognition that laws are upheld to avoid the breakdown of society ("law and order" stage).
Postconventional	Substage 5: Young adulthood	The individual recognizes that morality and the law may not be the same; in fact they may conflict with one another. Decisions are made by what is "best" for all concerned.
	Substage 6: Adulthood	Individuals follow self-chosen ethical principles, which may be in conflict with laws. Not all adults develop to this level.

(Wolraich, 1996)

PRENATAL ALCOHOL AND DRUG EXPOSURE

The National Survey on Drug Use and Health (combined data, 2006 and 2007) identified that up to 22% of pregnant women between 15 and 17 years of age used substances, whereas only 13% of non-pregnant teens were using. When all women are considered, 14% to 22% report some use of alcohol during pregnancy, and 1% of children are born with signs of prenatal alcohol damage. Mental retardation developmental, behavioral, and social deficits can be the result. Low birth weight, impaired attention, and delays in language and learning skills have been seen in children who were prenatally exposed to cocaine and marijuana.

Methamphetamine exposure has been associated with fetal growth restriction, decreased arousal, and poor quality of movement in infants. Heroin use has been associated with low birth weights, but the effects of increasing oral opioid abuse (see Chapter 8) have yet to be studied (National Institute on Drug Abuse, 2009). Little is known about the long-term consequences of prenatal drug exposure on areas of learning, cognitive, and emotional development. Legal drugs (such as tobacco) have been associated with low birth weight, premature birth, and intrauterine growth retardation. Studies have also suggested links between attention deficit disorder and prenatal tobacco exposure (Braun, Kahn, Froehlich, Auinger, & Lanphear, 2006; Cornelius & Day, 2000).

Fetal Alcohol Effects

Fetal alcohol effects and fetal alcohol syndrome cause the most dramatic impact on the child. Features of fetal alcohol syndrome have been documented since the 1970s, though vague references can be found in literature going back centuries. There is no reliable way in which to diagnose fetal alcohol effects or fetal alcohol syndrome, other than by a maternal history. In pronounced cases of fetal alcohol syndrome, facial malformations in association with mental retardation provide clues, but in less severe situations there may be no physical changes. Two characteristics appear to be consistent in all children with this disorder: poor impulse control and delayed or stunted moral development. Children with fetal alcohol effects or fetal alcohol syndrome tend to have difficulty in discerning right from wrong, and even when they can verbalize how they "should" behave, their impulsivity and poor insight lead to poor choices. Children with more significant impairments may demonstrate a myriad of problems, including growth retardation, developmental delays, attention deficit hyperactivity disorder, small head circumference (microcephaly), a shortened nose, dental abnormalities, cardiac abnormalities, and hearing impairment. Intellectual impairments can range from minimal to severe. Most children born with fetal alcohol effects or fetal alcohol syndrome will require some degree of special education services during the school years.

Cocaine Exposure

Cocaine use during pregnancy can precipitate miscarriage or premature delivery because of a direct positive effect on blood pressure and uterine contractions. Neonates born to cocaine-using women have fewer withdrawal symptoms than seen in opioids; they tend to be jittery, shrill, and to startle easily. Long-term effects are still being studied but early research indicates low birth weight, smaller head circumference, abnormal neonatal behaviors, and a potential for cerebral infarction at birth. Children with a history of cocaine exposure tend to be easily distracted and have a variety of visual-perceptual problems and fine motor difficulties.

Methamphetamine Exposure

Children born to mother's that use methamphetamine during pregnancy are three times more likely to be underweight (less than 10th percentile), which is thought to be related to a restriction of placental blood flow. Premature birth does not seem to be as problematic as seen in cocaine-exposed neonates. Long-term effects, however, appear to be similar, with early studies in learning delays and behavioral problems underway.

Opiate Exposure

Opiate-exposed neonates often have to endure withdrawal symptoms at birth. These can include restlessness, tremulousness, disrupted sleep, poor feeding, stuffy nose, vomiting, diarrhea, a high-pitched cry, fever, irregular breathing, and seizures. Heroin exposure can also cause sneezes, twitches, hiccups, and tearfulness. Symptoms may begin immediately or be delayed up to 4 weeks after delivery; they usually resolve at 1 month of age, but may persist until 3 months of age. Growth disturbances, hyperactivity, short attention spans, temper tantrums, slowed motor development, and impaired visual motor functioning have been reported in children born to opiate-dependent mothers.

Marijuana Exposure

Increased tremulousness, altered visual response patterns to light, and some withdrawal-like crying (irritability) have been noted in children born to women who smoked marijuana heavily during pregnancy. Little information is available on long-term consequences of marijuana use during pregnancy.

CHILD ABUSE AND NEGLECT

Although drug and alcohol use during pregnancy is arguably a form of child abuse and neglect, this section will address more direct effects seen in the mental health setting and their impact on child development. Areas to be covered include the failure-to-thrive infant, shaken baby syndrome, Munchausen syndrome by proxy, and reactive attachment disorders. For a more in-depth discussion of childhood sexual abuse, refer to Chapter 13.

Failure-to-thrive

Failure-to-thrive can be defined as a child who fails to gain weight as expected. Causes of failure-to-thrive include a lack of education in the parents, problems with breastfeeding or formula preparation, problems with digestion, swallowing difficulties, genetic conditions, and neglect. The primary issue in determining neglect is whether reasonable efforts by the parents would allow the child to grow adequately, and if the caregivers are making those efforts. Underweight children who grow and flourish in foster care settings are diagnostic of failure-to-thrive neglect. Deprivation of necessary nutrition in an infant and young child can result in inadequate brain development with lifelong consequences, such as poor language or intellectual development.

Shaken Baby Syndrome

Shaken baby syndrome occurs when there is violent shaking of a young child, leading to brain bruising, bleeding, cerebral edema, and other signs of pressure on the brain. Spinal cord injuries may also be present. Almost 90% of shaken babies and young children demonstrate retinal hemorrhages (in fact, there is little else that causes this physical finding outside of automobile accidents and child abuse). Twenty percent of victims die of complications associated with brain swelling. Long-term consequences include mental retardation, severe developmental delays, visual impairments, and neurological impairments. Perpetrators of shaken baby syndrome are likely to repeat the behaviors. Particularly tragic to parents is the child who dies, or is permanently injured, at the hands of a trusted family member or babysitter.

Munchausen Syndrome by Proxy

Munchausen syndrome by proxy is a rare form of child abuse that consists of the fabrication or production of illness symptoms in a child by the caregiver. The medical symptoms typically disappear if the child is removed from the environment. Suspicion is aroused when the caregiver presents the child repeatedly for medical care (not injuries) due to a variety of symptoms. Because much of pediatric care is based on the parents' reports, children may be diagnosed and treated with numerous medications, have invasive tests and procedures performed, and may undergo surgery before the diagnosis is suspected. The most common diagnoses seen are chronic vomiting and diarrhea, infections, severe allergies, seizures, and failure-to-thrive. In severe cases, parents have been known to systematically give their children poison, to inject foreign substances into an IV line, or to smear feces in a wound, thereby keeping it infected. Parent behaviors that may be suggestive of this syndrome include highly attentive parents who: seem to have excessive medical knowledge; appear to enjoy the hospital and health care arena and are interested in medical details; seem to require a great deal of attention from the staff; demonstrate symptoms similar to the child's; and appear to be unusually calm, despite the seriousness of the child's illness. Munchausen syndrome by proxy is not recognized in the *DSM-IV-TR* but is generally classified under factitious disorders and much has been written about the disorder. Perpetrators of Munchausen syndrome by proxy are not usually in lower socioeconomic groups; in fact, the disorder is more prevalent in educated parents with some healthcare experience. Diagnosis can be confirmed in a hospital setting by hidden cameras in the child's room (most large facilities have rooms set up for this purpose).

Reactive Attachment Disorder

The *DSM-IV-TR* defines reactive attachment disorder as a failure to develop appropriate social-relatedness, usually beginning before 5 years of age, and associated with grossly pathological care. There are two subtypes: inhibited and disinhibited. In the inhibited subtype of reactive attachment disorder, the child demonstrates a pattern of hypervigilant, ambivalent, or highly inhibited behaviors toward caregivers. The child may be resistant to comfort measures or appear to be watchful or suspicious of others. In the disinhibited type, the child will show diffuse and nondiscriminatory attachments with such behaviors as kissing strangers or climbing into the lap of persons just met. The disorder cannot be accounted for by more pervasive developmental problems (such as retardation or autism). The pathological care history may include a persistent disregard for the child's basic physical or emotional needs or repeated changes in caregivers that prevent formulation of stable attachments. This disorder is frequently seen in children with a long history of foster home placement, particularly when they have been moved often. Reactive attachment disorder treatment consists of a combination of family therapy and a stable, nurturing, permanent home and caregivers.

MENTAL RETARDATION

Mental retardation is defined by standardized tests that measure intelligence (IQ). Mild mental retardation is an IQ of 55 to 69, moderate measures from 40 to 54, severe from 25 to 39, and profound below 25. Borderline levels (70 to 80) may be diagnosed as mental retardation if functioning is poor in important life areas. Cognitive abilities have a significant impact on coping skills, decision-making, and other important areas. There are no consistent behaviors associated with mental retardation; some clients are aggressive or explosive, whereas others may be calm and passive. Clients who have mental retardation have a fourfold risk of developing other mental disorders, when compared to the general population. Deficits in communication occur proportionate to the degree of retardation. Causes of mental retardation vary considerably and include heredity (Down syndrome, fragile X-syndrome), environmental influences (failure-to-thrive), other mental disorders (autism), prenatal problems (alcohol exposure, fetal malnutrition, hypoxia, infections, or trauma), and medical conditions (head injury, lead poisoning). Occasionally, many family members will have greater or lesser degrees of retardation, suggesting familial traits; however, mental retardation can occur in a child born to parents with normal IQs and no other apparent cause. Clients who have Down syndrome are encountered frequently in the healthcare setting and warrant further discussion.

Down Syndrome

Described first in 1866 by Dr. John Langdon Down (but erroneously thought to be related to perinatal tuberculosis), Down syndrome has been seen and treated in healthcare settings, schools, and residential programs since that time. Identifying excess material on the 21st chromosome in the deoxyribonucleic acid (DNA) strand confirms the diagnosis of Down syndrome. Down syndrome can usually be recognized at birth because of specific physical characteristics that are seen:

- Flattened nasal bridge

- Brushfield spots (around the irises)

- Shortened, thick fingers

- Ear abnormalities

- Epicanthal eye folds

- Protruding tongue

Numerous other physical characteristics may also be seen. The degree of mental retardation in Down syndrome can vary from borderline to profound.

Medical problems are common in Down syndrome. Table 15-5 provides an overview of problems frequently seen in the healthcare setting. Neurological and cardiovascular problems are the most prominent and present the greatest challenge.

Clients who live with Down syndrome can be highly productive members of society. Formerly housed in institutions, they now live independently or with others in a variety of settings. Many clients are employed; some marry and raise families of their own and others need the support of residential or nursing facilities. Parents of babies with Down syndrome should be encouraged to think in terms of their child's future abilities and not to focus on potential disabilities or have lowered expectations.

PERVASIVE DEVELOPMENTAL DISORDERS

A pervasive development disorder is characterized by severe impairment in several areas of development. These disorders are usually evident in the first years of life and may be associated with some degree of mental retardation (though not required). Several types of pervasive development disorders can occur, but all have some combination of language or communication skill impairment, social interaction impairment,

TABLE 15-5: MEDICAL PROBLEMS ENCOUNTERED IN DOWN SYNDROME

System Affected	Related Disorders
Neurological	Seizures
	Hypotonia
	Attention deficit/ hyperactivity disorder
	Alzheimer's disease
Musculoskeletal	Joint abnormalities
	Hip instability
	Scoliosis
Cardiovascular	Congenital cardiac lesions
	Mitral valve disease
	Atrial ventricular or ventricular septal defect
	Pulmonary stenosis
Integumentary	Excessive neck skin folds
	Fissured tongue
	Dryness/coarseness/aging
Neurological	Sleep apnea
Hematological	Leukemia
	Polycythemia
Immunological	Increased infections
	Autoimmune disorders
Ear, Nose, Throat	Hearing loss or deafness
	Recurrent otitis media
	Sinus problems and infections
Eye	Brushfield spots (white and yellow nodules circling the iris)
	Conjunctivitis
	Cataracts
Dental	Retained deciduous teeth
	Delayed tooth eruption
	Atypical tooth size or shape
Reproductive	High rate of sterility in men
Gastrointestinal	Anomalies of the GI tract
	Choking problems
	Constipation
	Obesity
Endocrine	Thyroid disease
	Short stature

(Wolraich, 1996)

or stereotyped behaviors, interests, or activities. Comorbidity with other psychiatric disorders is extremely high. The two disorders encountered most often in the mental health care setting are autism and Asperger's syndrome.

Autism

Autism is a developmental disorder that is readily recognized early in life. Infants with this disorder are described as aloof or non-cuddly. Repetitive, stereotyped behaviors, such as rocking, spinning or twirling, may be seen. Language acquisition and usage is impaired. Individuals with this disorder may have some degree of mental retardation; some even demonstrate savant characteristics with incredible abilities in music, mathematics, or memorization skills. Hearing problems can occur, which may include deafness or hypersensitivity. Social interactions are dramatically affected – clients with autism have trouble making and keeping friends or they may have no interest in other people at all. Rigid adherence to routines and structure occurs, which may help the clients to maintain some sense of control in their environments. Autism has attracted significantly more public attention in recent years because of the increasing numbers of cases reported. What may be occurring is that there is a greater recognition of the autism-spectrum, and children are being identified with the developmental disorder even when symptoms are mild to moderate. Autism occurs more often in males than females (4 or 5:1) and it is equally distributed across all socioeconomic groups. Prevalence rates, as measured by the CDC, indicate that about 1 in every 150 children has an autism-spectrum disorder, with geographic variability noted across the country (overall prevalence rate is 2 to 6 per 1000 children). In 2006, about half of these children (224,595) were receiving special education services, as compared to only 22,664 children in 1994. Table 15-6 provides the *DSM-IV-TR* criteria for autism.

Early views on the causes of autism focused on poor parenting and environmental influences.

Today, it is seen as a neurobiological disorder with diverse physical causes. In many cases, no causative factor for the disorder can be identified. Many attempts have been made to correlate the development of autism with noxious agents, such as mercury in childhood immunizations, or to living next to a commercial orchard (exposure to insecticide sprays); however, none of these theories currently have any basis in research and only exist as case reports. The onset of autism is before 3 years of age, but most parents will say that their child "has been this way since birth." There is an increased risk of autistic disorders and other developmental problems among siblings with the disorder (5%). The nature of the impairments in social interaction may change over time, depending on the developmental age of the child.

Early identification is essential to maximize the child's abilities and provide supportive instruction. Speech therapy, hearing evaluations, occupational therapy, and individualized educational plans may be necessary. A thorough medical examination helps to rule out other disorders (seizure disorders can occur in up to 25% of individuals with autism). Concomitant psychiatric disorders often include obsessive-compulsive disorder, attention deficit hyperactivity disorder, intermittent explosive disorder, impulse control disorder, and other anxiety or mood disorders. The primary focuses of treatment are to promote the development of social and communication skills and to improve adaptive living skills to the maximum capabilities of the child. Counseling and education for families is also essential.

The medication risperidone (Risperdal®) has been approved by the FDA to treat moodswings, irritability, and aggression associated with autism. In adults, risperidone is dosed up to 12 mg daily; however, in children and adolescents, doses of 1 to 3 mg daily in divided doses is usually sufficient without as much risk for side effects. Other new-generation atypical antipsychotics are also used for the mood

TABLE 15-6: CRITERIA FOR AUTISM

1. A total of two or more items from (a) and at least one each from (b) and (c)

   a. Impairment in social interaction

      i. impaired use of nonverbal behaviors, such as eye contact, facial expression, body postures, or gestures

      ii. failure to develop age-appropriate peer relationships

      iii. lack of spontaneous seeking to share interests, achievements, or enjoyment with other people

      iv. lack of social or emotional reciprocity

   b. Impairments in communication

      i. delay or lack in a spoken language

      ii. impairment in the ability to initiate or sustain a conversation in the presence of normal speech abilities

      iii. stereotyped and repetitive use of language

      iv. lack of make-believe play or social imitative play appropriate to age

   c. Restricted patterns of behavior, interests, and activities

      i. preoccupation with abnormally intense or focused interests

      ii. apparently inflexible adherence to specific, nonfunctional routines or rituals

      iii. repetitive motor mannerisms (e.g., hand-flapping)

      iv. preoccupation with parts of objects

2. Delays or abnormal functioning before 3 years of age in at least one of the following areas: social interaction, language used in social communication, or symbolic or imaginative play activities

3. Disorder not better explained by another developmental disorder (e.g., childhood disintegrative disorder or Rett's disorder)

(American Psychiatric Association, 2000)

problems sometimes experienced in children with autism, including aripiprazole (Abilify®), olanzapine (Zyprexa®), ziprasidone (Geodon®), quetiapine (Seroquel®), and paliperidone (Invega®). The reader is referred to Chapter 5 for a more complete discussion of these medications.

Asperger's Syndrome

Asperger's syndrome is similar to autism in that children with the disorder express developmental problems early in life and there are pronounced social-relatedness problems. In all other ways, it is a markedly different disorder. The essential features of Asperger's syndrome are severe impairment in social interaction along with the development of hyperfocused, but restricted patterns of behaviors, interests, or activities. Language development is usually normal, if not precocious. Mental retardation rarely occurs. Variability in cognitive and intellectual functioning can occur, however, with erratic performances in reading, mathematics, science, music, art, or other abilities. *DSM-IV-TR* criteria for Asperger's syndrome are provided in Table 15-7. To diagnose Asperger's syndrome, there must be clinically significant distress in functioning abilities as well; however, there are no clinically significant delays in language, cognitive development, or in age-appropriate self-care skills, curiosity, or adaptive behaviors.

Children with Asperger's syndrome are often acutely aware of their social deficits, but puzzled as to how to behave or respond to others. They can grow into adults who are brilliant scientists, mathematicians, or musicians, but have few friends,

TABLE 15-7: CRITERIA FOR ASPERGER'S SYNDROME

1. Impairment in social interaction with at least two of the following:

    a. marked impairment in nonverbal behaviors such as eye-to-eye gaze, facial expression, body postures, or gestures

    b. failure to develop peer relationships appropriate to developmental level

    c. lack of spontaneous seeking to share enjoyment, interests, or achievements with other people

    d. lack of social or emotional reciprocity

2. Restricted repetitive and stereotyped patterns of behavior, interests, or activities with at least one of the following:

    a. preoccupation with an interest that is abnormal either in intensity or focus

    b. inflexible adherence to specific, nonfunctional routines or rituals

    c. repetitive motor mannerisms (twisting, rocking, or hand-flapping)

    d. preoccupation with parts of objects

(American Psychiatric Association, 2000)

which can result in loneliness and low self-esteem. Other psychiatric disorders are also more common in individuals with Asperger's syndrome, including obsessive-compulsive disorders, attention deficit hyperactivity disorder, and major depression. Treatment should also address other coexisting disorders. Counseling for clients with Asperger's syndrome is focused on teaching the client more adaptive social skills along with homework assignments to practice these skills in a real-world environment.

OTHER DEVELOPMENTAL DISORDERS

A number of other developmental disorders are identified in the *DSM-IV-TR,* including academic-based disorders (reading, writing, and arithmetic), communication disorders, disorders of feeding in early childhood, and elimination disorders. For the purpose of simplicity, these will be grouped into broad categories for discussion.

Reading, Writing, and Arithmetic Disorders

Disorders that involve reading, written words, or understanding mathematical concepts are frequently encountered in the academic setting (as opposed to the psychiatric). A learning disorder is

diagnosed when a client's achievement on standardized tests is substantially below that expected for age, schooling, and level of intelligence. The learning problems must also interfere with academic achievement or daily living activities that require those skills (such as filling out job applications or balancing a checkbook in an adult, or learning to count money in a child). Other conditions, such as generalized mental retardation, visual problems, or hearing loss, must be ruled out. Reading disorders are diagnosed 60% to 80% of the time in males, with a prevalence of 4% of all school-age children. Diagnosis usually does not occur until 1st grade, when it becomes more readily apparent. Reading disorders can take a variety of forms, which may include dyslexia (reversing letters or words), visual-perceptual problems, and reading comprehension problems. Mathematics disorders are identified later (2nd or 3rd grade) because of the more advanced skills required at those ages. Mathematics disorders are less common, occurring in about 1% of school-age children. Disorders of written expression (writing) are difficult to separate from other learning disorders, because writing skills are dependent upon a complex interaction among reading, comprehension, and motor coordination. The diagnosis is not given if the only problem noted is sloppy or poor handwriting. Tasks in which a child is asked to copy, write to dictation, or write spontaneously are better for uncovering this disorder. School testing and an individualized educational plan are usually necessary for children with these disorders.

Language and Communication Disorders

Communication disorders consist of expressive and receptive language disorders, phonological disorder, and stuttering. Expressive language disorders require that the child scores lower than expected on standardized tests that measure language development. Frequently, a child demonstrates word-finding or vocabulary errors, a limited range of vocabulary, a limited amount of speech, difficulty acquiring new words, simplified or shortened sentences, use of unusual word order, omissions of parts of sentences, and a slow rate of language development that is not consistent with his or her IQ. If the child also has a sensory deficit, severe environmental deprivation, or mental retardation, then the language delay must be more severe than expected for that disorder. Schoolwork suffers and grades are low in reading, language, and spelling because of the child's inability to express himself verbally or in writing. A mixed receptive-expressive language disorder is one in which standardized scores in both expressive and receptive language abilities are lower than expected. With this disorder, expressive language problems are always present, but the child also demonstrates difficulties in understanding language. Problems with understanding words, sentences, or phrases may exist. In mild cases, understanding complicated language structure may be all that is impaired. In severe cases, understanding basic vocabulary, discriminating sounds, associating sounds with symbols, storage, recall, and sequencing may all be affected. Because expressive abilities always rely on perception and understanding, a pure receptive language disorder does not exist (as may be seen in adults with cerebro vascular accidents).

A phonological disorder (formerly called a developmental articulation disorder) is a failure to use developmentally expected speech sounds. Common errors that are seen include mispronunciations of letters (*r, th, ch*) or substitutions of one sound for another (e.g., *t* for *k*). Lisping (*th* for *s*) is relatively common. Phonological development problems are more prominent in males than in females and present in about 2% of the population. Environmental factors should be considered when assessing a child's speech (learned patterns). About 75% of affected children spontaneously remit by 6 years of age. Speech therapy through the school system may be indicated for enduring problems.

Stuttering differs from phonological problems in that the pronunciation of the letters and words is not impaired, but there is a disturbance in the fluency and time patterning of the speech. There may be frequent repetitions or prolongations of sounds, syllables, or words. Blocking (silences between words), broken words (pauses within a word), word substitutions, or other disturbances may be seen. The extent and intensity of the disturbance varies, depending on the situation and is often more severe when the client is feeling under pressure or anxious. Stuttering may be absent when reading aloud, singing, or talking to pets or toys. Motor movements, such as eye-blinking or head-jerking, may accompany stuttering. It is three times higher in males than in females and occurs in 1% of children prior to puberty (0.8% post pubescent). Speech therapy and relaxation counseling can help clients to live with the disorder.

PICA

Several disorders may occur in young children that affect eating and feeding behaviors, which may in turn have a negative impact on development. These are differentiated from anorexia nervosa and bulimia nervosa in that there is no perception of being overweight or desire to lose weight, as seen in those disorders. Of most clinical interest is the unusual eating of nonnutritive substances on a persistent basis for at least 1 month that is known as pica. Very young children may eat paint (which can contain lead), plaster, hair, string, or cloth. Older children may consume sand, insects, leaves, pebbles, or animal dropping. Adolescents tend to eat clay, soil, or starch. Pica is also found in pregnant women and has been associated with iron deficiencies in that population. To be diagnosed as a disorder, the behavior may not be a part of a culturally sanctioned practice (some countries regularly encourage the consumption of clay with meat). Children with pica do not have any particular aversions to eating normal food as well. Pica is frequently associated with mental retardation and pervasive developmental disorders, although it may occur in other children as well. Although there are some reports of vitamin or other nutrient deficiencies, these are not consistent and a cause cannot always be found. Complications of pica include poisoning, bowel obstruction, intestinal perforations, and infections (e.g., parasitic). Some substances are harmless, and the behavior can be ignored. In other cases, increased supervision of the child may be necessary.

ELIMINATION DISORDERS

Two types of elimination disorders are seen in children: encopresis and enuresis. To be diagnosed as a psychiatric or behavioral disturbance, medical causes must first be ruled out. The essential feature of encopresis is the passing of feces (either voluntarily or involuntarily) into inappropriate places (clothing, closets, floor, or toy box). The behavior must occur at least once a month for 3 months or more, and the child must be older than 4 years of age. Encopresis is often the result of constipation or impaction, which may be due to psychological stress (anxiety, fear, defiance) or illnesses such as dehydration. Painful stool passage predisposes the child to avoidance behavior which, in turn, increases the withholding and causes constipation. Occasionally, a child is incontinent of liquid, runny stools secondary to fecal retention. Encopresis is seen in many children, but its association to severe distress (such as that experienced following sexual abuse) warrants close attention when obtaining a nursing history. Encopresis can be socially devastating to a child, resulting in repeated embarrassment and ostracizing by other children.

Treatment for encopresis involves bowel-retraining programs. The child is usually put on a daily laxative (such as mineral oil) and may also be given a fiber supplement daily. Educate the parents about high-fiber diets that include fruit juices (especially apple and grape), whole fruits, vegetables, and whole grain cereals. Also teach the parents to have their child sit on the toilet on a regular basis, usually right after breakfast, and to sit without straining for several minutes (if necessary, the child should be taken to the toilet every 4 hours until successful, but not left sitting more than 5 or 6 minutes each time). Extra clean clothes should be taken to the school and left at the school nurse's office. Alerting the health aid or school nurse and classroom teacher of the problem may help to diminish some of the stigma associated with encopresis.

Enuresis is the involuntary (or voluntary) passage of urine at inappropriate times or in inappropriate places. Enuresis is subdivided into nocturnal only, diurnal only, and both nocturnal and diurnal subtypes. Criteria to diagnose enuresis require that the "accidents" occur at least twice a week for 3 months or more in a child who is at least 5 years of age. The amount of impairment associated with enuresis is dependent upon the age, subtype, and how it impacts on peer relationships. A 6-year-old who wets the bed every night is not as devastating as a 12-year-old who wants to stay over at a friend's home or go camping. Prevalence rates for enuresis are relatively high: 5% to 10% of all children younger than 10 years of age. There is a significant familial component, with 75% of children having a family member with a history of the disorder. Enuresis is more likely in children with attention deficit hyperactivity disorder, developmental delays, sleep disorders, or urinary tract infections. Enuresis is less related to psychological distress than is encopresis.

When medical causes are ruled-out, treatment of enuresis is usually a combination of medications and behavior modification. Medications used include desmopressin (DDAVP®), a synthetic antidiuretic hormone, or imipramine (Tofranil®), a tricyclic antidepressant. Both are administered at bedtime. DDAVP is available orally (doses are usually 0.1 to 0.3 mg) or in a nasal spray (1 spray in each nostril). Imipramine is only available orally and is usually dosed at 10 mg. Doses higher than 20 mg place the child at risk for slowed cardiac conduction and an electrocardiogram reading is advised. Two types of behavior management are useful for treating enuresis. In the first, parents may purchase a pad that sets off an alarm when it becomes wet. The alarm is designed to wake the child, prompting a visit to the toilet. Hopefully, the child will eventually become conditioned to waking at that same time every night. The second method requires that the parents set an alarm clock and check on the child at increasingly earlier hours nightly, until they find the point at which the bed becomes wet during the night. They then must wake the child immediately before that "wetting time" every night and escort the child to the bathroom, until the child wakes up automatically. It is always prudent to restrict fluids within an hour of bedtime and to ask the child to urinate before retiring. Using pull-up diapers at night can be acceptable in young children, but they may be emotionally traumatic for the older child (in addition, they tend to give permission for wetting behaviors). Diurnal, or daytime, wetting is best treated by toileting routines of escorting (or sending) the child to the bathroom every 2 to 3 hours, including during the school day.

CASE STUDY: DEVELOPMENTAL DISORDERS

Matthew is an 8-year-old boy with autistic disorder who presents in the behavioral health care facility for an increase in aggressive behaviors. His mother reports that he was first recognized as autistic at 3 years old. He has difficulty relating to others, and prefers to play alone with his toy cars (stacking them and twirling their wheels), which he can do for hours. Lately, he has started to lick the backs of his hands repetitively and they are red and chapped. Whenever family members or schoolteachers ask him to stop playing or licking and attend to tasks-at-hand (such as schoolwork or a family meal), he starts to yell and rock back and forth. If he is touched, he strikes out violently against anyone he can reach. Matthew has difficulty in using language to express his needs, and at times he doesn't seem to understand what is being asked of him. In addition to the autism diagnosis, academic testing has revealed an IQ of 72. Medical findings are as follows: 4'10", 75 lb, blood pressure 110/58, heart rate 110; hands are chapped and reddened; nails are bitten to the quick; nocturnal enuresis 4 to 5 nights out of 7; rare diurnal enuresis; rare encopresis; sleep is decreased with an onset of 11 p.m. and awake by 5 a.m. daily; appetite is erratic; and increased motor activity and impulsive striking out. Matthew is placed on risperidone (Risperdal®) 0.25 mg twice a day and DDAVP nasal spray bilateral nares at bedtime. A toileting routine was also discussed with his parents to facilitate his staying dry at night.

Questions

1. How does this client demonstrate autism rather than Asperger's syndrome?

2. What parent education should be done regarding the use of risperidone?

3. What are some components of a toileting routine?

Discussion

Asperger's syndrome is characterized by severe social interaction problems, but usually does not include stereotypical behaviors or mental retardation or cognitive delays. Speech and language development are chiefly normal in Asperger's syndrome. Risperidone is used to treat moodswings, irritability, and aggression in children with autism. It can increase appetite causing weight gain, cause sleepiness, and put the child at risk for pseudo-parkinsonism side effects and tardive dyskinesia. Parents should be advised to monitor for tremors or involuntary motor movements. Toileting routines often include daily mineral oil or other mild laxatives and having the child sit on the toilet at the same time every day, usually right after breakfast, for 5 to 10 minutes.

NURSING CARE PLAN: DEVELOPMENTAL DISORDERS

Problem Listing

- Bedwetting 4 or 5 nights out of 7
- Sleep onset problems
- Red, chapped hands (potential for infection)
- Impulsive, aggressive behaviors
- Inflexibility with changes in routines

Priority Nursing Diagnosis

Risk for violence directed toward others related to poor impulse control, as evidenced by striking out at caregivers when redirected.

Long-term Goal

Client will learn alternative ways to communicate his needs, without resorting to aggression.

Short-term Objectives

1. Client will not strike out more than once a month.
2. Client will demonstrate personal time-outs when feeling upset prior to striking out.

Nursing Interventions

1. Educate parents to recognize the four stages of crisis escalation:
   a. Trigger (events that precipitate acting-out)
   b. Escalation (behaviors that indicate increasing tension)
   c. Acting-out (striking out or destructive behaviors)
   d. De-escalation (calming down)

2. Educate parents as to means of dealing with each stage as it occurs:
   a. Trigger – identify precipitants, then work to reduce or eliminate them
   b. Escalation – recognize signs of tension (e.g., pacing or rocking), then help the child to redirect his energy or to take a personal time-out
   c. Acting-out – place the child in safe time-out area; may use as needed medications if they are available
   d. De-escalation – talk with the child about what led to the time-out (e.g., "In this family we don't hit other people;" reassure the child, "You're a good boy and we love you.")

3. Ask parents to log acting-out behaviors for one week, then help them to analyze the triggers, how they responded to signs of escalation and acting-out, and how the process of de-escalation occurred.

4. Educate parents in ways to help their child transition between activities in order to reduce stress-responses (e.g., giving 5-minute warnings, getting eye contact prior to giving directions, and asking him to repeat directions.)

ADVANCED PRACTICE NURSING: PRESCRIBING MEDICATIONS FOR CHILDREN

Nurses with prescriptive privileges who see children and adolescents are at a higher risk for liability than are nurses who work exclusively with adults. Very few psychiatric drugs are studied or approved for children outside of attention deficit hyperactivity disorder (ADHD) treatment; however, many drugs are utilized. Additionally, *DSM-IV-TR* criteria for diagnosing psychiatric disorders are often slanted toward adults, (i.e., bipolar disorder, major depression, anxiety disorders) with only vague qualifiers for children. Children are more likely to have comorbid conditions; it is not uncommon for a child in a psychiatric setting to have 2 or 3 Axis I disorders, a learning disorder, and medical complications, such as enuresis, constipation, seizure disorder, or asthma. This is in addition to family dysfunctions, foster care placement or other psychosocial stressors, or trauma. It is no wonder that we have a shortage, especially in rural areas, of qualified psychiatric and mental health providers specializing in children and adolescent treatment.

The nurse clinician who chooses this specialty practice will find it extremely rewarding because children can demonstrate dramatic improvements in mood, affect, academic performance, and overall happiness. However, certain cautions should always be remembered. First, no child exists in a vacuum. That is, all children must be treated within the context of the family. This can be extremely complicating when children have multiple parents because of divorce, are being raised by extended families, or are in foster care or residential placement. The parent, legal guardian, or caregiver should always be involved from the beginning in obtaining an accurate history and in giving permission for the child to be treated, including with medica-

tions. It should also be remembered that noncustodial parents who retain legal rights (who have not had their rights terminated or do not have a protective order against them) also have the right to refuse treatment for the child and to have full disclosure of medical and psychiatric records. Only adolescents older than 14 years of age who are in addictions treatment (or receiving reproductive planning) can be treated confidentially without a parent's consent. Second, informed consent should always be obtained from the parent or legal guardian before prescribing medications. It is probably best to require that a parent or legal guardian attend all medication appointments; this differs from therapy appointments, during which family intervention is interspersed with individual treatment. Some agencies require written consent, whereas others are content with documentation in clinical notations. The prudent clinician obtains consent for medications from both parents or, if only one parent is available, ensures that the parent understands that the information should be shared with the other parent. Third, the nurse clinician should remember that the "patient" is the whole family and involve parents in decision-making as much as possible. A contractual relationship enhances compliance better than an authoritarian one. Ultimately, the parent or guardian is responsible for the child; if he or she isn't comfortable with a medication or treatment, then it should not be prescribed. Slow titration and lots of parent education helps to build up the parents' or guardian's comfort level with a medication intervention.

SUMMARY

A good basis in normal growth and development is the foundation for understanding developmental disorders and learning problems. In this chapter, both expected and problematic childhood development were explored. Several developmental disorders were presented and their relationship to childhood psychiatric illness was discussed. Child abuse, including prenatal substance abuse, was discussed along with the effects of substance abuse during pregnancy on the child and infant. One of these disorders, fetal alcohol syndrome/fetal alcohol effects, is particularly damaging to the child. Reactive attachment disorders are seen in children who have been unable to bond in a healthy manner during early childhood with their adult caregivers. Other, less overt, learning delays in such areas as reading and mathematics or language problems, such as stuttering and phonological disorders, were reviewed. A few unusual disorders were presented, including pica (the eating of non-nutritive substances) and Munchausen syndrome by proxy (intentional harm done to a child by a parent to gain attention and sympathy from others). More commonly seen in child behavioral health is enuresis, or the involuntary passing of urine (called incontinence in adults), and encopresis, the involuntary or voluntary withholding of feces with subsequent toileting accidents. Suggestions were provided to manage the problems, such as toileting routines. To enhance learning, the reader was provided with a case study and sample nursing care plan for a child with a developmental disorder.

EXAM QUESTIONS

CHAPTER 15
Questions 90-94

Note: Choose the one option that BEST answers each question.

90. The stage of growth and development entitled "Identity versus Role Confusion" usually emerges in

    a. early childhood.
    b. adolescence.
    c. adulthood.
    d. old age.

91. A jittery, shrill baby who startles easily may have been exposed prenatally to

    a. heroin.
    b. cocaine.
    c. ecstasy.
    d. marijuana.

92. Signs of heroin withdrawal in a neonate include

    a. a jittery, easily startled baby.
    b. jaundice and seizures.
    c. tremulousness, sneezes, and a high-pitched cry.
    d. irritability and light sensitivity.

93. Reactive attachment disorder is a failure to develop appropriate social relatedness and is associated with

    a. grossly pathological care.
    b. neurological delays.
    c. educational deprivation.
    d. sensory deprivation problems.

94. Diagnostic criteria for autism always includes impairments in

    a. social interaction and communication.
    b. thought processes and intelligence.
    c. emotional expression and range.
    d. reading and arithmetic abilities.

CHAPTER 16

BEHAVIOR DISORDERS AND TOURETTE'S DISORDER

CHAPTER OBJECTIVE

At the completion of this chapter, the reader will be able to describe disruptive behavior disorders and Tourette's disorder and their relevant treatments.

LEARNING OBJECTIVES

At the end of this chapter, the reader will be able to

1. differentiate ADHD from other psychiatric disorders.

2. discuss medication interventions and nursing management of the child with ADHD.

3. recognize motor and vocal tics and their relationship to Tourette's disorder.

INTRODUCTION

Parents and teachers are confronted daily with disruptive behaviors in children. At some point, normal defiance, energy, and tantrums exhibited by all children and adolescents become dysfunctional and begin to interfere with the child's peer and family relationships and academic progress. Disruptive behavior disorders, once thought to be only problematic in childhood, may persist into adulthood, causing occupational, social, and other problems. Closely associated with disruptive behavior is the chronic motor and vocal tic disorder called Tourette's disorder. Comorbidity of Tourette's dis-

order with psychiatric or behavioral problems, such as attention deficit disorder, obsessive-compulsive and other anxiety disorders, Asperger's syndrome, major depression, or bipolar disorder, is as high as 80%. In this chapter, disruptive behavior disorders will be examined, including attention deficit problems, oppositional-defiant disorder, conduct disorder, and Tourette's disorder. A case study that demonstrates some of the comorbidity commonly encountered in this area is presented along with a sample nursing care plan.

ATTENTION DEFICIT HYPERACTIVITY DISORDER

Attention deficit hyperactivity disorder (ADHD) is the most frequently encountered psychiatric diagnosis in children, with prevalence rates 4% across the country. The core features of ADHD have been described in the literature since the 1930s, although terminology has changed over time. Early diagnoses included minimal brain damage and minimal brain dysfunction, because it was believed that ADHD symptoms were similar to behaviors seen in clients with CNS injuries. In the 1950s the diagnosis was changed to "hyperactive child syndrome." The *DSM-II* altered the diagnosis to be "hyperkinetic reaction of childhood" in 1968, which was the prevailing standard until 1980. The *DSM-III* first recognized that ADHD was a disorder of attention as well as hyperactivity. In 1984, the *DSM-IV* further described ADHD utilizing the subtypes of "with hyperactivity," "without hyperactivity," and "combined presentation." Before the 1970s, it was believed that ADD/ADHD was a child-only disorder; today we know that this is not true. Approximately 4% of adults also meet criteria for ADHD, and between 40% and 60% of children diagnosed with the disorder will still be symptomatic as adults (WebMD, 2009a, 2009b).

Much of the difficulty in diagnosing ADHD arises from the fact that many of its symptoms are developmentally appropriate in certain contexts. For example, 4-year-old children are talkative, impulsive, and extremely active. A diagnosis of ADHD can only be made when the symptoms are determined to be at a level that is greater than expected for the average child. Table 16-1 provides the *DSM-IV-TR* criteria for diagnosing ADHD in children.

ADHD is classified in three subtypes: inattentive type, which is diagnosed when only criterion (a) is met; hyperactive/impulsive type, which is diagnosed when only criterion (b) is met; and combined type, which is diagnosed when six symptoms from both criteria (a) and (b) are met.

Features that are not part of the diagnostic criteria, but are certainly associated with ADHD, vary with developmental age and may include low frustration tolerance, temper outbursts (common), bossiness, stubbornness, demanding, mood lability, depressed moods, poor peer interactions, and low self-esteem. Peers may reject or refuse to play with children with ADHD. Academic achievement is usually markedly impaired, despite normal or above normal intellectual capabilities. This often contributes to a great deal of conflict between the child and the parents, leading to strained family dynamics. The hyperactive and impulsive symptoms often cause the child to get into trouble at school or in other settings. Lost recess time, in-school suspensions, frequent visits to the principal's office, or even suspensions and expulsions may result, which serve to further interrupt the learning process. Individuals with ADHD, predominately inattentive type have few behavior problems, but they tend to be withdrawn, socially passive, and neglected by peers.

Almost one-half of the children diagnosed with ADHD (hyperactive-impulsive or combined types) also have oppositional or defiant behaviors or conduct disorders. This co-occurrence is significantly higher for ADHD than for other psychiatric disorders. Almost one-third of children with ADHD will have another concomitant disorder. The most common diagnoses reported are anxiety disorders, mood disorders (both major depression and bipolar disorder), learning disorders, and communication disorders (American Psychiatric Association, 2000).

Adults who have ADD are usually not as physically hyperactive as children, although impulsivity tends to persist. They tend to have difficulty with organizational skills and appear to others to be scattered and forgetful. Table 16-2 presents some symptoms that may indicate ADHD in adults. Because of these problems, adults with ADHD have more financial problems and difficulty in maintaining employment, more marital and relationship problems, and more psychological distress overall.

Causes of ADHD are not known. It has been found to be more common among first-degree biological relatives, lending credibility to genetic factors. In some children, there may be a history of child abuse or neglect, lead or other toxin exposures, brain infections, prenatal drug or alcohol exposure, or mental retardation. Prematurity and low birth weights have been associated with ADHD, though there is no research evidence to support this claim. Medications that treat ADHD work by improving the production of the neurotransmitter dopamine, and secondarily norepinephrine, from the presynaptic neurons in the brain, leading some to

TABLE 16-1: CRITERIA FOR ATTENTION DEFICIT HYPERACTIVITY DISORDER IN CHILDREN

1. Either (a) or (b)

   a. Six (or more) of the following symptoms of inattention have been present for at least 6 months at a degree that is maladaptive and developmentally inconsistent:

      i. fails to give close attention to details or makes careless mistakes in work or other activities

      ii. has difficulty sustaining attention during tasks or play activities

      iii. does not seem to listen when spoken to directly

      iv. does not follow through on instructions and fails to finish tasks once started

      v. has difficulty in organizing tasks or activities

      vi. avoids, dislikes, or is reluctant to engage in tasks that require mental effort (such as school work)

      vii. loses things necessary for activities or tasks

      viii. is easily distracted by external stimuli

      ix. is often forgetful in daily activities

   b. Six or more of the following symptoms of hyperactivity-impulsivity have persisted for at least 6 months at a level that is maladaptive:

      i. fidgets with hands or feet or squirms in seat

      ii. leaves the seat in the classroom or in other situations where it is inappropriate (e.g., church, dinner table)

      iii. runs about or climbs excessively in inappropriate situations

      iv. has difficulty playing or engaging in leisure activities quietly

      v. is often "on the go" or acts as if "driven by a motor"

      vi. often talks excessively

      vii. often blurts out answers before questions have been completed

      viii. has difficulty taking turns

      ix. often interrupts or intrudes on others

2. Some symptoms have to be present prior to age 7

3. Some form of impairment from the symptoms presenting in two or more settings (e.g., home and school, home and grandparents home)

4. Symptoms clearly interfering with social and family relationships, academic performance, or occupational functioning

5. Symptoms cannot be better accounted for by another disorder

(American Psychiatric Association, 2000)

hypothesize that ADHD is an abnormality in dopamine activity in the brain.

ADHD is two to three times more common in males than in females, although the predominately inattentive type has fewer gender distinctions. Most parents first observe ADHD symptoms when their child is a toddler; however, occasionally, parents will report that even as an infant the child was restless and "squirmy," or a "difficult baby."

There are no laboratory tests or other physical findings that diagnose or suggest ADHD. Physical examinations should be completed to rule-out other causes of overactivity (e.g., thyroid disease) or mood lability (e.g., diabetes mellitus).

Administering structured assessments to parents, select teachers, and other involved adults is done to evaluate for the disorder. Direct observations are also helpful, but children with ADHD are frequently able to behave well or pay attention for short periods of time and during one-on-one appointments (such as in an office setting). Parent history is the best source of diagnostic information. Other psychiatric disorders, such as major depression or childhood-onset schizophrenia, may mimic the inattentive components of ADHD. Table 16-3 provides a comparison of some of the similarities and differences between ADHD and other psychiatric disorders seen in children.

TABLE 16-2: SYMPTOMS OF ATTENTION DEFICIT DISORDER IN ADULTS

Chronic lateness and forgetfulness

Anxiety

Low self-esteem

Employment problems

Difficulty controlling anger

Impulsiveness

Substance abuse or addiction

Poor organization skills

Procrastination

Low frustration tolerance

Chronic boredom

Difficulty concentrating when reading

Mood swings

Depression

Relationship problems

(WebMD, 2009b)

TREATMENT INTERVENTIONS FOR ADHD

There are three core categories of intervention in the treatment of ADHD. These are client education, behavior management, and medications. The following is a detailed discussion of each of these interventions.

Client Education

Educating the client, whether adult, child, or parents, becomes a priority when a diagnosis of ADHD is established; clients need to understand that ADHD is believed to be related to chemical and neurological alterations in the brain and not a result

TABLE 16-3: DIFFERENTIAL DIAGNOSIS OF ADHD AND OTHER PSYCHIATRIC DISORDERS

Disorder	Hyperactivity or Restlessness	Impulsivity	Decreased Attention Span or Poor Concentration	Decreased Sleep	Appetite Changes	Cognitive Impairments (hallucinations, delusions, disorganized thoughts)	Mood Changes (sadness, grouchiness, irritability, anxiety)	Physical Complaints (GI upset, headaches)
ADHD Combined	Yes	Yes	Yes	Yes	No	No	May occur	No
ADHD Inattentive	No	No	Yes	No	No	No	Not usually	No
ADHD Hyperactive-Impulsive	Yes	Yes	No	Yes	No	No	May occur	No
Major Depression	May occur	Not likely	Yes	Yes	Yes	May occur	Yes	May occur
Anxiety Disorders	Yes	Not likely	Yes	No	Yes	No	Yes	Yes
Childhood Schizophrenia	Not likely	May occur	Yes	No	No	Yes	No	Not likely

of poor parenting practices or a weak character. ADHD is a well-publicized disorder and clients may have preconceived ideas about the diagnosis, based on accurate and inaccurate media reports and the opinions of family members. Additionally, ADHD is a disorder of deficits and not one of non-compliance. That is to say that individuals with the disorder are not intentionally hyperactive or inattentive; rather, they are as much at a loss to understand why they behave in such ways as are others in their lives. Repeatedly punishing a child for impulsive behaviors succeeds only in frustrating both the child and the parent and may result in significant self-esteem problems in adulthood. Children with ADHD want to do well and to please their parents and teachers, but they are unable to force themselves to be asymptomatic (in many ways this is similar to asking an epileptic person to stop having seizures merely by force of will power). Clients also have a responsibility to learn as much as possible about the disorder in order to serve as advocates with school systems, employers and, occasionally, with various social service or government agencies. Support groups are an invaluable way for clients to receive ongoing education and interactions with others who may be having similar problems. Children and Adults with Attention Deficit Disorders is a support and advocacy program that also functions as a legislative watchdog for bills that may have a significant impact on the education of a child with ADHD or on americans with disabilities in the workplace. Their Web site (www.chadd.org) contains a wealth of information for parents and adults with ADHD.

Behavior Management

A second and equally important component of ADHD treatment in children is training parents in behavior management. Utilizing basic techniques of positive and negative reinforcers, negative consequences, and ignoring some behaviors, parents can motivate their children to function at a maximum level. Clients with ADHD often do not feel in con-

trol of themselves. Implementing behavior management techniques improves a sense of self-control that contributes to feeling proud of one's accomplishments and improved self-esteem. Parents should be assisted in identifying target behaviors that need modification, such as having tantrums, acting-up in the classroom, or refusing to do homework. Vague and ill-defined problems (e.g., "being bad" or "poor attitude") should be avoided. After problem behaviors are identified, the parent and child, together, determine positive reinforcers that will be awarded the child on a daily or weekly basis when the problem behaviors are avoided. Rewards have to be meaningful to the child; for example, monetary rewards may not be as intrinsically rewarding as special favors, such as a later bedtime or a trip to the ice cream parlor. Conversely, the parent and child need to have negative consequences for the continuance of the problematic behavior. Negative consequences should be clear, concise, and nonnegotiable; being "grounded" from television or videogames or having an early bedtime are good choices for the younger child, whereas suspending phone privileges or preventing visits with friends are more appropriate for the adolescent. Negative reinforcement refers to the removal of noxious stimuli when a problem behavior improves; for example, keeping the child under continuous supervision during homework is a negative reinforcer that is removed when the homework is completed or the child learns to work independently. Some behaviors also can be ignored. Behaviors that are essentially harmless (e.g., whining or nonphysical tantrums) may be inadvertently positively reinforced when a parent responds to the behavior. Ignoring the behavior prevents its reinforcement and it will eventually extinguish. Naturally, behaviors that could potentially be harmful to the client or others must be dealt with immediately.

Time-outs are an effective means of managing acting-out behaviors. The purpose of a time-out is to assist children in learning to calm themselves and it should not be perceived as a punishment. Timing is crucial – the time-out should begin immediately when acting-out occurs (not 4 hours later or "when your father gets home") and it should end when the child is calm and rational. During a time-out, the child should not receive any form of attention from the parents, including attempts to "make the child understand." Attention itself will serve as a positive reinforcer. As soon as the time-out is over, the parent should reconnect with the child through eye contact and praise the child for calming down; then the parent and child need to discuss the events that led up to the time-out and how they might be avoided in the future. For a young child this may be as simple as the statement, "Johnny, you're a good little boy and I love you very much. In this family we don't hit and call names." Older children can be asked to verbalize or write down the problem, why it occurred, and what could have been done differently. Personal time-outs are a useful tool to teach a child. The child, in recognition of increasing tension, initiates a personal time-out. The rules for a personal time-out are that the child may state "I need a break" and leave the situation without being pursued by the parent or sibling involved. When sufficiently calm, the child can return to the situation to discuss it more rationally. Clinicians vary in opinions on where a time-out should be taken. A chair in the busiest room of the house is never a good idea. Because a time-out is a chance to learn self-control and calm down, playing quietly with toys can be productive; therefore, sending a child to his bedroom is probably the best option. It also communicates a message to the child that undesirable behaviors will not be tolerated in the general family environment.

Environmental structure and predictability are also very important for children and adults with ADHD, perhaps because the client feels so out of control in general. Transitions (changing from one activity to another) are extremely difficult for those with ADHD. Families should make as much effort as possible to keep household routines consistent; getting up, eating meals, doing homework, allowing for play or relaxation time, and going to bed at the same time every day assists in this process. Parents can expect children with ADHD to have some worsening in behavior after weekends, extended vacations, or visitation with noncustodial parents. Children also act-out more at school when regular classroom teachers are gone and substitutes are in their place.

Educational Interventions

Although intellect is not usually a problem, children with ADHD often require individualized educational plans under the category of emotional handicap. Teachers and schools may need to make special accommodations for the child, including such things as extra study-hall time, in-class tutors, or physical rearrangements of the classroom (to reduce opportunities for distraction). Parents have to be active in the learning process and supervise homework assignments vigilantly. Frequently, homework scores and grades are used to determine the effectiveness of treatment interventions.

MEDICATION INTERVENTIONS FOR ADHD

Medications have been used for ADHD since the 1950s when methylphenidate (Ritalin®) was first introduced. It is important to explain to parents that medications do not cure ADHD; rather, they treat the symptoms of the disorder by altering neurotransmitters, primarily dopamine and to a lesser extent norepinephrine. The same medications are used regardless of the ADHD subtype. The FDA has approved two groups of medications for ADHD: stimulants and the norepinephrine reuptake inhibitor, atomoxetine (Strattera®); however, off-label medication usage includes alpha-adrenergics, some antidepressants, and the pro-histamine modafinil (Provigil®). An overview of ADHD medications is provided in Table 16-4.

TABLE 16-4: MEDICATIONS USED TO TREAT ATTENTION DEFICIT HYPERACTIVITY DISORDER (1 OF 2)

Category	Generic Name	Trade Name	Sedation	Weight Gain	Ortho-static blood pressure	Insomnia	GI Upset	Dry Mouth, Constipation	Comments
Stimulants	methyl-phenidate	Ritalin® Ritalin SR®	–	–	–	+++	+++	+	Short duration at 3-4 hr May induce tic disorder
	dexmethyl-phenidate	Focalin® Focalin XR®	–	–	–	++	++	+	More specific than Ritalin 12 hr duration for XR
	methyl-phenidate	Metadate ER® Metadate CD® Concerta® Daytrana®	– – –	– – –	– – –	++ +++ ++	++ ++ +	+ + +	Duration of 6-8 hr Duration of 12 hr Transdermal skin patch 16 hour activity Apply in a.m. Remove in p.m.
	dextroam-phetamine	Dexedrine®	–	–	–	++	++	+	Duration of 4-6 hr
	Combination of dextro-amphetamine sulfate and saccharate, and amphetamine sulfate and aspartate	Adderall® Adderall XR®	–	–	–	+++	++	+	Duration of 4-6 hr for immediate release, 10-12 hr for extended release Sprinkle tablets for children who can't swallow pills
	lisdexam-fetamine	Vyvanse®	–	–	–	++	+++	+	Bound with lysine. Activates in blood. 12 hr duration
Norepin-ephrine Reuptake Inhibitor	atomoxetine	Strattera®	+	+	+	+	++	+	Caution for suicidal thoughts Once-a-day dosing; takes 4 weeks to be fully effective

continued on next page

TABLE 16-4: MEDICATIONS USED TO TREAT ATTENTION DEFICIT HYPERACTIVITY DISORDER (2 OF 2)

Category	Generic Name	Trade Name	Sedation	Weight Gain	Ortho-static blood pressure	Insomnia	GI Upset	Dry Mouth, Constipation	Comments
Alpha-adrenergics	clonidine	Catapres® Catapres TTS®	+++	–	+++	–	–	–	Treats hyperactive & impulsive symptoms Very sedating, Good as a bedtime adjunct. Suppresses motor tics
	guanfacine	Tenex®	++	–	+++	–	–	–	Treats tics; good for impulsivity
Anti-depressants	bupropion	Wellbutrin® Wellbutrin SR®, XL®	–	–	–	+	–	–	Acts on dopamine system Better for adolescents or adults with ADHD; no abuse potential
	imipramine	Tofranil®	+++	++	++	–	–	+++	Primary use is enuresis. Cardiac conduction delays are possible
Pro-histamine	modafinil	Provigil®	–	–	–	–	–	+	Monitor for Stevens-Johnson rash and other allergic reactions
+++ High ++ Moderate + Low – Negligible									

Stimulants

Stimulants are highly treatment-effective for improving focus, concentration, attention span, and reducing distractibility and overactivity. They work by promoting the release of dopamine from the neurotransmitters in the brain, thus slowing or regulating chemical conduction at the neuron level. Dexamphetamine, mixed dexamphetamine salts, and lisdexamfetamine also boost the release of norepinephrine in the brain. Stimulants are all amphetamine-like agents. Some children tolerate one type of stimulant better than another. Young children may do better with shorter acting agents (Focalin®, Ritalin®, Adderall®), whereas older children and adolescents usually prefer long-acting medicines (Adderall XR®, Concerta®, Metadate CD®, Vyvanse®). One transdermal skin patch, Daytrana® is popular with younger children and some teens. It is applied early in the morning, and then is removed after suppertime. Children who are sensitive to tape adhesive may have local skin reactions to Daytrana®. Stimulant medications work within 15 to 20 minutes and are completely metabolized and eliminated by the body in the same day. They provide flexibility in dosing, with some parents choosing to utilize them only on school days. Side effects of stimulant medications, even at therapeutic doses, may include jitteriness, GI upset, decreased appetite, and insomnia. Weight loss can be significant in some children; weight should be checked at each follow-up appointment or at least every 3 months. Indications that the medication is dosed too high are cognitive dulling, a flattened affect, or agitation and mood lability. Overdosage can result in toxicity symptoms (hallucinations, tachycardia, and cardiac arrhythmias). Occasionally, children may develop motor tics at any dosage. Formerly, tic development was an indication to discontinue or change the medication. Today, clinicians are not as concerned about motor tics as they tend to resolve spontaneously by 10 to 12 years of age. Serum levels are not necessary when utilizing stimulant medications because dosages are based on clinical response and side effects.

Norepinephrine-reuptake inhibitor

Atomoxetine (Strattera®) was launched in 2003 to treat ADHD in a different way from stimulants. Originally studied as an antidepressant (but not approved for this use), Strattera® is a norepinephrine reuptake inhibitor. This means that it slows down the reuptake of norepinephrine by the post-synaptic neurons, allowing more norepinephrine to be available. It is highly effective in reducing hyperactive-impulsive symptoms and moderately effective in improving inattention symptoms. It may also be useful for modulating the moodiness and irritability experienced by some children. Strattera® is not immediately effective; it requires a titration over 4 to 5 days, and then it takes 2 to 4 weeks to achieve a steady state. Dosing is based on the weight of the child. Common side effects reported include GI upset (the product is mildly

corrosive to mucous membranes), activation, tachycardia (rarely) and, occasionally, drowsiness. It may be dosed once a day in the morning or at bedtime. The capsule should not be opened. Since its launch, there have been a few case reports of elevated liver enzymes and jaundice in children taking Strattera®. Pooled analyses of over 2200 children taking Strattera® have indicated an increase risk of suicidal thoughts (0.4%) over placebo; as a result, Strattera® now has a Black Box Warning (as do all antidepressants) to monitor for signs of suicidal thoughts or behaviors in children for whom it is prescribed.

Alpha-adrenergics

Alpha-adrenergics are medications that have an off-label use in treating the overactivity, hyper-arousal, and impulsivity associated with ADHD, combined and hyperactive-impulsive types. They do little to help with focus or concentration. Alpha-adrenergics are more commonly used as antihypertensives in adults. They appear to work by reducing norepinephrine levels, primarily in the frontal cortex of the brain. Two medications are prescribed: guanfacine (Tenex®) and clonidine (Catapres®, Catapres TTS® Transdermal). Side effects of these medications include drowsiness or sedation and dizziness. Doses should be titrated slowly and blood pressure checks should be done on follow-up appointments. Children rarely have blood pressure drops on the dosages used for ADHD. There are no long-acting forms of these medications. Dosing is usually required three to four times per day. Alpha-adrenergics may be prescribed in combination with stimulants. They are also effective in suppressing motor tic activity and are frequently used for that purpose.

Antidepressants

Antidepressants have some usefulness in ADHD treatment. Tricyclic antidepressants (TCAs), such as imipramine or desipramine, have been shown to be helpful, probably because of their potent norepinephrine effects. TCAs have to be used with caution, however, because of concerns about cardiac conduction delays. Serum monitoring and electrocardiograms are indicated. SSRIs do not demonstrate any significant positive effects on ADHD. They are useful, however, for children with concomitant depression or anxiety disorders. Buproprion (Wellbutrin SR® and XL®, Zyban®) has serotonin and dopamine activity and is moderately to highly effective in ADHD treatment. It is a good choice for adolescents, adults, or clients with substance-abuse problems. Side effects of antidepressant medications are generally low, with sedation and tremors prominent in TCAs and insomnia or GI upset with SSRIs.

The pro-histamine drug modafinil (Provigil®) that was discussed in Chapter 12 for fatigue associated with obstructive sleep apnea, narcolepsy, and shift-work sleep disorder was once researched for the treatment of ADHD. More effective than placebo, clinical approval was delayed because of the unexpected occurrence of a rash suspected to be Stevens-Johnson syndrome in the clinical trials. Modafinil appears to have very specific dopaminergic activity in the prefrontal cortex, but not as widespread as seen in stimulants. Modafinil interferes less with normal sleep patterns and does not seem to trigger neurological motor or vocal tics making it a helpful option for treating ADHD in combination with Tourette's or other Tic disorders. Armodafanil (Nuvigil®) was released in 2009 to provide a longer duration of effect, with the same benefits of modafinil.

OPPOSITIONAL DEFIANT DISORDER

Oppositional defiant disorder occurs in up to half of all children with ADHD. It is characterized by a recurrent pattern of negative, defiant and hostile behavior toward authority figures (and sometimes peers) to a degree that is not develop-

TABLE 16-5: CRITERIA FOR OPPOSITIONAL-DEFIANT DISORDER

1. A pattern of negative, hostile and defiant behavior lasting at least 6 months with four or more of the following:
 	
   a.   often loses temper;
 	
   b.   often argues with adults;
 	
   c.   often defies adults or refuses to comply with requests or rules;
 	
   d.   often deliberately annoys people;
 	
   e.   often blames others for his or her mistakes or poor behavior;
 	
   f.   often touchy or easily annoyed by others;
 	
   g.   often angry and resentful;
 	
   h.   often spiteful or vindictive.
 	
(American Psychiatric Association, 2000)

mentally appropriate. The *DSM-IV-TR* criteria for oppositional defiant disorder are presented in Table 16-5.

Like all psychiatric disorders, the symptoms must be at a level that is detrimental to the child and interferes with functioning (social or family relationships, academic achievement). The behaviors seen cannot be attributed to another psychiatric disorder, such as major depression or a psychotic disorder.

Children with oppositional defiant disorder are unpleasant to live with because they are frequently argumentative and defiant. Parents describe them as stubborn, resistant to redirection, inflexible, or argumentative. Testing limits is common, as is verbal aggression and a refusal to take responsibility for one's actions. It is important to note, however, that this disorder is also a disorder of deficit and the child may not be happy with his or her behaviors. Low self-esteem and depression can occur easily in children with an oppositional defiant disorder, and they always seem to be in conflict with others. Oppositional defiant disorder symptoms usually begin before 8 years of age, initially in the home setting. The symptoms will later generalize to other places such as school. Oppositional defiant disorder is more common in families with at least one member who has a history of major depression, and in families with significant conflict or marital discord.

Treatment for oppositional defiant disorder consists of individual and family therapy that focuses on the dynamics in the family and ways to structure the environment so that the child is not dominating all family interactions. Behavior modification techniques are also useful. Medications are not particularly helpful, although an underlying depressive disorder should be carefully considered and antidepressants may be of some benefit.

CONDUCT DISORDER

The main features of a conduct disorder are repetitive and persistent patterns of behavior, in which the rights of others or social rules are consistently violated. Diagnostic criteria for conduct disorder are provided in Table 16-6.

Conduct disorders are specified as mild, moderate, and severe, depending on the number of problems and degree of harm to others. Children or adolescents with this disorder often act aggressively toward others and they display little empathy or concern for the feelings of others. They may feel justified in their behaviors because they may perceive others as having hostile intentions (a paranoid disorder should be ruled out when diagnosing con-

TABLE 16-6: CRITERIA FOR CONDUCT DISORDER

1. A persistent pattern of behavior in which the rights of others, or major societal norms or rules, are violated. At least three of the following must be seen over the previous 12 months (with at least one in the past 6 months):

Aggression to people and animals

    a. bullies, threatens, or intimidates others

    b. initiates physical fights

    c. has used a weapon that can cause physical harm

    d. has been physically cruel to people

    e. has been physically cruel to animals

    f. has stolen while confronting a victim (e.g., mugging)

    g. has forced someone into sexual activity

Destruction of property

    h. has engaged in fire-setting with the intent of causing damage

    i. has deliberately destroyed other's property

Deceitfulness or theft

    j. has broken into someone else's house, building, or car

    k. often lies or "cons" others

    l. has stolen items of nontrivial value (e.g., shoplifting)

Serious violation of rules

    m. stays out at night regardless of parental curfew (before age 13)

    n. has run away from home overnight at least twice (or once if a lengthy period of time)

    o. often truant from school (beginning before age 13)

(American Psychiatric Association, 2000)

duct disorder). Feelings of guilt or remorse are often absent. Poor frustration tolerance, reckless-ness, irritability, and temper outbursts are associated features, as are promiscuity, gang activity, and drug use. Suicide ideation and attempts occur at a higher than average rate.

Children with conduct disorder are more likely to have parents with antisocial personalities and to be raised in homes that are harsh, abusive, or lack supervision. In certain environmental situations, some behaviors consistent with conduct disorder may be socially adaptive (inner-city high-crime areas, war-ravaged countries) and the diagnosis should only be made when the behavior is indica-tive of an underlying dysfunction within the client. Children with conduct disorder are at risk for developing other psychiatric disorders or of dis-playing adult criminal behaviors.

Treatment for conduct disorder almost invari-ably involves the court system. Court-ordered counseling may have some impact on future behav-iors. Psychiatric assessment should be done to rule-out any other mental health disorders that may be responsive to medication intervention. Children and adolescents with severe conduct disorders often have one or more residential placements in mental health or juvenile detention facilities.

CHRONIC MOTOR OR VOCAL TIC DISORDER

Motor tics are sudden, rapid, and recurrent motor movements that occur involuntarily several times a day, nearly every day, throughout a period of more than 1 year. Vocal tics are explosive vocaliza-tions, also involuntary, that occur nearly every day for more than a year. Motor and vocal tics typically have an onset prior to 18 years of age, and may not be caused by the direct effects of a medication, drug, or neurological disorder. Transient tics (motor or vocal tics lasting less than 1 year) occur in children at a rate as high as 18% (Bruun, Cohen, & Leekman, 2009).

Multiple motor and vocal tics lasting more than 1 year is known as Tourette's disorder.

TOURETTE'S DISORDER

In 1825, a French doctor named Itard described the case of a woman who developed motor and vocal tics starting at 7 years of age and lasting until her death as a recluse in her 90s. Dr. George Gilles de la Tourette described nine of his patients (includ-ing Dr. Itard's patient) who had uncontrollable motor or vocal outbursts, thus first treating the dis-order that now bears his name.

Tourette's disorder is a neuropsychiatric condi-tion that occurs in approximately 4 of every 10,000 children in the United States. It is higher in boys than in girls, and the onset is usually about 6 to 7 years of age, although it may onset as early as 2 years old or as late as adolescence. The disorder may be life long, or it may spontaneously remit. The severity, frequency, disruptiveness, and vari-ability of the tics can wax and wane over time, and the characteristics of the tics can change without warning. Common simple motor symptoms include eye blinking, facial scrunching, grimacing, neck jerking, head turning, tongue protrusion, or licking. Complex tics may involve stooping, walk-ing, twirling, or other multi-step activities. Vocal tics may be expressed as grunts, squeaks, squeals, sniffs, snorts, coughs, barks, throat clearing, or whole words or phrases. Coprolalia is a rare, com-plex vocal tic, involving the uttering of obscenities, that is present in fewer than 10% of individuals with Tourette's disorder (American Psychiatric Association, 2000). Chronic tic symptoms can be extremely embarrassing to the client and lead to fears of rejection or humiliation in social situations.

Tourette's disorder has been associated with a number of other psychiatric problems (Table 16-7); in particular, anxiety disorders (50%), ADHD (50% to 75%), and OCD (25%). Children with Tourette's disorder often present a complicated

TABLE 16-7: CO-OCCURRENCE OF TOURETTE'S DISORDER WITH OTHER PSYCHIATRIC DISORDERS

Disorder	% co-occurrence
Any psychiatric disorder	80%
Attention deficit hyperactivity disorder	50%-75%
Obsessive-compulsive disorder	25%
Other anxiety disorders	50%
Major depression	49%
Oppositional defiant disorder	58%
Bipolar disorder	14%
Speech and language disorder	24%
Enuresis	33%
(Coffey et al., 2000)	

clinical picture. The causes of Tourette's disorder are unclear. Genetic studies are underway, and some evidence of genome markers was first identified in 1999. The role of several neurotransmitters has also been implicated. Dopamine receptor hypersensitivity has been the primary hypothesis for tic disorder and Tourette's disorder (Coffey, 2002).

Therapy is not indicated for the specific treatment of tic disorders or Tourette's disorder; however, counseling is extremely useful for the comorbid conditions, especially when self-esteem problems and depression occur. Mild cases may benefit from education, support, and monitoring.

MEDICATION INTERVENTIONS FOR TIC DISORDERS

Pharmacotherapy is essential for tics that have a significant impact on functioning or that cause emotional distress. First line treatment recommendations are the alpha-adrenergic medications guanfacine (Tenex®) and clonidine (Catapres®); if either of these medications is ineffective or poorly tolerated, then new-generation antipsychotics are the most effective treatment, primarily risperidone (Risperdal®), aripiprazole (Abilify®), olanzapine (Zyprexa®), or ziprasidone (Geodon®). Older antipsychotics, such as haloperidol (Haldol®) and pimozide (Orap®), are highly effective but much greater in side effects. TCAs have been useful in tic disorders, combined with ADHD. SSRIs help with Tic disorders combined with depression or anxiety, but they have little direct action on the tics themselves. Anxiolytics such as clonazepam (Klonopin®) may be used for short-term treatment. The use of stimulants to treat comorbid conditions (such as ADHD) in a child with a tic disorder should be addressed with caution, as stimulants may precipitate worsening of vocal or motor tics.

ADVANCED PRACTICE NURSING: CHILDREN'S MEDICATION ALGORITHM PROJECT FOR ADHD

In 2006, the Children's Medication Algorithm Project (CMAP) recommendations for the medication treatment of non-complicated ADHD (ADHD without co-morbid conditions) were revised. After diagnostic assessment and family consultation, non-medication interventions are recommended, followed by the initiation of a stimulant medication, either in the methylphenidate or dexamphetamine family. In this author's experience, ADHD clients with more defiance and oppositional behaviors tend to respond well to dexamphetamine salts (Adderall, Adderall XR®) or lisdexamfetamine (Vyvanse®) although these products may also trigger more agitation because of their norepinephrine activity. Methylphenidate products (Concerta®, Focalin XR®) are highly effective for the classic ADHD symptoms, but have a lesser effect on some of the defiance and moodiness problems that may be seen. Side effects of the two groups are similar. The CMAP recommendation for unsuccessful stimulant treatment in stage 1 is to switch to a product from the alternate family; for example, if methylphenidate product is ineffective, change to dexamphetamine and vice versa. For partial or incomplete response, stage 3 treatment is to use atomoxetine (Strattera®), instead of the stimulant; stage 3A treatment is to add atomoxetine to the stimulant. Stage 4 treatment for a partial or non-responder is to add buproprion or a TCA to the stimulant. (Stage 5 is to change to the opposite product, buproprion or a TCF, with the stimulant). Lastly, the CMAP advises to add an alpha-agonist (guanfacine or clonidine) as a second or third agent. If there is still a poor response, clinical consultation is often advisable. The CMAP does not advise using modafinil or new-generation atypical antipsychotics at any point, but in clinical practice these are often used for very treatment-resistant children (and adults) with ADHD. Clients with co-morbidity present particular challenges because antidepressants can activate hyperactivity and stimulants can increase anxiety and motor tics. Clinical approaches for the medication treatment of comorbid conditions are provided in Table 16-8 to serve as a guide to the prescribing APRN; they are presented as First (1) option, Second (2) option, and Third (3) option.

CASE STUDY: DISRUPTIVE BEHAVIOR DISORDER

Isaac is a 7-year-old boy who was referred for an evaluation at the end of first grade for problems with hyperactivity and temper tantrums. His mother reports that he gets angry over something every day, sometimes several times a day, and starts screaming, throwing things, hitting, or kicking. He does not harm himself during these episodes. The examiner notes that Isaac is running up and down the halls while in

TABLE 16-8: MEDICATION APPROACHES TO COMORBID ADHD CONDITIONS	
ADHD & Obsessive-compulsive disorder	1) Atomoxetine; then 2) Stimulant plus SSRI
ADHD & Other anxiety disorders	1) Atomoxetine; then 2) Stimulant plus SSRI
ADHD & Tourette's disorder	1) Atomoxetine; then 2) Modafinil, then 3) Low dose stimulant plus any other, including Alpha-agonist
ADHD & Major depression	1) Stimulant plus SSRI
ADHD & Oppositional defiant disorder	1) Stimulant in dexamphetamine family; then 2) Stimulant plus SSRI
ADHD & Bipolar disorder	1) New generation atypical antipsychotic plus low dose stimulant; then 2) Antiepileptic plus low dose stimulant; then 3) Any combination of antipsychotic and antiepileptic, plus low dose stimulant
ADHD & Enuresis	1) Stimulant plus low dose TCA at night or DDAVP
ADHD & Insomnia	1) Short-acting stimulant plus antihistamine; then 2) Stimulant plus trazodone; then 3) Stimulant plus alpha-agonist clonidine at night; then 4) Stimulant plus melatonin, Rozerem®

the waiting room. In the office, he is talkative and loud but quite cheerful, and he is interested and curious about his surroundings. He plays with Legos® for a few minutes, trucks for a few minutes, and then scribbles a picture and announces he is ready to leave. He scatters the toys around the office without putting anything away. He also tries to play with the office computer and phone and open the desk drawers. He even grabs an apple off of the desk and starts to eat it. Isaac's mother reports that his grades are very poor and he will have to attend summer school to be advanced to second grade. His citizenship grades are also poor, with comments about out-of-seat behaviors, pushing or touching others, and frequently inter-rupting the teacher. During the session, the exam-iner also notices animal sounds (squeaking, grunting, and throat clearing) of which the child seems unaware. Every few minutes, Isaac rolls his head back and rapidly blinks, then scrunches up his nose and sniffs. The mother states he has been doing this since he was 4 years old. The medical history reveals a normal prenatal period with a full-term delivery weight of 9 lb, 11 oz. There are no allergies or current medications. He is sleeping fine at present. His language development has been nor-mal, but some mild phonological problems persist and he is receiving speech therapy at school. Toilet training has been problematic – he is dry all day but wets the bed nearly every night and his mother puts him in Pull-ups® to sleep. He is of average weight and height for his age. A social history reveals an intact family with both biological par-ents and five children. Isaac is the youngest of four boys and one girl (ages range from 7 to 17). His father is a full-time mechanical engineer and his mother works part-time in a daycare center. He is diagnosed with the following: ADHD, Tourette's disorder, phonological disorder, and enuresis. He is prescribed Abilify 2 mg every morning plus Concerta® 18 mg every morning.

Questions

1. What are the ADHD symptoms this child is exhibiting?

2. What are the Tourette's disorder symptoms this child is exhibiting?

3. What is the rationale for using aripiprazole (Abilify®) in this child?

Discussion

Hyperactivity, short attention-span, distractibility, talkativeness, loud play, and not working at his potential are all signs of ADHD. Sniffing, throat clearing, head rolling and blinking are combined vocal and motor tics that are required to make the diagnosis of Tourette's disorder. Abilify® is a med-ication that works by altering dopamine levels in the brain, which are thought to be associated with Tourette's disorder. Abilify® may also help to reduce the aggression and irritability exhibited by this child.

NURSING CARE PLAN: DISRUPTIVE BEHAVIOR DISORDER

Problem Listing

- Bed-wetting

- Hyperactivity

- Speech problems

- School failure

- Chaotic home life

- Low frustration tolerance

- Problems with social skills

- Risk of harm due to impulsivity

- Aggressive acting-out

- Short attention span

- Potential for low self-esteem

- Poor academic performance

Priority Nursing Diagnosis

Poor frustration tolerance and self-control related to inability to control self, as evidenced by daily tantrums and aggressive acting-out.

Long-term Goal

Client will demonstrate improved self-control and a reduction in tantrums.

Short-term Objectives

1. Client will stop hitting others.

2. Client's temper tantrums will be reduced from daily to 1 to 2 per month.

3. Parents will report better management and prevention of temper outbursts.

Nursing Interventions

1. Assist the parents in making a list of triggers that precipitate tantrums.

2. Discuss ways in which precipitants can be reduced or eliminated (e.g., not taking the child into the store if he usually has tantrums there).

3. Educate the parents as to effective use of time-outs.

4. Educate the client as to the use of personal time-outs.

5. Help the client learn to recognize signs of increasing tension and frustration.

6. Demonstrate and ask the parents to practice safe, therapeutic holds that may be necessary to prevent harm to others during tantrums.

7. Discuss the importance of providing support and reassurance to the client after a tantrum occurs, while discussing how things could have been handled differently.

8. Help the parents to identify ways to restructure the home environment in order to increase a sense of predictability and routines.

SUMMARY

Caring for a child, adolescent, or adult with a disruptive behavior disorder can be quite challenging. Because 40% to 60% of children with ADHD will likely have this neurobiological disorder well into adulthood, the impairments they experience will have an impact on their education and career decisions as adults. Adults with untreated or unrecognized ADHD have more difficulties with relationships, employment, legal problems, and substance abuse than do ADHD adults under good management or non-ADHD adults. Children with oppositional defiant disorder are difficult to live with on a daily basis, but there is a tendency for this disorder to dissipate after adolescence through normal growth and development. Conduct disorder is thought to be a precursor for the development of adult antisocial personality disorder (discussed in Chapter 13). The development of socially acceptable moral standards appears to be lacking. Children and adults with this problem are often charismatic and charming, but are self-centered and think only of their own needs, often at the expense of others. They have little remorse or guilt over their actions. Often, legal intervention is required to manage conduct disorder problems. Chronic motor and tic disorder (Tourette's disorder) is a neurobiological illness that is highly comorbid with other psychiatric problems. Along with motor and/or vocal tics, the client may demonstrate social relatedness problems (Asperger's syndrome, high-functioning autism), anxiety disorders, learning difficulties, ADHD, depressive disorders, or bipolar disorder. Working with clients who have Tourette's disorder can be difficult, but very rewarding.

EXAM QUESTIONS

CHAPTER 16
Questions 95-100

Note: Choose the one option that BEST answers each question.

95. A person with ADHD

    a. listens well but is noncompliant.

    b. completes assigned schoolwork with minimal supervision.

    c. has difficulty organizing or finishing assigned tasks.

    d. should be put into special education classes at school.

96. A feature that is not part of the diagnostic criteria for ADHD, but is a common finding is

    a. high self-esteem.

    b. positive peer interactions.

    c. low frustration tolerance.

    d. mood stability.

97. A child with oppositional defiant disorder will demonstrate a pattern of

    a. hyperactive and impulsive behaviors.

    b. negative, defiant, and hostile behaviors.

    c. disorganized and confused behaviors.

    d. criminal behaviors such as stealing.

98. ADHD management consists of the three core interventions of

    a. medications, school conferences, and physical exams.

    b. individual therapy, group therapy, and school conferences.

    c. family counseling and individualized educational plans.

    d. client education, behavior management training, and medications.

99. Side effects of stimulant medications may include

    a. a loss of appetite, insomnia, and tic development.

    b. an increased appetite along with improved sleep patterns.

    c. decreased concentration and attention span.

    d. pacing, tremors, and other signs of extrapyramidal syndrome.

100. Motor tics are described as

    a. hand tremors with intentional movement.

    b. sudden, rapid, and recurrent motor movements.

    c. tonic-clonic movements with poor muscle control.

    d. a sudden loss of muscle tone and weakness.

This concludes the final examination.

Please answer the evaluation questions found on page v of this workbook.

APPENDIX A

CULTURE-BOUND SYNDROMES

(Reprinted with permission from the *Diagnostic and Statistical Manual of Mental Disorders, Fourth Edition, Text Revision.* Copyright 2000. American Psychiatric Association.)

amok: "A dissociative episode characterized by a period of brooding followed by an outburst of violent, aggressive, or homicidal behavior directed at people and objects." The syndrome is described as primarily prevalent in males. Symptoms may include "persecutory ideas, automatism, amnesia, exhaustion, and a return to premorbid state."
Malaysia, Laos, Philippines, Polynesia (cafard or cathard), *Papua New Guinea, and Puerto Rico* (mal de pelea), *and among the Navajo* (iich'aa)

ataque de nervios: "Commonly reported symptoms include uncontrollable shouting, attacks of crying, trembling, heat in the chest rising into the head, and verbal or physical aggression. Dissociative experiences, seizurelike or fainting episodes, and suicidal gestures are prominent in some attacks but absent in other. A general feature...is a sense of being out of control." Attacks frequently occur in response to a stressful event.
Latinos for the Caribbean, Latin Americans, Latin Mediterraneans

bilis and **colera** (also called **muina**): "Symptoms can include acute nervous tension, headache, trembling, screaming, stomach disturbances, and, in more severe cases, loss of consciousness. Chronic fatigue may result from the acute episode. The underlying cause...is thought to be strongly experienced anger or rage. The major effect is to disturb core body balances."
Latino populations

boufee delirante: "A sudden outburst of agitated and aggressive behavior, marked confusion, and psychomotor excitement...sometimes accompanied by visual and auditory hallucinations or paranoid ideation."
West Africa, Haiti

brain fag: "A condition experienced by high school or university students in response to the challenges of schooling...somatic symptoms are usually centered around the head and neck and include pain, pressure or tightness, blurring of vision, heat, or burning."
West Africa

dhat: "Severe anxiety and hypochondriacal concerns associated with the discharge of semen, whitish discoloration of the urine, and feelings of weakness and exhaustion."
India, Similar to **jiryan** *(India),* **sukra prameha** *(Sri Lanka),* and **shen-k'uei** *(China)*

falling-out or **blacking-out:** "sudden collapse, which sometimes occurs without warning but sometimes is preceded by feelings of dizziness or "swimming" in the head...eyes are usually open but the person claims an inability to see. The person usually hears and understands what is occurring around him or her but feels powerless to move."
Southern United States, Caribbean groups

ghost sickness: "A preoccupation with death and the deceased...symptoms can be attributed to ghost sickness, including bad dreams, weakness, feelings of danger, loss of appetite, fainting, dizziness, fear, anxiety, hallucinations, loss of consciousness, confusion, feelings of futility, and a sense of suffocation."
American Indian Tribes

hwa-byung (wool-hwa-byung): "Anger syndrome" "Symptoms include insomnia, fatigue, panic, fear of impending death, dysphoric affect, indigestion, anorexia, dyspnea, palpitations, generalized aches and pains, and a feeling of a mass in the epigastrium."
Korea

koro: "An episode of sudden and intense anxiety that the penis (or, in females, the vulva and nipples) will recede into the body and possibly cause death" "Koro at times occurs in localized epidemic form in east Asian areas."
Malaysian origin, South and East Asia: Chinese **(shuk yang, shook yong, suo yang);** *Assam* **(jinjinia bemar);** *Thailand* **(rok-joo)**

latah: "Hypersensitivity to sudden fright, often with echopraxia, echolalia, command obedience, and dissociative or trancelike behavior. More frequent in middle-aged women."
Malaysian or Indonesian origin, Siberian groups **(amurakh, irkunii, ikota, olan,myriachit,** *and* **menkeiti);** *Thailand* **(bah tschi, bah-tsi, baah-ji)**; *Ainu, Sakhalin, Japan* **(imu)**; *Philippines* **(mali-mali, silok).**

locura: "A severe form of chronic psychosis… symptoms exhibited by persons with locura include incoherence, agitation, auditory and visual hallucinations, inability to follow rules of social interaction, unpredictability, and possible violence."
Term used by Latinos in the United States, Latin America

mal de ojo: "A Spanish phrase translated into English as "evil eye." Children are especially at risk. Symptoms include fitful sleep, crying without apparent cause, diarrhea, vomiting, and fever in a child or infant. Sometimes seen in adults (especially females).
Mediterranean cultures and throughout the world

nervios: "Both a general state of vulnerability to stressful life experiences and to a syndrome brought on by difficult life circumstances. Common symptoms include headaches and "brain aches," irritability, stomach disturbances, sleep difficulties, nervousness, easy tearfulness, inability to concentrate, trembling, tingling sensations, and **mareos** (dizziness with occasional vertigo-like exacerbations)."
Common idiom of distress in Latin America and Latinos in the United States, Greeks in North America **(nevra)**

pibloktoq: "An abrupt dissociative episode accompanied by extreme excitement of up to 30 minutes' duration and frequently followed by convulsive seizures and coma lasting up to 12 hours." "During the attack the individual may tear off his or her clothing, break furniture, shout obscenities, eat feces, flee from protective shelters, or perform other irrational or dangerous acts."
Arctic and Subarctic Eskimo communities

qi-gong psychotic reaction: "An acute, time-limited episode characterized by dissociative, paranoid, or other psychotic or nonpsychotic symptoms that may occur after participation in the Chinese folk health-enhancing practice of qi-gong."
Chinese

rootwork: "a set of cultural interpretations that ascribe illness to hexing, witchcraft, sorcery, or the evil influence of another person. Symptoms may included generalized anxiety and gastrointestinal complaints (e.g., nausea, vomiting, diarrhea), weakness, dizziness, the fear of being poisoned, and sometimes fear of being killed (voodoo death)."
Southern United States in both African American and European American populations, Caribbean or Latino societies **(mal puesto, brujeria)**

running syndromes: "Conditions characterized by a sudden onset of a high level of activity, a trancelike state, potentially dangerous behavior in the form of running or fleeing, and ensuing exhaustion, sleep, and amnesia for the episode."
Native Peoples of the Arctic **(pibloktoq)**, *Miskito of Honduras and Nicaragua* **(grisi siknis)**, *Navajo "frenzy" witchcraft, Western pacific Cultures* **(amok)**

sangue dormido: "sleeping blood" "Pain, numbness, tremor, paralysis, convulsions, stroke, blindness, heart attack, infection, and miscarriage."
Portuguese Cape Verde Islanders and their immigrants

Shenjing shuairuo: "A condition characterized by physical and mental fatigue, dizziness, headaches, other pains, concentration difficulties, sleep disturbance, and memory loss. Other symptoms include gastrointestinal problems, sexual dysfunctions, irritability, excitability, and various signs suggesting disturbance of the autonomic nervous system."
Chinese

shen-k'uei, shenkui: "A label describing marked anxiety or panic symptoms with accompanying somatic complaints for which no physical cause can be demonstrated. Symptoms include dizziness, backache, fatigability, general weakness, insomnia, frequent dreams and complaints of sexual dysfunction. Symptoms are attributed to excessive semen loss."
Taiwan, China

shin-byung: "Anxiety and somatic complaints (general weakness, dizziness, fear, anorexia, insomnia, gastrointestinal problems), with subsequent dissociation and possession by ancestral spirits."
Korean

spell: "A trance state in which individuals "communicate" with deceased relative or with spirits. At times....associated with brief periods of personality change."
African Americans, European Americans

susto "fright" or "soul loss", a.k.a. **espanto, pasmo, tripa ida, perdida del alma, chibih:** "an illness attributed to a frightening event that causes the soul to leave the body and results in unhappiness and sickness. Symptoms may appear any time from days to years after the fright is experienced. It is believed that in extreme cases, susto may result in death. Typical symptoms include appetite disturbances, inadequate or excessive sleep, troubled sleep or dreams, feeling of sadness, lack of motivation to do anything, and feelings of low self-worth or dirtiness. Somatic symptoms include muscle aches and pains, headache, stomachache, and diarrhea. Ritual healings are focused on calling the soul back to the body and cleansing the person to restore bodily and spiritual balance."
Latinos in the United States, Mexico, Central America, South America

taijin kyofusho: "This syndrome refers to an individual's intense fear that his or her body, its parts or its functions, displease, embarrass, or are offensive to other people in appearance, odor, facial expressions, or movements."
Japan

zar: "A term applied to the experience of spirits possessing an individual. Persons possessed by a spirit may experience dissociative episodes that may include shouting, laughing, hitting the head against a wall, singing, or weeping. Individuals may show apathy and withdrawal, refusing to eat or carry out daily tasks, or may develop a long-term relationship with the possessing spirit. Such behavior is not considered pathological locally."
Ethiopia, Somalia, Egypt, Sudan, Iran, other North African and Middle Eastern societies

APPENDIX B

NURSING ASSESSMENT AND DATA BASE (ADULT)

NURSING ASSESSMENT AND DATA BASE
ADULT

Client's Name: _____ Date: _____ MRN #: _____

Legal Status: ( ) Voluntary ( ) Involuntary: ( ) 24 hr immediate detention: Begins: _____
                                                         Ends: _____
                               ( ) 72 hr emergency detention: Begins: _____
                                                          Ends: _____
                               ( ) Temporary or Regular Commitment

Date of Birth: _____

Reason for Admission:

Previous Psychiatric Treatment:
Where?   When?

Medical Assessment:

BP: _____ HR: _____ RR: _____ Temp: _____ Ht: _____ Wt: _____

Allergies:

Medical History:

Integumentary:
Musculoskeletal:
Cardiac:
Respiratory: Cigarettes? _____ How many? _____
Gastric:
Urological:
Neurological:
Other:

Surgery History:

Alcohol or Drug Use:
What?   Last Used?

Current signs of alcohol/drug withdrawal?

263

NURSING ASSESSMENT AND DATA BASE (pg.2)
ADULT

Client's Name: _____ Date: _____ MRN #: _____

Review of Systems:

Sleep problems?

Nutritional concerns?

Acute or chronic pain?

Medication side effects?

Reproductive issues?

Other physical health issues:

Psychosocial History:

With whom does client live? _____

Identified significant other: _____ Phone: _____
       Release of Info signed? ( ) Yes ( ) No: reason _____

Children? ( ) Live with client: Ages? _____
       ( ) Live elsewhere: With whom? _____

Employment status: ( ) Employed: Where? _____
             ( ) Unemployed: Chief source of income_____
             ( ) Disabled: Type of disability _____
School status: ( ) High school, GED or higher education
             ( ) Less than high school education: Learning disabilities? _____
             ( ) Currently in school: Where? _____

Health Care Insurance coverage? Type: _____
       Does this policy cover prescription medications? ( ) Yes ( ) No ( ) Don't know

Support Systems:

Who does client identify as chief source of support? _____
Religious affiliation? ( ) Yes   Type: _____
          ( ) No

Mental Status Assessment:

Overall Appearance:

Behavior:

Mood and Affect:

NURSING ASSESSMENT AND DATA BASE (pg.3)
ADULT

Client's Name: _____Date: _____ MRN #: _____

Thought Processes and Organization:

Thought Contents:

    Primary focus of thoughts:

    Any hallucinations or delusions?

    Any suicidal thoughts/urges?

        Plan:

    Any homicidal thoughts/urges?

        Directed toward:

        Duty to warn? ( ) No ( ) Yes Whom:_____

    Memory impairments:

    Concentration problems:

Insight into illness:

Judgment:

Strengths: (Attributes that will assist client in recovery.)

Problem Listing: (Identify problems the client is experiencing.)

_____   _____

Nurse's Signature   Date

RESOURCES

American Academy of Child and Adolescent
Psychiatry
http://www.aacap.org

American Academy of Family Physicians
http://www.aafp.org

American Institute on Domestic Violence
http://www.aidv-usa.com

American Nurses Association
http://www.nursingworld.org

American Nurses Credentialing Center
http://www.nursingworld.org/ancc

American Psychiatric Nurses Association
http://www.apna.org

American Psychological Association
http://www.apa.org

American Red Cross
http://www.redcross.org

Autism Collaboration
http://www.autism.org

Centers for Disease Control and Prevention
http://www.cdc.gov

Children and Adults with Attention-
Deficit/Hyperactivity Disorder (CHADD)
http://www.chadd.org

Domestic Abuse Intervention Programs
http://www.theduluthmodel.org

EMDR Institute, Inc.
http://www.emdr.com/efficacy.htm

Federal Emergency Management Agency (FEMA)
http://www.fema.gov

Focused Treatment Systems (FTS): Alcohol
Withdrawal Treatment Manual
http://www.sagetalk.com

International Society of Psychiatric-Mental
Health Nurses
http://www.ispn-psych.org

MayoClinic.com
http://www.mayoclinic.com

Motivational Interviewing
http://www.motivationalinterview.org

National Alliance on Mental Illness (NAMI)
http://www.nami.org

National Council on Alcoholism and Drug
Dependence, Inc.
http://www.ncadd.org

National Institutes of Health (NIH)
http://www.nih.gov

National Institute of Mental Health (NIMH)
http://www.nimh.nih.gov

National Institute on Alcohol Abuse and Alcoholism
http://www.niaaa.nih.gov

National Institute on Drug Abuse
http://www.drugabuse.gov

National Tourette Syndrome Association
http://www.tsa-usa.org/Medical/guideto
diagnosis.html

National Women's Health Information Center
http://www.womenshealth.gov

Psychiatric/Mental Health Nursing Practice
http://www.apna.org/i4a/pages/index.cfm?
pageid=3343

Santa Clara University: Markula Center for
Applied Ethics
http://www.scu.edu/ethics

Substance Abuse and Mental Health Services
Administration (SAMHSA): Mental Health: A
Report of the Surgeon General
http://mentalhealth.samhsa.gov/cmhs/
surgeongeneral

Substance Abuse and Mental Health Services
Administration (SAMHSA): Mental Health
Information Center
http://mentalhealth.samhsa.gov

Substance Abuse and Mental Health Services
Administration (SAMHSA), Office of
Applied Studies
http://www.oas.samhsa.gov

Texas Department of State Health Services: Mental
Health Programs and Initiatives
http://www.dshs.state.tx.us/mhprograms

U.S. Census Bureau
http://www.census.gov

U.S. Drug Enforcement Administration
http://www.usdoj.gov/dea/index.htm

World Health Organization
http://www.who.int/en

GLOSSARY

accommodation: Used by Piaget, refers to learning new information based on previous experiences. For example, a child learns that dogs are animals then he accommodates to include cats, horses, and cows as also being animals.

acting-out: A term used in mental health care to describe any aggressive or self-injurious behavior committed by another, usually in response to increasing levels of anxiety or tension, but may also be a result of hallucinations or delusions.

affective flattening: Used to describe emotions, refers to a blunting of emotional expression often seen in the disorder of schizophrenia.

agnosia: Inability to recognize familiar objects, usually as a result of brain injury or dementia.

agoraphobia: Pathological fear of being in public places. Can vary in intensity from mild (unable to be in large crowds) to extreme (unwilling to leave the house).

agranulocytosis: Serious and sometimes fatal illness characterized by a significant reduction in white blood cells. Can be caused by illnesses or medications.

alogia (poverty-of-speech): Paucity of speech content that reflects a lack of abstraction in thoughts. Clients with this problem often respond minimally to questions and are unable to elaborate or provide details or embellishments.

amenorrhea: Absence of menstrual cycles. May be associated with normal changes related to menopause or may be induced by disorders, such as anorexia nervosa or medications.

amnesia: Defect in memory; an inability to recall parts or wholes of certain events or situations.

anorexia: Loss of appetite. May refer to self-restricting behaviors (anorexia nervosa) or may be caused by medical conditions (cancer treatment) or psychiatric disorders (depression).

anticholinergic: Refers to a medication action; anticholinergic drugs block nerve transmission through parasympathetic pathways resulting in reduced activity of the gastrointestinal and urinary tract and reduced secretions, such as saliva or tears.

aphasia: Partial or total loss of the ability to speak, usually as a result of brain injury.

apraxia: Impaired ability to carry out purposeful movements, usually as a result of brain injury.

assimilation: Term used by Piaget to indicate how children learn; refers to learning new information by comparing it to previously learned data. For example, a child learns that a fly is an insect, and then assimilates to include ants, beetles, and wasps as insects as well.

ataxia: Staggering gait or unsteadiness. Commonly seen in acute alcohol, sedative, or opioid intoxication. Also seen in other toxic reactions (heavy metal poisoning and lithium toxicity).

avolition: Inability to initiate actions seen in individuals with neurological disorders (e.g., Parkinson's disease) or in schizophrenia. A tendency to have little motivation or activity level.

battered woman syndrome: Phenomenon of emotional exhaustion experienced by women who are in a domestic violence situation from which they feel they are unable to escape. Depression, hopelessness, helplessness, and suicidal thoughts may occur. Depersonalization experiences are common. Victim may become delusional or homicidal.

beneficience: Act of being kind or doing good.

blood dyscrasias: Any abnormal condition of the blood.

bradykinesia: Abnormal slowing of motor movements as seen in disorders such as Parkinson's disease. Related to medical disorders, severe psychiatric disturbances, or older antipsychotic medications.

catalepsy (waxy flexibility): State of prolonged rigid posture usually encountered in catatonic schizophrenia. Others can move the extremities and the client will hold them statue-like until they are moved again.

cataplexy (sleep paralysis): Sudden and complete state of paralysis brought on by shock or experienced during the phase of sleep encountered immediately prior to waking. Associated with rapid eye movement sleep stages.

catatonia: State of stupor and muscular rigidity encountered in the catatonic subtype of schizophrenia. The client does not move for long periods of time.

choreiform movements: Writhing, wormlike movements, usually of the upper extremities or neck, that are associated with tardive dyskinesia, but may also be caused by neurological disorders.

circumstantial thoughts: Thought patterns, reflected by speech, that do not get directly to the point but rather talk around the main topic for a period of time before eventually returning to finish the sentence or main idea.

cognitive: General term that refers to mental acts, such as reasoning, perception, intuition, and knowledge.

cognitive behavior therapy: Therapy model that teaches individuals to examine their preconceived ideas about events or situations, then examine how those ideas influence perceptions and interpretations, emotional responses and behaviors. The ultimate goal is to relearn how to interpret life events.

compulsions: Irrational urge to perform an action repeatedly, often without a logical reason to do so. It is often associated with obsessive thoughts.

concomitant: Occurring at the same time, or in conjunction with.

coprolalia: Rare form of vocal tic that is characterized by the expression, usually explosively, of socially unacceptable words or phrases such as curse words.

cross-tolerance: Phenomenon that is seen in substance-dependent clients, in which addictions to one substance can induce very high tolerance levels for similar substances. Most likely is related to elevated liver enzymes.

culture-bound syndromes: Psychologically driven behaviors or patterns of behavior that vary between cultures. May be representative of distinct disorders, but most likely they are a result of learned responses and differences in defining a psychiatric disturbance.

decompensate: Term used when a client with a psychiatric disorder is becoming symptomatic again after a period of relative stability.

defense mechanisms: Coping strategies utilized by clients in times of stress. First categorized and labeled by Sigmund Freud to explain behavioral reactions based on unconscious drives.

delirium tremens: Usually refers to alcohol withdrawal that is accompanied by vivid hallucinations, anxiety, and tremors. Commonly referred to as "D.T.'s," delirium tremens often precede seizures.

delusions: Abnormal and false beliefs associated with a brain-based disorder. Can be expressed in a variety of ways (physical beliefs and paranoid beliefs) but all are real to the person experiencing them.

disinhibition: Loss of inhibitions usually caused by the effects of a substance (e.g., alcohol, drugs). Can also be associated with a brain injury or a disorder such as dementia. Disinhibited individuals will behave in ways in which they would normally be too embarrassed or reserved to do.

duty-to-warn: Legal term resulting from the 1976 case of Tarakoff v. The Regents of the University of California, in which the University was found negligent for not directly warning Ms. Tarakoff that her life had been threatened (thus denying her the opportunity to protect herself) when they had information revealed in a therapy session that she was going to be murdered. Mental health practitioners now have an individual duty to warn others when a threat has been made, even without the consent of the client.

dysmenorrhea: Irregular or abnormal menstrual cycles that are caused by medical illness or medication side effects.

dysphasia: Disorder of language that is caused by a learning disability or a brain lesion. May affect either expressive or receptive/expressive abilities to communicate.

dysphagia: Disorder of swallowing that may have medical or psychological causes.

dysphoria: Feeling of being ill at ease; commonly used in the mental health field to refer to an individual who looks sad or depressed.

dystonia: Neurological disorder that causes skeletal muscles to go into a spasm and contract. Psychiatrically, it is usually associated with the side effects of traditional antipsychotic medications. Dystonic reactions frequently involve the head, neck, trunk, or ocular muscles.

echolalia: Tendency to repeat words spoken by another. Usually seen in mental retardation or other developmental delays, brain injuries, and schizophrenia.

echopraxia: Involuntary repetition of the actions of others. Usually seen in mental retardation or other developmental delays, brain injuries, and schizophrenia.

encephalopathy: General term that refers to any degenerative disease of the brain. Is often associated with chronic exposure to toxins, including alcohol.

encopresis: Voluntary or involuntary passing of feces after 4 years of age in socially unacceptable places or at inappropriate times.

enuresis: Voluntary or involuntary passing of urine after 5 years of age in socially unacceptable places or at inappropriate times.

enzymes: Biological proteins that act as catalysts to trigger or accelerate chemical reactions.

erotomania: Abnormally strong sexual desire or an obsession with another person that is accompanied by an unfounded belief that the other person returns those affections.

escalate: Term used in mental health care to indicate an increasing level of tension and anxiety by the client. Can be a precursor to acting-out.

euphoria: Feeling of exaggerated happiness or well-being often accompanied by increased activity. May be induced by drugs or associated with the mania phase of a bipolar disorder.

executive functioning: Term that refers to the brain's ability to dictate or rule or organize the person's thoughts and behaviors. May be impaired from illnesses, injuries, or drugs.

extrapyramidal syndrome: Side effects of antipsychotic medications related to low dopamine levels in the extrapyramidal tract of the brain that is characterized by tremors, shuffling gait, stiff muscles, and a masklike facial expression.

failure to protect: Legal term used when a parent has knowledge that a dependent (child or adult) is endangered, but fails to act on the knowledge and allows the dependent to come to harm. Often used in child abuse and neglect cases.

fight-or-flight: Primitive physiological response to a perceived threat to the self that is characterized by increased adrenalin (epinephrine) levels, increased corticosteroids, a release of endogenous opiates, and other changes that prepare the organism to fight for protection or to run away.

flashbacks: Sudden reoccurrence of a memory or an experience that is unwanted by the individual; may be triggered by an event or situation similar to the original experience. Flashbacks occur in individuals with posttraumatic stress disorder, acute stress disorder, or following ingestion of a hallucinogenic agent.

flight-of-ideas: Description of thought processes that are unable to stay focused or on topic; one idea will cause the client to think of another idea and so forth until the individual loses track of the original thread of the conversation.

flooding: Experience in which clients are suddenly exposed to an extreme anxiety provoking phenomenon from which they are unable to flee. May be part of a therapy plan in treating specific phobias or obsessive compulsive disorder.

folie á deux: Also called a shared delusional disorder, refers to the adoption of the false beliefs of another, usually based on a close relationship or proximity.

galactorrhea: Abnormal and excessive expression of breast milk. Galactorrhea is seen in nonpregnant clients in the psychiatric setting as a result of medications that elevate serum prolactin levels (traditional antipsychotics and risperidone).

general adaptation syndrome: Term coined by Hans Selye to describe the stages of adaptation to stress experienced by the human organism. Incorporates elements of alarm, resistance, and exhaustion. Alarm is associated with fight-or-flight responses; resistance is associated with chronic anxiety and somatoform disorders; and exhaustion is associated with depression, dissociative disorders, and posttraumatic stress.

grandiosity: Feeling that one has special abilities or traits that elevates one above the common man. May include a sense of entitlement or be demonstrated as arrogance.

grimacing: Scrunching up of the face, as seen with pain. In the psychiatric setting this is usually recognized either as a symptom of schizophrenia or as an indication of tardive dyskinesia associated with traditional antipsychotic medications.

guarded: Refers to a client who presents as evasive or paranoid and is unwilling to share any personal information.

guided imagery: Form of relaxation therapy in which a client is taught to imagine a calm, serene place and pretend that he or she is there.

habituation: Development of a tolerance for a substance that indicates the beginnings of a physiological addiction; a need for increasing amounts of the substance to accomplish the same effects.

hallucinations: Experience of false sensory perceptions: visual, auditory, olfactory, tactile, or gustatory.

holistic: Used in nursing and healthcare to mean the whole person: physical, emotional, and spiritual.

hypervigilance: Position of heightened alertness or awareness that is often accompanied by an exaggerated startle response and frequently seen in posttraumatic stress disorder or in paranoid delusions.

hypomania: State of elevated moods and activity that represent a change from the baseline of the individual and that may be accompanied by impulsive behaviors or a decreased need for sleep. Does not require hospitalization and psychosis may not be present.

ideas of reference: Type of delusion in which clients believe that mundane or irrelevant experiences in the world have a personal connection to them; such as the belief that the news reporter is secretly trying to send you a personal message regarding an impending terrorist attack. Also includes beliefs of telepathic abilities or thought insertion by others.

incest: Sexual abuse of a minor perpetrated by a family member.

insight: Act of developing awareness into the self that includes understanding one's own motivations, drives, impulses, and urges.

intellectual quotient: Standardized test that is usually referred to as IQ, which measures the intellectual capability of a client and is used for educational planning. IQ tests have some cultural bias for non-English speaking persons.

intrusive thoughts: Experience of having unwanted thoughts come into the mind repeatedly and that usually requires an inordinate amount of effort to overcome.

lacrimation: Fluid running from the tear ducts as seen in weeping, but without the emotional context of sadness.

lanugo: Fine, usually blond hair found on the bodies and faces of newborn babies that is lost within a few days to weeks. Lanugo can occur in clients with severe anorexia nervosa.

maladaptive: Coping mechanisms or behaviors employed by the client that do not help the client to cope adequately and may be very detrimental. Examples include excess alcohol consumption, risk-taking behaviors, and self-mutilation.

maleficience: Act of wrongdoing or causing harm to another.

mania: Presence of an abnormally elevated, expansive, or irritable mood that is a clear change from baseline and that causes impairment in social relationships or occupational or educational functioning. Clients with mania may sleep little and they may have psychotic symptoms or require hospitalization.

melatonin: Naturally occurring hormone that is produced by the body in response to daylight. Melatonin levels have an association to mood problems seen in seasonal affective disorder and to jet lag.

mutism: Inability or refusal to speak in the absence of damage to the vocal cords or the brain. May be seen in children or adults who have been severely traumatized.

myopathy: Degenerative condition of the skeletal muscles causing problems with strength and stability. Can be related to neurological disorders, toxins, or infections.

negativism: Persistent and pronounced pessimistic outlook on life that is characterized by chronic disgruntlement.

neologisms: Phenomenon seen in schizophrenia and other brain-based disorders in which an individual makes up words that are not in the standard dictionary.

neuroleptic malignant syndrome: Life-threatening syndrome in which muscle tissue breaks down at an alarming rate and is accompanied by hyperthermia and elevated blood pressure and heart rates. Causes of this syndrome are unknown, but it is thought to be associated with traditional antipsychotic mediations. Rates are higher in older adult women with other medical problems and in clients taking both an antipsychotic and lithium.

neurons: Part of the physical makeup of the gray matter of the brain, a neuron is composed of a cell body with a large nucleus. Neurons transmit waves of electrical potential by using chemical elements called neurotransmitters.

neuropsychiatric: Term used to describe a disorder that has psychiatric or psychological expressions, but is associated with physical or neurological alterations.

neurosis: First used by Freud, a neurosis is a psychological disorder that does not alter the individual's perception of reality; primarily used for personality disorders and some anxiety disorders.

neurotransmitter: Chemical messengers that move from one neuron to another and carry electrical action potential. The neurotransmitters most important in psychiatry are serotonin, dopamine, norepinephrine, acetylcholine, and gamma-amino-butyric acid.

obsession: Recurrent, unwanted thought that the individual can usually recognize as illogical or irrational (unless it occurs in children, then there is less insight), but is unable to resist or prevent from occurring.

orientation: Used in nursing and healthcare to refer to an awareness of one's identity, surroundings, location, and time. Disorientation is seen in delirium and dementia disorders and in acute substance intoxication.

PANDAS: Acronym that stands for pediatric autoimmune neuropsychiatric disorders associated with Streptococcal infection. PANDAS are usually sudden onset obsessive-compulsive or tic disorders that occur following a positive strep throat culture.

paradoxical reaction: Unexpected reaction to a medication that is opposite of the intended reaction. Often seen in children (e.g., an antihistamine causes agitation and hypomania), but benzodiazepines can cause paradoxical reactions in adult clients as well.

paranoia: Delusion that is characterized by an irrational belief that one is endangered, being followed, or being watched by others or by governmental agencies.

pharmacodynamics: Refers to what a drug is designed to do or the action of drugs on the physiology of the body (e.g., certain antidepressants block the reuptake of serotonin in the neurons).

pharmacokinetics: How a drug moves through the body. It involves absorption and distribution, metabolism, and excretion.

pica: Abnormal desire or compulsion to consume non-nutritive material (chalk, dirt, paint, or hair). May be associated with nutritional deficiencies, especially in pregnancy, or may have no known cause. More common in individuals with mental retardation or developmental delays.

piloerection: Commonly known as "goosebumps," an autonomic response to cold or fear that causes small muscles in the skin to contract and pull the hair upright. Also seen in opioid withdrawal.

polygenic polydipsia: Compulsive urge to drink fluids, particularly water, to a degree that overwhelms the body's ability to eliminate excess fluid via the kidneys, resulting in dangerously low sodium and potassium levels through a dilutional effect. Thought to be related to the activities of certain medications on the thirst-control mechanisms in the brain, polydipsia can constitute a medical emergency.

poverty-of-speech (alogia): Paucity of speech content that reflects a lack of abstraction in thoughts. Clients with this problem often respond minimally to questions and are unable to elaborate or provide details or embellishments.

poverty-of-thoughts: Inability to think abstractly or to embellish or add details to thoughts.

priapism: Painful, unremitting erection associated with the medication trazodone. Although rare, it can constitute a medical emergency.

prions: Protein in the brain, the abnormal form of which is thought to be responsible for viral infections such as Creutzfeldt-Jakob syndrome (mad cow disease).

pseudodementia: Phenomenon in which an individual with major depression presents with memory deficits similar to those seen in a dementia disorder. It is characterized by a fairly rapid onset and an erratic and fluctuating course.

pseudoparkinsonism: Symptoms of Parkinson's disease that are caused by some medications, in particular antipsychotics, which have a nonspecific dopamine-blocking effect in the brain. The symptoms are reversed when the medication is withdrawn. Includes tremors, shuffling gait, stiff muscles, and a masklike facial expression.

psychoanalysis: Type of therapy first implemented by Freud and based on the premise that unconscious sexual tensions drive behaviors and that change is accomplished by uncovering early childhood experiences.

psychomotor retardation: Severely slowed movements of the body that are accompanied by slowed or abnormal mental processes.

psychosis: General term used in psychiatry to indicate a client who is suffering from hallucinations, delusions, or gross disorganization of thought processes. Psychosis is a descriptor and not a diagnosis.

relaxation training: Type of therapy commonly practiced by nurses that involves teaching the client to use a combination of deep breathing and muscle contractions and relaxations to achieve a calmer state. Often used in combination with guided imagery.

repression: Involuntary burying of memories into the subconscious, usually related to a traumatic event or situation. The client is unaware of these memories unless there is a triggering stimulation associated with the original trauma.

restraint: Act of physically restricting the freedom of an client using manual, mechanical, or chemical means (forced medications). Designed to prevent harm to the client or to others. Would constitute assault and battery if not in a clinically supervised setting.

rhabdomyolysis: Breakdown of skeletal muscle that is usually associated with neuroleptic malignant syndrome.

rhinorrhea: Excessive runny nose commonly seen in opioid withdrawal.

ruminative: Inability to stop thinking about something. May be associated with intrusive thoughts (thoughts that come unbidden), but differs from obsessions in that ruminations often have a real-life, rational basis.

saliorrhea: Excessive salivation often seen as a side effect to the antipsychotic clozapine.

seclusion: Restriction of a client's right to freedom by placing him or her in a locked or secure room. Constitutes illegal confinement if not done in a clinically supervised setting.

self-mutilation: Act of cutting, burning, or otherwise intentionally harming oneself, usually as a result of overwhelming emotional distress. Self-mutilation brings about a sense of relief and calm, which may be related to stimulation of endogenous opiates.

somatic: Of, or relating to, the physical human body (as opposed to the mind). Somatic disorders are those that involve some perception of a physical symptom or problem.

speedball: Lethal combination of heroin and cocaine or amphetamine that is snorted or injected to get high. Cardiac arrest can result.

stereotypical behaviors: Rigid, fixed, or non-productive repetitive behaviors, such as rocking, hand-flapping, or clapping, that are often seen in developmental delays or mental retardation.

Stevens-Johnson syndrome: Painful, excoriating rash that can result as a side effect from some medications. Of concern in the mental health setting are the antiepileptics used for bipolar disorder (Lamictal®, Tegretol®).

stupor: State of extreme mental dullness, cloudiness, or decreased consciousness in which the individual can be aroused with a great deal of effort, but has little awareness of his or her surroundings.

sundowning: Phenomenon that is seen in dementia disorders, particularly of the Alzheimer's type, in which confusion and disorientation worsens as the evening progresses and improves with daylight.

synesthesia: Experience while under the influence of an hallucinogenic agent that smells can be heard, sounds tasted, or music felt (a disorganization of sensory perceptions).

tangential: Thought process problem in which thoughts branch off from one to another and the central theme or idea is lost.

tardive dyskinesia: Potentially irreversible side effect of antipsychotic medications (particularly the traditional ones) that is characterized by smooth and rhythmic muscular contractions of the head, neck, or trunk; tongue thrusting; subvocalizations (such as grunting); or hand and finger movements.

teratogenic: Having to do with risk or harm to an unborn fetus. Teratogenic drugs are those that cause birth defects.

tic: Sudden and somewhat explosive motor or vocal spasm that occurs rapidly and without warning. Tics can exacerbate and remit spontaneously. They are more common in children or they may be a side effect of stimulant medications.

time-out: Distinct period of time away from a triggering event or situation that allows the individual to regain a sense of self-control before returning to confront the situation.

torsades de pointes: Potentially lethal ventricular tachycardia, in which electrical conduction in the heart follows an abnormal, circular pattern. Torsades de pointes can occur when depolarization of the heart muscle occurs during the critical part of repolarization, also referred to as the R-on-T phenomenon.

waxy flexibility (catalepsy): State of prolonged rigid posture that is usually encountered in catatonic schizophrenia. Others can move the extremities and the client will hold them statue-like until they are moved again.

word salad: Disorder of thought processes, in which words within a sentence have no logical connection to one another and the sentence does not make any sense. Seen in disorganized schizophrenia.

REFERENCES

Alcoholics Anonymous (3rd ed.). (1976). New York: Alcoholics Anonymous World Services, Inc.

American Academy of Pediatrics: Committee on Drugs. (1998). Neonatal drug withdrawal. *Pediatrics, 101*(6), 1079-1088.

American Bar Association. (n.d.). Commission on Domestic Violence. *Survey of Recent Statistics: Prevalence of Domestic Violence.* Retireved July 12, 2010 from http://new.abanet.org/domesticviolence/Pages/Statistics.aspx

American Institute on Domestic Violence. (2001). *Domestic violence targets the heart of American business.* Retrieved July 12, 2010, from http://www.aidv-usa.com/myths.html

American Nurses Association. (2005). *Code of ethics for nurses.* Retrieved September 5, 2009, from http://www.nursingworld.org/MainMenu Categories/EthicsStandards/CodeofEthicsfor Nurses.aspx

American Psychiatric Association. (2000). *Diagnostic and statistical manual of mental disorders* (4th ed., text revision). Washington, DC: APA.

American Psychiatric Nurses Association. (1995). *Psychiatric-mental health nursing practice.* Retrieved September 5, 2009, from http://www.apna.org/i4a/pages/index.cfm?pageid=3343

American Psychiatric Nurses Association. (2009). *About advanced practice psychiatric nurses.* Retrieved September 5, 2009, from http://www.apna.org/i4a/pages/index.cfm?pageid=3857

American Red Cross. (2009). *Emergency disaster response and preparedness.* Retrieved September 29, 2009, from http://www.redcross.org/portal/site/en/menuitem.d229a5f06620c60 52b1ecfbf43181aa0/?vgnextoid=cc0795e5ded 8e110VgnVCM10000089f0870aRCRD&vgne xtchanel=5002af3fbac3b110VgnVCM100000 89f0870aRCRD

Bayard, M., McIntyre, J., Hill, K., & Woodside, J., Jr. (2004). *Alcohol withdrawal syndrome.* Retrieved September 20, 2009, from http://www.aafp.org/afp/20040315/1443.pdf

Braun, J.M., Kahn, R.S., Froehlich, T., Auinger, P., & Lanphear, B.P. (2006). Exposures to environmental toxicants and attention deficit hyperactivity disorder in U.S. children. *Environmental Health Perspectives, 114*(12), 1904-1909.

Bruun, R.D., Cohen, D.J., & Leckman, J.F. (2009). *Guide to the diagnosis and treatment of Tourette syndrome.* Retrieved May 27, 2009, from http://www.tsa-usa.org/Medical/guide todiagnosis.html

Centers for Disease Control and Prevention. (2006). *Understanding intimate partner violence: Fact sheet.* Retrieved September 29, 2009, from http://www.cdc.gov/Violence Prevention/pdf/IPV-FactSheet.pdf

Centers for Disease Control and Prevention. (2009). *Alzheimer's disease.* Retrieved March 14, 2009, from http://www.cdc.gov/aging/healthy brain/alzheimers.htm

Children's Medication Algorithm Project (CMAP). (2005). *Texas Department of State Health Services: Texas medication algorithm procedure manual.* Retrieved on July 22, 2010 from http://www.dshs.state.tx.us/mhprograms/CMAP over.shtm

Coffey, Barbara (2002). *Tics and Tourette's disorder.* Presented March 16, 2002, at the Conference on Child and Adolescent Psychopharmacology. March 15-17. Massachusetts General Hospital and Harvard Medical School (sponsors).

Coffey, B., Biederman, J., Smoller, J., Geller, D., Sarin, P., Schwartz, S., & Kim, G. (2000). Anxiety disorders and tic severity in juveniles with Tourette's disorder. *Journal of the American Academy of Child and Adolescent Psychiatry, 39*(5), 562-568.

Cornelius, M. & Day, N. (2000). The effects of tobacco use during and after pregnancy on exposed children. *Alcohol Research & Health, 24*(4), 242-249.

Costello, E.J., Angold, A., Burns, B., Stangl, D.K., Tweed, D.L., Erkanli, A., & Worthman, C.M. (1996). The Great Smoky Mountains study of youth: Goals, design, methods, and the prevalence of DSM-III-R disorders. *Archives of General Psychiatry, 53*(12), 1129-1136.

Decker, H.S. (2008). Psychoanalysis in Central Europe: The Interplay of Psychoanalysis and Culture. In E.R. Wallace, IV & J. Gach (Eds.) *History of psychiatry and medical psychology* (pp. 587-628). New York: Springer Science and Business Media.

DePetrillo, P. & McDonough, M. (1999). *The Alcohol Withdrawal Treatment Manual.* Retrieved September 21, 2009, from http://www.sagetalk.com

Dittmann, S., Forsthoff, A., Thoma, H., & Grunze, H. (2002). Clozapine as an add-on in the maintenance treatment of rapid cycling bipolar disorder. *Clinical Approaches in Bipolar Disorders, 1*(1), 31-33.

Domestic Abuse Intervention Project. (2003) *Domestic Abuse Intervention Programs.* Retrieved September 29, 2009, from http://www.theduluthmodel.org

Eli Lilly & Company. (2010). *Zyprexa prescribing Information.* Retrieved February 7, 2010, from http://pi.lilly.com/us/zyprexa_relprevv.pdf

Federal Emergency Management Agency. (2009). *Number of declarations per calendar year since 1999.* Retrieved September 20, 2009, from http://www.fema.gov/government/grant/pa/stat1.shtm

Fleming, L. & O'Brien, P. (2008). Anxiety and Dissociative Disorders. In P.G. O'Brien, W.Z. Kennedy, & K.A. Ballard (Eds.), *Psychiatric mental health nursing: An introduction to theory and practice* (pp. 335-352). Sudbury, MA: Jones and Bartlett.

Folstein, M.F., Folstein, S.E., & McHugh, P.R. (1975). *Mini-Mental State: Manual of Rating Scales for the Assessment of Geriatric Mental Illnesses.* Schneider, L.S., Tariot, P.N., & Olin, J.T. (Eds.). (2000). Wilmington, DE: AstraZeneca Pharmaceuticals LP.

Foucha v. Louisiana, 504 U.S. 71 (U.S. Supreme Court, 1992).

Greenberg, G.A. & Rosenheck, R.A. (2008). Jail incarceration, homelessness, and mental health: A national study. *Psychiatric Services, 59*(2), 170-177.

Headlee, R. & Corey, B.W. (1948). *Psychiatry in nursing.* New York: Rinehart

Hughes, D. (2002). *Sudden onset of obsessive-compulsive disorder may point to PANDAS.* Retrieved May 16, 2009, from http://www. neurologyreviews.com/apr02/pandas.html

Iavicoli, L.G. (2005). Mandatory reporting of domestic violence: the law, friend or foe? *Mount Sinai Journal of Medicine 72*(4), 228-231.

Indiana Medicaid Drug Utilization Review Board Newsletter. (2008). *Serotonin Syndrome Risk in Patients on Multiple Proserotonergic Therapies.* Retrieved October 5, 2010, from http://provider.indianamedicaid.com/media/ 19729/200804.pdf

Jackson v. Indiana, 406 U.S. 715 (U.S. Supreme Court, 1972).

Johnston, L.D., O'Malley, P.M., Bachman, J.G., & Schulenberg, J.E. (2009). *Teen marijuana use tilts up, while some drugs decline in use.* University of Michigan News Service: Ann Arbor, MI. Retrieved June 14, 2010 from http://www.monitoringthefuture.org

Keltner, N.L., Schwecke, L.H., & Bostrom, C.E. (Eds.). (2007). *Psychiatric nursing* (5th ed.). St. Louis, MO: Mosby/Elsevier.

Kübler-Ross, E. (1969). *On death and dying.* New York: Simon and Schuster.

Levin, A. (2008). Suicide among soldiers still rising as stress piles up. *Psychiatric News, 43*(12), 1-27.

Markley, V. (2008). Major depressive disorder. In P.G. O'Brien, W.Z. Kennedy, & K.A. Ballard (Eds.), *Psychiatric mental health nursing: An introduction to theory and practice* (pp. 311-321). Sudbury, MA: Jones and Bartlett.

Marshall, M., Lewis, S., Lockwood, A., Drake, R., Jones, P., & Croudace, T. (2005). Association between duration of untreated psychosis and outcome in cohorts of first-episode patients: A systematic review. *Archives of General Psychiatry, 62*(9), 975-983.

Maslow, A.H. (1943). A theory of human motivation. *Psychological Review, 50*(4), 370-396.

Mayo Clinic staff (2008). *Postpartum depression.* Retrieved September 21, 2009, from http://www.mayoclinic.com/health/postpartum-depression/DS00546

Miller, W.R. (1983). Motivational interviewing with problem drinkers. *Behavioural Psychotherapy, 11*(2), 147-172.

Nasrallah H.A. & Smeltzer D.J. (2002) *Contemporary diagnosis and management of the patient with schizophrenia.* Newtown, PA: Handbooks in Health Care

National Alliance on Mental Illness. (2006). *Depression: What is depression.* Retrieved September 21, 2009, from http://www.nami. org/Template.cfm?Section=By_Illness&templa te=/ContentManagement/ContentDisplay.cfm &ContentID=7725

National Institute of Mental Health. (2008). *Science update: Study probes environment-triggered genetic changes in schizophrenia.* Retrieved January 24, 2009, from http://www.nimh.nih.gov/science-news/ 2008/study-probes-environment-triggered-genetic-changes-in-schizophrenia.shtml

National Institute of Mental Health. (2009). *Suicide in the U.S.: Statistics and prevention.* Retrieved April 29, 2009, from http://www.nimh.nih.gov/ health/publications/suicide-in-the-us-statistics-and-prevention/index.shtml

National Institute on Alcohol Abuse and Alcoholism (2008). *Data and statistical tables.* Retrieved April 6, 2009, from http://www.niaaa. nih.gov/Resources/DatabaseResources/Quick Facts

National Institute on Drug Abuse. (2009). *Prenatal exposure to drugs of abuse.* Retrieved May 23, 2009, from http://www.drugabuse.gov/tib/ prenatal.html

Nulman, I., Rovet, J., Stewart, D., Wolpin, J., Pace-Asciak, P., Shuhaiber, S., & Koren, G. (2002). Child development following exposure to tricyclic antidepressants or fluoxetine throughout fetal life: A prospective, controlled study. *American Journal of Psychiatry, 159*(11), 1889-1895.

O'Brien, P.G., Kennedy, W.Z., & Ballard, K.A. (Eds.). (2008). *Psychiatric mental health nursing: An introduction to theory and practice.* Sudbury, MA: Jones and Bartlett.

Physicians' desk reference (63rd ed.). (2009). New York: Thomson Reuters.

Pratt, L.A. & Brody, D.J. (2008). *NCHS data brief: Depression in the United States household population, 2005-2006.* Retrieved April 29, 2009, from http://www.cdc.gov/nchs/data/data briefs/db07.htm

President's Advisory Commission on Consumer Protection and Quality in the Health Care Industry. (1997). *Consumer Bill of Rights and Responsibilities.* Retrieved October 5, 2010, from http://www.hcqualitycommission. gov/cborr

Prochaska, J.O. & DiClemente, C.C. (1983). Stages and processes of self-change of smoking: Toward an integrative model of change. *Journal of Consulting and Clinical Psychology, 51*(3), 390-395.

Rodriguez, M.A., McLoughlin, E., Nah, G., & Campbell, J. (2001). Mandatory reporting of domestic violence injuries to the police. *Journal of the American Medical Association, 286*(5), 580-583.

Selye, H. (1956). *The stress of life.* New York: McGraw-Hill.

Stahl, S. (2000). *Stahl's essential psychopharmacology: Neuroscientific basis and practical applications* (2nd ed.). New York: Cambridge University Press.

Stahl, S. (2009). *Stahl's essential psychopharmacology: The prescriber's guide* (3rd ed.). New York: Cambridge University Press.

State of Florida Department of Children and Families Mental Health Program Office. (2002). *History of the Baker Act: Its development and intent.* Retrieved January 28, 2009, from http://www.dcf.state.fl.us/programs/ samh/MentalHealth/laws/histba.pdf

Substance Abuse and Mental Health Services Administration (SAMHSA). (1999). *Mental health: A report of the Surgeon General.* Retrieved October 5, 2009, from http://mental health.samhsa.gov/cmhs/SurgeonGeneral

Substance Abuse and Mental Health Services Administration (SAMHSA). (2005). *Disasters and substance abuse or dependence: A fact sheet from the National Center for PTSD.* Retrieved May 29, 2009, from http://www. samhsa.gov/csatdisasterrecovery/outreach/disas tersAndSubstanceAbuseOrDependence.pdf

Substance Abuse and Mental Health Services Administration (SAMHSA). (2006). *Results from the 2005 National Survey on Drug Use and Health: National findings* (Office of Applied Studies, NSDUH Series H-30, DHHS Publication No. SMA 06-4194). Retrieved April 22, 2009, from http://www.oas. samhsa.gov/NSDUH/2k5NSDUH/2k5results. htm#High

Substance Abuse and Mental Health Services Administration (SAMHSA). (2008). *Results from the 2007 National Survey on Drug Use and Health: National findings.* Retrieved April 6, 2009, from http://www.oas.samhsa.gov/ nsduh/2k7nsduh/2k7Results.pdf

Suehs, B., Argo, T.R., Bendele, S.D., Crismon, M.L., Trivedi, M.H., & Kurian, B. (2008). *Texas Medication Algorithm Project procedural manual: Major depressive disorder algorithms.* Retrieved May 9, 2009, from http://www.dshs.state.tx.us/mhprograms/pdf/TIMA_MDD_Manual_080608.pdf

Sullivan, J.T., Sykora, K., Schneiderman, J., Naranjo, C.A., & Sellers, E.M. (1989). Assessment of alcohol withdrawal: The revised Clinical Institute Withdrawal Assessment for Alcohol Scale (CIWA-Ar). *British Journal of Addiction, 84*(11), 1353-1357.

Taylor, C.M. (2008). Introduction to psychiatric-mental health nursing. In P.G. O'Brien, W.Z. Kennedy, & K.A. Ballard (Eds.), *Psychiatric mental health nursing: An introduction to theory and practice* (pp. 3-20). Sudbury, MA: Jones and Bartlett.

U.S. Census Bureau. (2003). *Disability Status: 2000 – Census 2000 Brief.* Retrieved January 24, 2009, from http://www.census.gov/prod/2003pubs/c2kbr-17.pdf

U.S. Census Bureau. (2008). 2005-2007: *American Community Survey 3-year estimate.* Retrieved from http://factfinder.census.gov/servlet/DatasetMainPageServlet?_program=ACS

U.S. Conference of Mayors. (2004). *Hunger and Homelessness Survey: A status report on hunger and homelessness in America's cities.* Retrieved July 12, 2010 from http://www.usmayors.org/hungersurvey/2004/onlinereport/HungerAndHomelessnessReport2004.pdf

U.S. Department of Justice, Office of Justice Programs. (2007). *Dangers to children living at meth labs.* Retrieved April 21, 2009, from http://www.ojp.usdoj.gov/ovc/publications/bulletins/children/pg5.html

U.S. Drug Enforcement Administration. (2006). News release. *Operation Somalia express: Largest khat enforcement ever.* Retrieved September 21, 2009, from http://www.usdoj.gov/dea/pubs/pressrel/pr072606.html

Vermani, M., Milosevic, I., Smith, F., & Katzman, M. (2005). Herbs for mental illness: Effectiveness and interaction with conventional medicines: Some herbs do work as claimed; all have the potential for downside activity as well. *Journal of Family Practice, 54*(9), 789-800. Retrieved March 2, 2009, from http://findarticles.com/p/articles/mi_m0689/is_9_54/ai_n15653055/?tag=content;col1

Vornik, L.A. & Brown, E.S. (2007). Substance-abuse comorbidity in bipolar disorder: General considerations and treatment approaches. *Clinical Approaches in Bipolar Disorders, 6*(1), 3-11.

WebMD. (2009a). *ADD & ADHD health center: ADHD Overview.* Retrieved October 4, 2009, from http://www.webmd.com/add-adhd/default.htm

WebMD. (2009b). A*DHD guide: Attention deficit hyperactivity disorder: ADHD in adults.* Retrieved May 27, 2009, from http://www.webmd.com/add-adhd/guide/adhd-adults

Weiner, D.B. (2008a). Philippe Pinel in the Twenty-First Century: The Myth and the Message. In E.R. Wallace, IV & J. Gach (Eds.) *History of psychiatry and medical psychology* (pp.305-312). New York: Springer Science and Business Media.

Weiner, D.B. (2008b). The Madman in the Light of Reason. Enlightenment Psychiatry: Part II. Alienists, Treatises, and the and the Psychologic Approach in the Era of Pinel. In E.R. Wallace, IV & J. Gach (Eds.) *History of psychiatry and medical psychology* (pp.281-304). New York: Springer Science and Business Media.

Wolraich, M. (Ed.). (1996). *Disorders of development and learning: A practical guide to assessment and management* (2nd ed.). St. Louis, MO: Mosby.

World Health Organization. (2004). *Prevention of mental disorders: Effective interventions and policy options.* Retrieved January 24, 2009, from http://www.who.int/mental_health/evidence/en/prevention_of_mental_disorders_sr.pdf

World Health Organization. (2007). *Mental health and substance abuse: Facts and figures.* Retrieved January 24, 2009, from http://www.searo.who.int/en/Section1174/Section1199/Section1567_6741.htm

Yalom, I. & Leszcz, M. (2005). *The theory and practice of group psychotherapy* (5th ed.). New York: Basic Books.

INDEX

Western Schools® offers over 2,000 hours to suit all your interests – and requirements!

Cardiovascular
Cardiovascular Nursing: A Comprehensive Overview
Cardiovascular Pharmacology
A The 12-Lead ECG in Acute Coronary Syndromes

Clinical Conditions/Nursing Practice
A Advanced Assessment
Ambulatory Surgical Care (2nd ed.)
Asthma: Nursing Care Across the Lifespan
Clinical Care of the Diabetic Foot
A Complete Nurses Guide to Diabetes Care (2nd ed.)
Chronic Obstructive Lung Disease
Diabetes Essentials for Nurses
Essentials of Patient Education
Fibromyalgia in Women
Genetic & Inherited Disorders of the Pulmonary System
Helping the Obese Patient Find Success
Holistic & Complementary Therapies
Home Health Nursing (3rd ed.)
Humor in Health Care: The Laughter Prescription (2nd ed.)
Management of Systemic Lupus Erythematosus
Multiple Sclerosis: Nursing Strategies to Improve Patient Outcomes
Orthopedic Nursing: Caring for Patients with Musculoskeletal Disorders (2nd ed.)
Pain & Symptom Management
Pain Management: Principles and Practice
A Palliative Practices: An Interdisciplinary Approach
— Issues Specific to Palliative Care
— Specific Disease States and Symptom Management
— The Dying Process, Grief, and Bereavement.
Pharmacologic Management of Asthma
Pneumonia in Adults
Pulmonary Rehabilitation
Seizures: A Basic Overview
Wound Management and Healing

Critical Care/ER/OR
Acute Respiratory Distress Syndrome (ARDS)
Adult Acute Respiratory Infections
Auscultation Skills (4th ed.)
— Heart Sounds
— Breath Sounds
Basic Nursing of Head, Chest, Abdominal, Spine and Orthopedic Trauma
A Case Studies in Critical Care Nursing
Critical Care & Emergency Nursing
Hemodynamic Monitoring
Lung Transplantation
A Practical Guide to Moderate Sedation/Analgesia
Principles of Basic Trauma Nursing
Traumatic Brain Injury

Geriatrics
Alzheimer's Disease: A Complete Guide for Nurses
Alzheimer's Disease and Related Disorders
Cognitive Disorders in Aging
Depression in Older Adults
Early-Stage Alzheimer's Disease
Geriatric Assessment
Healthy Aging
Nursing Care of the Older Adult (2nd ed.)
Psychosocial Issues Affecting Older Adults (2nd ed.)
Substance Abuse in Older Adults

Infectious Diseases
Avian (H5N1) Influenza (2nd ed.)
H1N1 Flu (2nd ed.)
Hepatitis C: The Silent Killer (2nd ed.)
HIV/AIDS
Infection Control Training for Healthcare Workers
Influenza: A Vaccine-Preventable Disease
MRSA
Pertussis: Diagnosis, Treatment, and Prevention
Tuberculosis Across the Lifespan
West Nile Virus (3rd ed.)

Oncology
Cancer Nursing
Chemotherapy and Biotherapies
Lung Cancer (UPDATED 1st ed.)

Pediatrics/Maternal-Child/Women's Health
A Assessment and Care of the Well Newborn
Birth Control Methods and Reproductive Choices
Birth Defects Affecting the Respiratory System
Childhood Obesity
Diabetes in Children
Effective Counseling Techniques for Perinatal Mood Disorders
Fetal and Neonatal Drug Exposure
Induction of Labor
Manual of School Health (3rd ed.)
Maternal-Newborn Nursing
Menopause: Nursing Care for Women Throughout Mid-Life
A Obstetric and Gynecologic Emergencies
— Obstetric Emergencies
— Gynecologic Emergencies
Pediatric Health & Physical Assessment
Perinatal Mood Disorders: An Overview
Pregnancy Loss
Respiratory Diseases in the Newborn
Women and Cardiovascular Disease
Women's Health: Contemporary Advances and Trends (3rd ed.)

Professional Issues/Management/Law
Documentation for Nurses
Ethical Issues in Children's Health Care
Medical Error Prevention: Patient Safety
Management and Leadership in Nursing
Ohio Nursing Law Affecting Daily Practice
Surviving and Thriving in Nursing

Psychiatric/Mental Health
A ADHD in Children and Adults
Adoptive Families: Trends and Therapeutic Interventions
Asperger's Syndrome
Attention Deficit Hyperactivity Disorders Throughout the Lifespan
Basic Psychopharmacology
Behavioral Approaches to Treating Obesity
A Bipolar Disorder
A Child/Adolescent Clinical Psychopharmacology (2nd ed.)
A Childhood Maltreatment
A Clinical Psychopharmacology
A Collaborative Therapy with Multi-stressed Families
Counseling Substance Abusing or Dependent Adolescents
Depression: Prevention, Diagnosis, and Treatment
Disaster Mental Health
A Ethnicity and the Dementias
A Evidence-Based Mental Health Practice
Group Work with Substance Abusing & Dually Diagnosed Clients
A Growing Up with Autism
Harm Reduction Counseling for Substance Abusing Clients
Identifying and Assessing Suicide Risk in Adults
A Integrating Traditional Healing Practices into Counseling
A Integrative and Comprehensive Trauma Treatment
A Integrative Treatment for Borderline Personality Disorder
Intimate Partner Violence: An Overview
A Mental Disorders in Older Adults
A Mindfulness and Psychotherapy
A Multicultural Perspectives in Working with Families
Multidimensional Health Assessment of the Older Adult
A Obsessive Compulsive Disorder
Post-Divorce Parenting: Mental Health Issues and Interventions
Posttraumatic Stress Disorder: An Overview
A Problem and Pathological Gambling
Psychiatric Nursing: Current Trends in Diagnosis (2nd ed.)
Psychiatric Principles & Applications
A Psychosocial Adjustment to Chronic Illness in Children and Adolescents
A Psychosocial Aspects of Disaster
A Schizophrenia
Schizophrenia: Signs, Symptoms, and Treatment Strategies
Serious Mental Illness: Comprehensive Case Management
Substance Abuse (UPDATED 1st ed.)
Suicide
A Trauma Therapy
A Treating Explosive Kids
A Treating Substance Use Problems in Psychotherapy Practice
A Treating Victims of Mass Disaster and Terrorism
Understanding Attachment Theory
Understanding Loss & Grief: Implications for Healthcare Professionals

Visit our website at www.WesternSchools.com for course descriptions and additional CE offerings!